W9-CES-199

LIBRARY-LRC
TEXAS HEART INSTITUTE

Prevention of Cardiovascular Disease: A Continuum

Guest Editor

PRAKASH DEEDWANIA, MD

CARDIOLOGY CLINICS

www.cardiology.theclinics.com

Consulting Editor

MICHAEL H. CRAWFORD, MD

February 2011 • Volume 29 • Number 1

SAUNDERS an imprint of ELSEVIER, Inc.

W.B. SAUNDERS COMPANY
A Division of Elsevier Inc.

1600 John F. Kennedy Blvd. ● Suite 1800 ● Philadelphia, PA 19103-2899

http://www.theclinics.com

CARDIOLOGY CLINICS Volume 29, Number 1
February 2011 ISSN 0733-8651, ISBN-13: 978-1-4557-0426-2

Editor: Barbara Cohen-Kligerman
Developmental Editor: Jessica Demetriou

© **2011 Elsevier Inc. All rights reserved.**

This journal and the individual contributions contained in it are protected under copyright by Elsevier, and the following terms and conditions apply to their use:

Photocopying
Single photocopies of single articles may be made for personal use as allowed by national copyright laws. Permission of the Publisher and payment of a fee is required for all other photocopying, including multiple or systematic copying, copying for advertising or promotional purposes, resale, and all forms of document delivery. Special rates are available for educational institutions that wish to make photocopies for non-profit educational classroom use. For information on how to seek permission visit www.elsevier.com/permissions or call: (+44) 1865 843830 (UK)/(+1) 215 239 3804 (USA).

Derivative Works
Subscribers may reproduce tables of contents or prepare lists of articles including abstracts for internal circulation within their institutions. Permission of the Publisher is required for resale or distribution outside the institution. Permission of the Publisher is required for all other derivative works, including compilations and translations (please consult www.elsevier.com/permissions).

Electronic Storage or Usage
Permission of the Publisher is required to store or use electronically any material contained in this journal, including any article or part of an article (please consult www.elsevier.com/permissions). Except as outlined above, no part of this publication may be reproduced, stored in a retrieval system or transmitted in any form or by any means, electronic, mechanical, photocopying, recording or otherwise, without prior written permission of the Publisher.

Notice
No responsibility is assumed by the Publisher for any injury and/or damage to persons or property as a matter of products liability, negligence or otherwise, or from any use or operation of any methods, products, instructions or ideas contained in the material herein. Because of rapid advances in the medical sciences, in particular, independent verification of diagnoses and drug dosages should be made.

Although all advertising material is expected to conform to ethical (medical) standards, inclusion in this publication does not constitute a guarantee or endorsement of the quality or value of such product or of the claims made of it by its manufacturer.

Cardiology Clinics (ISSN 0733-8651) is published quarterly by Elsevier Inc., 360 Park Avenue South, New York, NY 10010-1710. Months of issue are February, May, August, and November. Business and Editorial Offices: 1600 John F. Kennedy Blvd., Ste. 1800, Philadelphia, PA 19103-2899. Customer Service Office: 3251 Riverport Lane, Maryland Heights, MO 63043. Periodicals postage paid at New York, NY and additional mailing offices. Subscription prices are $282.00 per year for US individuals, $458.00 per year for US institutions, $139.00 per year for US students and residents, $345.00 per year for Canadian individuals, $569.00 per year for Canadian institutions, $400.00 per year for international individuals, $569.00 per year for international institutions and $196.00 per year for Canadian and international students/residents. To receive student/resident rate, orders must be accompanied by name of affiliated institution, data of term, and the *signature* of program/residency coordinator on institution letterhead. Orders will be billed at individual rate until proof of status is received. Foreign air speed delivery is included in all *Clinics* subscription prices. All prices are subject to change without notice. **POSTMASTER:** Send address changes to *Cardiology Clinics*, Elsevier Health Sciences Division, Subscription Customer Service, 3251 Riverport Lane, Maryland Heights, MO 63043. **Customer Service: 1-800-654-2452 (U.S. and Canada); 314-447-8871 (outside U.S. and Canada). Fax: 314-447-8029. E-mail: journalscustomerservice-usa@elsevier.com (for print support); journalsonlinesupport-usa@elsevier.com (for online support).**

Reprints. For copies of 100 or more, of articles in this publication, please contact the Commercial Reprints Department, Elsevier Inc., 360 Park Avenue South, New York, NY 10010-1710. Tel.: 212-633-3812; Fax: 212-462-1935; E-mail: reprints@elsevier.com.

Cardiology Clinics is also published in Spanish by McGraw-Hill Interamericana Editores S. A., P.O. Box 5-237, 06500, Mexico D. F., Mexico; in Portuguese by Reichmann and Alfonso Editores Rio de Janeiro, Brazil; and in Greek by Dimitrios P. Lagos, 8 Pondon Street, GR115-28 Ilissia, Greece.

Cardiology Clinics is covered in *MEDLINE/PubMed (Index Medicus), Excerpta Medica, The Cumulative Index to Nursing and Allied Health Literature* (CINAHL).

Printed in the United States of America.

Contributors

CONSULTING EDITOR

MICHAEL H. CRAWFORD, MD
Professor of Medicine, University of California,
San Francisco; Lucie Stern Chair in Cardiology
and Chief of Clinical Cardiology, University
of California, San Francisco Medical Center,
San Francisco, California

GUEST EDITOR

PRAKASH DEEDWANIA, MD, FACC, FAHA
Professor of Medicine and Chief, Division of
Cardiology, Department of Medicine, Veterans
Affairs Central California Health Care
System/University of California, San Francisco,
Fresno Program, Fresno, California

AUTHORS

DEEPAK L. BHATT, MD, MPH, FACC, FAHA
Chief of Cardiology, Division of Cardiology,
Veterans Affairs Boston Healthcare System;
Director, Integrated Interventional
Cardiovascular Program, Brigham and
Women's Hospital and Veterans Affairs
Boston Healthcare System; Senior
Investigator, TIMI Study Group; Associate
Professor of Medicine, Harvard Medical
School, Boston, Massachusetts

ENRIQUE V. CARBAJAL, MD
Associate Professor of Medicine, Division
of Cardiology, Department of Medicine,
Veterans Affairs Central California Health
Care System/University of California,
San Francisco, Fresno Program, Fresno,
California

KUANG-YUH CHYU, MD, PhD
Associate Clinical Professor of Medicine,
Department of Medicine, University
of California, Los Angeles, Los Angeles,
California

MICHAEL H. DAVIDSON, MD, FACC
Clinical Professor of Medicine, Pritzker
School of Medicine, University of Chicago;
Executive Medical Director, Radiant
Research, Chicago, Illinois

PRAKASH DEEDWANIA, MD, FACC, FAHA
Professor of Medicine and Chief, Division of
Cardiology, Department of Medicine, Veterans
Affairs Central California Health Care
System/University of California, San Francisco,
Fresno Program, Fresno, California

JOANNE M. FOODY, MD
Associate Professor, Division of Cardiology,
Brigham and Women's Hospital,
Harvard Medical School, Boston,
Massachusetts

RAJEEV GUPTA, MD, PhD
Department of Medicine, Fortis Escorts
Hospital; Department of Medicine, Rajasthan
University of Health Sciences, Jaipur, India

KUMARAN KOLANDAIVELU, MD, PhD
Cardiovascular Fellow, Division of Cardiology,
Brigham and Women's Hospital, Boston;
Postdoctoral Fellow, Division of Health Sciences
and Technology, Massachusetts Institute
of Technology, Cambridge, Massachusetts

JOEL A. LARDIZABAL, MD
Division of Cardiology, Department
of Medicine, University of California,
San Francisco (Fresno Medical Education
Program), Fresno, California

L. VERONICA LEE, MD
Clinical Research and Development,
Lantheus Medical Imaging, North Billerica,
Massachusetts

PREDIMAN K. SHAH, MD
Professor of Medicine, Department
of Medicine, University of California,
Los Angeles, Los Angeles, California

SUNDARARAJAN SRIKANTH, MD
Division of Cardiology, Veterans Affairs
Central California Health Care System/
University of California, San Francisco,
Fresno Program, Fresno, California

**KRISHNASWAMI VIJAYARAGHAVAN,
MD, MS, FACP, FACC**
Medical Director, Cardiovascular
Research and Education, Scottsdale
Healthcare, Scottsdale; Professor
of Medicine, Midwestern University,
Glendale, Arizona

PETER W.F. WILSON, MD
Professor of Medicine (Cardiology),
Professor of Public Health (Epidemiology,
Global Health), Atlanta VAMC
Epidemiology and Genetics Section,
Emory Clinical Cardiovascular Research
Institute, Atlanta, Georgia

Contents

Observational studies with incidence of cardiovascular disease (CVD) events have typically provided the information that is used. Prediction of risk is dependent on accurate and precise baseline measurements in persons without coronary disease at baseline. Follow-up of 5 to 10 years is a typical interval of interest for the prediction of coronary disease events in adults who are asymptomatic at the baseline. Performance criteria for risk estimation include discrimination, calibration, and reclassification, and newer heart disease risk factors and biomarkers can be evaluated in the context of existing risk estimation approaches.

Cardiovascular disease prevention is a continuum that encompasses the life-course. This article discusses preventive strategies focusing on policy and clinical initiatives including primordial prevention (lifestyle changes involving smoking, diet and exercise), primary prevention (risk factor control), and secondary prevention (acute and chronic disease management). Combined use of all the three strategies can have an immediate and large impact on reducing CVD morbidity and mortality.

In the United States heart disease causes more than one-third of all deaths and most of these occur in women, not men, although women and health care professionals alike continue to view death from heart disease as a threat primarily to middle-aged men. The disparity between genders in the incidence of cardiovascular disease (CVD) may be the result of significant differences in both cardiovascular risk factors and presentation between men and women. This article reviews recent data regarding unique sex-specific characteristics of both risk for, and presentation of, CVD in women.

The majority of individuals with diabetes die from cardiovascular disease (CVD) and related complications. The risk of CVD is 2 to 4 fold greater in diabetes and largely magnified by co-morbidities that aggregate along with it. Sufficient evidence-based data now exist to support multifactorial risk intervention with specific targets for goal-directed therapy for both primary and secondary prevention. These interventions have shown survival benefit in addition to prevention of vascular complications. Prevention of diabetes and delaying its onset should also be an important aspect in future health care strategy and research to confront the oncoming tsunami of CVD related to diabetes.

Platelets are central to the pathogenesis of coronary heart disease (CHD). An ever-growing number of antiplatelet therapies used in different doses and combinations have helped manage atherothrombosis, both acutely and in primary and secondary prevention. Despite modern therapy, nearly 800,000 individuals suffer annually from an initial coronary event in the United States alone; almost 500,000 experience a recurrent event. This review provides a current appraisal of antiplatelet drug use in CHD prevention and discusses key barriers to achieving its full potential in real-world practice.

Cardiovascular disease (CVD) still ranks as the top cause of mortality worldwide. Lipid-modifying therapy has revolutionized the treatment of the disease and is partly responsible for the recent decline in deaths due to CVD. Treatment strategies have evolved since the introduction of the earlier lipid-lowering agents (fibrates, niacin, bile acid resins) to the advent of statins, which have become the standard drugs in cholesterol therapy. The strategy of using high-intensity statin therapy as the initial treatment approach in high-risk individuals, rather than focusing on specific cholesterol levels alone, remains a subject of debate.

A low level of high-density lipoprotein (HDL) is an acknowledged risk factor for coronary heart disease (CHD). HDL cholesterol (HDL-C) exerts its primary cardioprotective effect through a reverse cholesterol transport process, and suppression of this process has been the focus of the development of novel therapeutic agents for increasing HDL-C levels. Several strategies can be used to increase HDL-C levels to target cardiovascular risk reduction. This article presents a review of the biologic actions of HDL that can serve as a potential basis for antiatherosclerotic activity and discusses strategies for targeting HDL for CHD risk reduction.

Atherosclerosis is a chronic immunoinflammatory disease involving medium and large arteries, resulting from a complex interaction between genetic and environmental risk factors. Acute atherosclerotic vascular disease largely results from thrombosis that supervenes on a disrupted atherosclerotic plaque. A healthy lifestyle coupled with management of modifiable risk factors reduces the adverse clinical consequences of atherothrombosis. Reducing low-density lipoprotein cholesterol levels using statins and other agents is the primary pharmacologic approach to stabilize atherosclerosis, but a large residual risk burden remains, stimulating the search for additional therapies for atherosclerosis management. This review focuses on new and emerging therapeutic strategies targeting atherosclerosis.

The renin-angiotensin-aldosterone system (RAAS) plays a significant role in pathophysiology of multiple disease states. RAAS blockade is beneficial in patients with hypertension, acute myocardial infarction, chronic heart failure, stroke, and diabetic renal disease. RAAS blockade with the combination angiotensin-converting enzyme inhibitors (ACEIs) and angiotensin receptor blockers (ARBs) has demonstrated conflicting results in recent clinical trials. This article reviews the latest evidence of isolated ACEI or ARB use, their combination, and the role of aldosterone blockers and direct renin inhibitors in patients at risk, and makes recommendations for their use in the prevention of morbidity and mortality in cardiovascular disease.

Chronic coronary artery disease (CAD) is a highly prevalent and complex health problem in the United States. The goals of treatment in patients with stable CAD are to reduce symptoms and thus improve quality of life, reduce myocardial ischemia, and, more importantly, reduce the risk of myocardial infarction and death. In this article, the authors review the evidence regarding the role of medical versus interventional strategies in reducing the risk of future coronary events in patients with stable CAD.

Cardiology Clinics

VISIT OUR WEB SITE!
Access your subscription at:
www.theclinics.com

Foreword

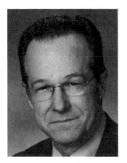

Michael H. Crawford, MD
Consulting Editor

Increasingly cardiologists are being called upon to advise higher risk individuals regarding the prevention of atherosclerotic cardiovascular disease. For most of us this was not something we learned a lot about during our training. Consequently, it is difficult to put new trials into prospective, yet our patients read trial reports on various news services and want our advice. The last time an issue of *Cardiology Clinics* was dedicated to the prevention of cardiovascular disease was August 2003. Since then much has happened surrounding this topic. Major trials have been completed and reported such as REVERSAL, PROVE-IT, TNT, RITA 3, ICTUS, COURAGE, JUPITER, and many more. Clearly it was time to update our readers on the current state of prevention strategies.

In November of 2004 and May of 2005 Dr Prakash Deedwania guest edited two issues of *Cardiology Clinics* on diabetes and cardiovascular disease. I was delighted when he agreed to put together this issue on Prevention. He has assembled a group of international experts to author this issue and has put considerable personal effort into its content. Appropriately, he has focused the issue on what is new in

Prevention. Also, the issue emphasizes interventions to prevent cardiovascular disease. Various pharmacologic strategies are covered in detail, but coronary interventions and emerging therapies are discussed as well. Appropriate prevention strategies hinge on risk prediction, which is the subject of the first article. Finally, two special risk groups are considered in separate articles, one focusing on diabetics and one on women.

This issue is a practical treatise on how to prevent atherosclerotic cardiovascular disease at the end of the first decade of the 21st century. It is a must read for everyone caring for patients at risk for or with heart and vascular disease.

Michael H. Crawford, MD
Division of Cardiology, Department of Medicine
University of California
San Francisco Medical Center
505 Parnassus Avenue, Box 0124
San Francisco, CA 94143-0124, USA

E-mail address:
crawfordm@medicine.ucsf.edu

Cardiol Clin 29 (2011) ix
doi:10.1016/j.ccl.2010.12.002
0733-8651/11/$ – see front matter © 2011 Elsevier Inc. All rights reserved.

Preface
Cardiovascular Disease Prevention: The Continuum of Primary and Secondary Prevention

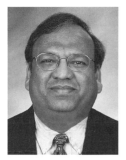

Prakash Deedwania, MD
Guest Editor

"Superior doctors prevent the disease;
  Mediocre doctors treat the disease before
it is evident;
  Inferior doctors treat the full blown disease"
  Adapted from Huang Dee: Nai-Ching (2600
BC, First Chinese Medical Tex)

Cardiovascular diseases (CVD, coronary heart disease, stroke) are the leading cause of death and disability in the world. Although CV mortality has declined in developed nations and high-income countries, CV risk and related complications are on the rise in developing nations. Careful implementation of effective preventive strategies that are simple and easy to apply on a population-wide scale is essential to curb the epidemic of CVD.

It is now well recognized that the risk of CVD can be estimated by evaluation of established risk factors, which include smoking, hypertension, type II diabetes, hypercholesterolemia and other dyslipidemias, obesity, and sedentary lifestyle. However, it is important to recognize that although most of the current risk scoring methods provide risk estimates for a 5- to 10-year period, the risk of CVD is a lifelong phenomenon and risk estimates need to be developed for the total lifespan of a given individual.

CVD prevention is a continuum and should include primordial prevention (lifestyle changes involving diet and exercise), primary prevention (risk factor control), and secondary prevention (acute and chronic disease management). Combined use of all three strategies can have an immediate and significant impact in reducing CVD morbidity and mortality. During the past two decades a number of large observational studies as well as randomized controlled clinical trials (RCTs) have demonstrated that interventions designed for primary and secondary prevention of CVD are highly effective in reducing the subsequent risk of CV events. Based on a number of cost-effectiveness analyses, it is evident that both primary and secondary prevention strategies can be cost effective and save many lives. However, despite the available evidence, many recent surveys in the United States and Europe indicate that preventive strategies are not widely applied and implemented,

Cardiol Clin 29 (2011) xi–xiii
doi:10.1016/j.ccl.2010.12.001
0733-8651/11/$ – see front matter © 2011 Elsevier Inc. All rights reserved.

thus leaving a large proportion of the population at risk. Although the precise reasons for lack of universal application of preventive strategies are not known, it is postulated that inadequate health care financing/resources, physician inertia, and lack of access to health care could be major contributors.

It is also important to recognize that primordial prevention strategies are urgently needed to prevent the oncoming tsunami of obesity, diabetes, and CVD. Primordial prevention generally requires inexpensive public health measures such as smoking control policies, legislative control of saturated and trans fat (as recently implemented in New York City), salt and alcohol consumption controls, as well as promotion of increased physical activity through better urban planning (for example, providing walking/bicycle paths) and public health education.

It is with these issues in mind and the importance of CVD prevention that I conceived this special issue of *Cardiology Clinics* focused on prevention of CVD. Although it is really impossible to provide a comprehensive manual of all preventive strategies in a single volume, a concerted effort has been made to include the most pertinent and up-to-date information for CV risk assessment and the role of various primary and secondary prevention strategies for CV risk reduction. The authors represent an outstanding group of international authorities in their field.

The first article by Wilson provides a comprehensive state-of-the-art overview about the importance of and methods to evaluate the risk of CV disease and related events. The article by Gupta and Deedwania provides an overview of various interventions needed for CVD prevention. In this article emphasis has been placed on the fact that CVD prevention is a continuum over the entire lifespan, beginning with primordial prevention and followed by primary and secondary preventive strategies. Furthermore, the need for implementation of effective preventive strategies at all stages of CVD and on a global basis is emphasized. The next article deals with the important issue of heart disease in women and emphasizes the fact that although CVD is the leading cause of death in women, not enough emphasis has been placed on screening and recognition of CVD in women. This article also emphasizes the need for a more concerted effort to implement preventive strategies in women.

It is now well recognized that type II diabetes is a CHD risk equivalent and CV complications are the leading cause of death and disability in

diabetes. A number of recent studies have provided conflicting data on the importance of tight glycemic control and aggressive blood pressure reduction in diabetes. The article on primary and secondary prevention in diabetes provides a comprehensive overview of these trials and summarizes the recommendations from various guidelines for the clinician. Subsequent articles deal specifically with various treatment strategies for primary and secondary prevention of CVD. The article on antiplatelet therapy emphasizes the critical role of platelets in CVD and provides an overview of all available antiplatelet agents in prevention of coronary events.

Lipid-lowering therapy with statins has been perhaps the most effective intervention for both primary and secondary prevention of CVD. Several articles in this issue not only describe the unquestionable benefit of statin therapy for prevention of CVD but also emphasize the need for intensive lipid-lowering therapy in high-risk patients and the importance of the residual risk related to decreased levels of HDL cholesterol. The article by Davidson provides an overview of conventional and newer evolving therapies for raising HDL cholesterol. This is further discussed in the article by Chyu and Shah in which they also describe several novel and evolving therapies for prevention of atherosclerosis and forecast that someday it might be conceivable to have a vaccine against atherosclerosis.

A number of studies in the last decade have emphasized the role of the renin-angiotensin-aldosterone system (RAAS) in CVD. The article by Vijayaraghavan and Deedwania provides a comprehensive overview of a large number of studies that have documented the evidence for the beneficial role of RAAS blockade in prevention of CVD. The final article in this issue deals with perhaps the most controversial issue regarding the role of medical therapy versus interventional strategies to prevent coronary events in patients with stable CAD. Although the number of coronary interventions in the United States has steadily increased in the past decade, there is little evidence to support their role in the prevention of coronary events. Recently, evidence has emerged from well-conducted RCTs documenting the fact that optimal medical therapy (which should include comprehensive risk factor reduction) is as effective as any coronary intervention in reducing the risk of myocardial infarction and death.

It is my hope that the compendium of articles in this issue provides the clinician with the latest information regarding the best strategies for CV risk assessment and prevention of CVD.

I would like to thank Michael Crawford, the consulting editor of *Cardiology Clinics*, for inviting me to compile this issue dedicated to prevention of CVD. I would also like to express my gratitude to all of the contributors and collaborators for providing their input and articles in a timely manner. A final thanks goes to my family and friends, who are always supportive of my academic endeavors.

Let us remind ourselves of the old axiom, "An ounce of prevention is worth a pound of cure."

Prakash Deedwania, MD
Division of Cardiology
Department of Medicine
Veterans Affairs Central California Health Care System
University of California, San Francisco
Fresno Program
2615 East Clinton Avenue
Fresno, CA 93703, USA

E-mail address:
deed@fresno.ucsf.edu

Prediction of Cardiovascular Disease Events

Peter W.F. Wilson, MD

KEYWORDS

- Coronary heart disease • Risk factors • Prediction
- Biomarkers

Prediction of cardiovascular disease has evolved because long-term observational studies have included detailed information on elements of risk prior to the development of clinical disease. Storage of information, computerization, and exportability of risk prediction tools has facilitated this process. Estimation of vascular disease risk includes accurate and precise baseline measurements, determination of outcomes, statistical programming, algorithm development, and performance evaluation.

ORIGINS OF VASCULAR DISEASE RISK ESTIMATION

Initial efforts to predict cardiovascular disease (CVD) events were related to the development of logistic regression data analysis and its adaptation to the prediction of coronary heart disease (CHD) events, with a focus on the first occurrence of myocardial infarction or CHD death. Prospective studies that originated in the late 1940s considered the role of factors such as age, sex, high blood pressure, high blood cholesterol, diabetes mellitus, and smoking as risk factors for heart disease. Logistic regression methods become available on large-frame computers in the 1950s and 1960s.[1,2] This process involved assembling data for a population sample that had been followed prospectively for the occurrence of a dichotomous event such as clinical CHD.

This approach involves identification of persons free of the vascular event of interest, obtaining baseline data on factors that might affect risk for the outcome, and following the participants prospectively for the development of the clinical outcome under investigation.[3] The original Framingham participants returned for new examinations and assessment of new cardiovascular events every 2 years, and cross-sectional pooling methods were developed using logistic regression in the original Framingham cohort to assess risk over time.

BASELINE MEASUREMENTS

Longitudinal studies of vascular disease usually have standardized measurements at baseline, and adjudicated outcomes that are consistent over the follow-up interval. It is possible to undertake multivariable analyses of factors that might be associated with a vascular disease outcome in a cross-sectional study,[4] but it is preferable to have a prospective design to fully understand the role of factor that might increase risk for developing a vascular disease event. A prospective design is necessary because critical risk factors may change after the occurrence of CHD, and such a design allows the inclusion of fatal events as outcomes. Standardized measurements are important to use when assessing the role of factors that might increase risk for vascular disease outcomes. For example, blood pressure levels are typically measured in the arm using an appropriate size arm cuff, inflating and deflating the arm cuff according to a protocol, maintaining the level of the arm near the level of heart, taking measurements in subjects who have been sitting in a room at ambient temperature for a specified number of minutes, using a sphygmomanometer that has been

The author has nothing to disclose.
Atlanta VAMC Epidemiology and Genetics Section, Emory Clinical Cardiovascular Research Institute, 1462 Clifton Road NE, Room 505, Atlanta, GA 30322, USA
E-mail address: peter.wf.wilson@emory.edu

Cardiol Clin 29 (2011) 1–13
doi:10.1016/j.ccl.2010.10.004
0733-8651/11/$ — see front matter © 2011 Elsevier Inc. All rights reserved.

standardized, and having determinations made by properly trained personnel. There are many ways that blood pressure can be measured inaccurately, including inconsistent positioning of the patient, varying the time the subject is at rest before taking measurement, varying credentials of the examiner (eg, nurses vs doctors), and rounding errors when recording the measurements.[5]

Lipid standardization has been in helping to assure accuracy and precision of lipid measurements used to help assess risk for cardiovascular events, and measurements are typically obtained in the fasting state. The Lipid Research Clinics Program that was initiated in the 1970s led to the development of a Lipid Standardization Program at the Centers for Disease Control with monitoring of research laboratories that measure cholesterol, high-density lipoprotein (HDL) cholesterol, and triglycerides.[6–8] This program updated the laboratory methodologies and techniques over time to accommodate newer methods of measurement.[9–11] Laboratory determinations have several potential sources of variability, including preanalytical, analytical, and biologic sources.[12,13] Preanalytical sources of error include fasting status, appropriate use of tourniquets during phlebotomy, room temperature, and sample transport conditions. Laboratory variability is minimized by using high-quality instrumentation and reliable assays, performing replicate assays, and employing algorithms to repeat assays if the difference between replicates exceeds specified thresholds. Other methods to ensure accuracy and precision with laboratory determinations include external standards, batching samples, and minimizing the number of lots for calibration. Sources of biologic variability include fasting status, time of day, season of the year, and intervening illnesses.[12]

Another key risk factor is diabetes status. Many of the older studies did not have fasting visits for each clinical visit and an expert-derived diagnosis of diabetes mellitus was employed based on the available glucose information, medication use, and chart reviews. The American Diabetes Association has changed the criteria for diabetes over the last few decades. For example, diabetes was considered present in 1979 if fasting glucose level was 140 mg/dL or greater or if a casual glucose level was greater than 200 mg/dL.[14] These criteria were revised in 1997 so that a fasting glucose level of 126 mg/dL or greater was considered to be diagnostic of diabetes mellitus.[15]

CARDIOVASCULAR DISEASE OUTCOMES

First CVD events have been studied the most. Total CHD (angina pectoris, myocardial infarction, and coronary heart disease death), or hard CHD (myocardial infarction and coronary heart disease death) are the outcomes that have been studied most frequently, but others have reported on the risk of hard CHD and have included persons with a baseline history of angina pectoris,[16] and the European CHD risk estimates have focused on the occurrence of CHD death.[17] In addition, investigators have developed risk algorithms for the occurrence of stroke, intermittent claudication, cardiac failure, and other outcomes.[18–21]

HISTORY OF CORONARY HEART DISEASE RISK ESTIMATION

Initial research on CHD prediction used logistic regression analyses, and the relative risk effects for each of the predictor variables were provided.[22] Time-dependent regression methods and the addition of HDL cholesterol levels as an important predictor led to improved prediction models for CHD,[23] employing score sheets and regression equation information with intercepts to estimate absolute risk for coronary heart disease over an interval that typically spanned 8 to 12 years of follow-up.

Score sheets to estimate CHD risk were highlighted in a Framingham CHD risk publication in 1991 that predicted total CHD,[24] and a variety of first cardiovascular events.[21] The outcome of interest was prediction of a first vascular disease event using the independent variables age, sex, high blood pressure, high blood cholesterol, diabetes mellitus, smoking, and left ventricular hypertrophy on the electrocardiogram. Risk equations with coefficients were provided to allow estimation of CHD risk using score sheets, pocket calculators, and computer programs.[24]

A 1998 Framingham CHD risk estimation article showed little difference in the overall predictive capability of Total CHD when total cholesterol was replaced by low-density lipoprotein (LDL) cholesterol, which suggested that an initial lipid screening with total cholesterol, HDL cholesterol, age, sex, systolic blood pressure, diabetes mellitus, and smoking had good overall predictive capabilities without lipid subgroup measurements.[25]

A workshop was convened by the National Heart, Lung, and Blood Institute in 2001 to assess the performance of estimating first CHD events in middle-aged Americans. In summaries of the workshop proceedings D'Agostino and colleagues[26] and Grundy and colleagues[27] compared the predictive results for CHD in several studies using Framingham equations or using equations that employed the same variables as the Framingham equation but used study-specific predictions. The summary findings included the following: (a) relative risks for the individual variables were similar to the Framingham experience, (b) the Framingham equations predicted CHD quite well when applied to other populations, and the c-statistic for the Framingham prediction was usually very similar to the c-statistic from the study-specific predictor equation, and (c) in African Americans and Japanese American men from the Honolulu Heart Study, the Framingham equation prediction had much lower discrimination capability.[26]

CORONARY HEART DISEASE RISK ALGORITHM DEVELOPMENT

In the modern era, risk estimates for CHD are usually derived from proportional hazards regression models according to methods developed by Cox.[28] The variables that are significant in the individual analyses are then considered for inclusion in multivariable prediction models using a fixed design or a stepwise model that selects the variables for inclusion using an iterative approach. Pair-wise interactions can be considered for inclusion in the model, but it may be difficult to interpret those results and interactions may be less generalizable when tested in other population groups.

Traditional candidate variables considered for this analysis have often included systolic or diastolic blood pressure, blood pressure treatment, cholesterol level, diabetes mellitus, current smoking, and body mass index. Including information related to treatment, such as blood pressure medication, should be used with caution in this situation because the risk algorithm is typically being developed from an observational study with a prospective design, not from a clinical trial in which treatments are randomly assigned.

A validation group is used to test the usefulness of the risk prediction algorithm. One approach uses an internal validation sample within the study. By this method a fraction of the data are used for model development and the other fraction of the data are used for validation. An alternative to this approach is to take a very large fraction of the persons in the study and successively develop models from near-complete data sets. External validation of a risk prediction model is especially useful, testing the use of the model in other population samples and providing the first indication of whether it is possible to generalize the risk prediction model to other venues.

PERFORMANCE CRITERIA FOR VASCULAR DISEASE RISK ALGORITHMS

A variety of statistical evaluations are now available to evaluate the usefulness of CHD risk prediction, and they are discussed successively in this section.

Relative Risk

For each risk factor, proportional hazards modeling yields regression coefficients for a study cohort. The relative risk of a variable is computed by exponentiating the regression coefficient in the multivariable regression models. For example, this measure estimates the difference in risk for someone with a given risk factor such as cigarette smoking compared with the risk for someone who does not smoke.

Discrimination

Discrimination is the ability of a statistical model to separate those who experience clinical CHD events from those who do not. The c-statistic is the typical performance measure, analogous to the area under a receiver-operator characteristic curve, and is a composite of the overall sensitivity and specificity of the prediction equation (**Fig. 1**).[29] The c-statistic represents an estimate of the probability that a model assigns a higher risk to those who develop CHD within a specified follow-up than to those who do not. The error associated with c-statistic estimates can be estimated.[29,30] Values for the c-statistic range from 0.00 to 1.00, and 0.50 reflects discrimination

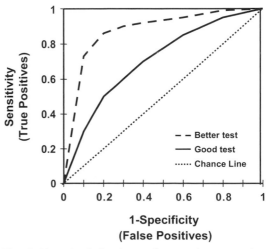

Fig. 1. Hypothetical schema for receiver-operating characteristic curves and disease prediction based on sensitivity and specificity of multivariable prediction models.

by chance. Higher values generally indicate a good level of agreement between observed and predicted risks. The average c-statistic for the prediction of CHD is typically in around 0.70.[3,26]

Calibration

Calibration measures how closely predicted estimates agree with actual outcomes. To present calibration analyses the data are often separated into deciles of risk, and observed rates are tested for differences from the expected across the deciles using a version of the Hosmer-Lemeshow chi-square statistic.[26]

Recalibration

An existing CHD prediction model can be recalibrated if it provides relatively good ranking of risk for the population being studied, but the model systematically over- or underestimates CHD risk in the new population. For example, recalibrating the Framingham risk prediction equation would involve inserting the mean risk factor values and average incidence rate for the new population into the Framingham equation. Kaplan-Meier estimates can be used to determine average incidence rates.[31] This approach was undertaken for Framingham risk equations that were applied to the CHD experience of Japanese American men in the Honolulu Heart Study, and for Chinese men and women.[26,31] In each of these instances the Framingham risk equation provided relatively good discrimination but did not provide reliable estimates of absolute risk. A schematic of such an approach is shown in **Fig. 2**, where the left panel shows that CHD risk is systematically overestimated when the Framingham equation is applied to another population. After calibration, the estimation fits the observed experience much more closely and the Hosmer Lemeshow chi-square is much lower.

Reclassification

Specialized testing in subgroups has been used to reclassify risk for vascular disease. An example of such an approach is the use of exercise testing to upgrade, downgrade, or not change estimates of vascular disease risk in patients being evaluated for angina pectoris.[32] CHD algorithms may do a reasonably good job in prediction of CHD risk, and the inclusion of a new variable may have minimal effects on c-statistic estimates.[33–36] Methods developed to assess this approach have used a multivariable estimation procedure and have tested the utility of a new test to increase, decrease, or not change risk estimates.[32] Pencina

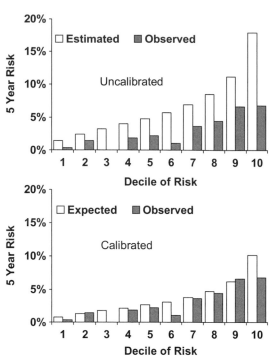

Fig. 2. Hypothetical example of uncalibrated and calibrated estimated and observed CHD risk according to deciles of CHD risk.

and colleagues[37] have recently published an updated method to assess reclassification, which takes into account the potential reclassification of both cases and noncases.

Reclassification has practical applications, as shown in **Fig. 3**, where an initial probability of CHD is estimated from a multivariable prediction

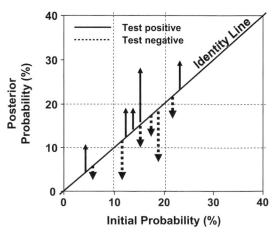

Fig. 3. Example of reclassification strategy and risk of disease according to initial and posterior probabilities. Gridlines represent potential levels that are associated with reclassification of risk.

equation, and additional information then provides an updated estimation of risk, which is commonly called the posterior estimate. If the new information did not provide any added value the risk estimate would be the same as for the initial calculation, and the risk estimate would lie close to the identity line. The schematic shows the hypothetical effects for a small number of patients. For some individuals the test was positive, increasing the posterior risk estimates. On the other hand, negative tests moved the risk estimates downward for some individuals. The magnitude of effects can be shown graphically by the length of the vertical lines and how they differ from the identifier line. Finally, it is important to evaluate a posterior risk estimate that would reclassify the individual to a lower or higher risk category. For example, **Fig. 3** shows 7 persons with an initial probability of developing disease in the 10% to 20% range. Risk was increased in 3 persons and decreased in 4 persons with new variable information, but some of the risk differences did not differ appreciably from the initial estimates. Risk was reclassified into a higher category in only 1 person and reclassified to a lower category in 2 persons. Some investigators have used performance measures such as the Bayes Information Criteria as another method to interpret potential effects of reclassification.[34]

PRESENT VASCULAR DISEASE RISK ESTIMATION

The current starting point for using a CHD risk prediction equation in persons being screened for CHD is a medical history and clinical examination with standardized collection of key predictor (independent) risk factors: age, sex, fasting lipids (total-, LDL-, HDL-cholesterol, total/HDL ratio), systolic blood pressure, history of diabetes mellitus treatment, fasting or postprandial glucose levels, and use of tobacco and other substances.[3,16] With this information it is possible to estimate risk of CHD over a 10-year interval using score sheets or computer programs.

Risk for several other vascular disease end points can be estimated, and examples of these algorithms for CHD, stroke, cardiac failure, and other outcomes are shown in **Table 1**. Most of the predictive models use the core variables that are employed for prediction of CHD.

Specialized models have been developed for persons with type 2 diabetes, which consider additional potential predictor variables. The experience of diabetic patients who participated in the United Kingdom Prospective Diabetes Study has been used to develop this prediction algorithm. The investigators have reported that the key predictor variables for initial CHD events were age, diabetes duration, presence of atrial fibrillation, glycosylated hemoglobin level, systolic blood pressure level, total cholesterol concentration, HDL-cholesterol concentration, race, and smoking status.[38]

European groups have developed strategies to estimate risk of CHD using European data. Investigators from the Prospective Cardiovascular Munster (PROCAM) in Germany (PROCAM) have followed a cohort for the development of CHD, and their results are generally similar to what has been estimated from Framingham data.[16] Their analyses were restricted to men. The factors significantly associated with the development of a next CHD event included age, LDL cholesterol, smoking, HDL cholesterol, systolic blood pressure, family history of premature myocardial infarction, diabetes mellitus, and triglycerides. Italian investigators[39] undertook prediction analyses in middle-aged men who were followed 10 years for CHD events, and found that age, total cholesterol, systolic blood pressure, cigarette smoking, HDL cholesterol, diabetes mellitus, hypertension drug treatment, and family history of CHD were associated with initial CHD events. The Italian team also tested the utility of Framingham and PROCAM in estimating equations in Italy. In general they found that both Framingham and PROCAM overestimated CHD risk in Italian men, and after calibration of the Framingham equations it was possible to reliably predict CHD events in their study cohort.[39] Risk scores have also been developed in the United Kingdom (QRISK) and Scotland (ASSIGN), with consideration of the effects of social deprivation. The QRISK algorithm predicts total cardiovascular disease (QRISK) using age, sex, smoking status, systolic blood pressure, ratio of total serum cholesterol to HDL cholesterol, body mass index, family history of CHD in first-degree relatives younger than 60 years, area measure of deprivation, and existing treatment with antihypertensive agents.

The EuroSCORE algorithm is currently the most popular CHD prediction algorithm in Europe. EuroSCORE predicts CHD death outcomes and includes a data from a large number of studies across Europe to generate the predictions. The factors used in the prediction include age, sex, smoking, systolic blood pressure, and the ratio of total cholesterol/HDL cholesterol. Unfortunately, not enough of the participating centers had data on CHD morbidity, and a prediction algorithm for total CHD based on experience across Europe is still in development.

Table 1
Examples of coronary heart disease and other CVD event prediction algorithms

	Authors,[Ref] Year of Publication							
	Wilson et al,[3] 1998	ATP III,[93] 2001	Assmann et al,[16] 2002	EuroSCORE,[17] 2003	Wolf et al,[18] 1991	Murabito et al,[19] 1997	Butler et al,[20] 2008	D'Agostino et al,[86] 2008
Source	Framingham	Framingham	PROCAM	Europe	Framingham	Framingham	Health ABC	Framingham
Outcome	Total CHD	Hard CHD	Hard CHD	CHD Mortality	Stroke	Intermittent claudication	Cardiac failure	Total CVD
Age interval	5 years	5 years	5 years	5 years	Intervals vary	5 years	5 years	5 years
Inclusion criteria	No CHD	No CHD	Possible CHD	No CHD	Possible CHD	Possible CHD	Possible CHD	No CVD
Sex	Men, women	Men, women	Men	Men, women	Men, women	Men, women	Men, women	Men, women
BP levels	JNC category	BP systolic	BP systolic	BP systolic	BP systolic	JNC category	BP systolic	BP systolic
BP therapy	No	Yes	No	No	Yes	No	No	Yes
Cholesterol	Yes	Yes	No	Yes	No	Yes	No	Yes
HDL cholesterol	Yes	Yes	Yes	No	No	No	No	Yes
LDL cholesterol	Optional	No	Yes	No	No	No	No	No
Cigarettes	Yes	Yes	Yes	Yes	Yes	Yes	No	Yes
Number/day	No	Yes	Yes	No	No			No
Glycemia	DM patients included	DM patients excluded	Diabetes status	Diabetes status	Diabetes status	Diabetes status	Glucose level	Diabetes status
Other factors	—	—	—	—	LVH-ECG, atrial fibrillation	—	Heart rate, LVH-ECG, albumin, creatinine	—
Baseline CVD included	ECG-LVH	No	MI history	No	CHD	No	CHD	No

Abbreviations: BP, blood pressure; DM, diabetes mellitus; ECG, electrocardiogram; JNC, Joint National Committee (on prevention, detection, evaluation, and treatment of high blood pressure); LVH, left ventricular hypertrophy; MI, myocardial infarction.

The development of CVD risk algorithms evolves according the measurement of risk factors, determination of the CVD outcomes, comparisons made with other groups, and whether calibration is used. **Table 2** shows how such evidence is used to estimate CVD risk and how successively greater evidence and confidence in predictions is achieved for investigations that use the methods shown in the lower rows in this table. As an example, Chinese investigators developed calibrated vascular disease risk scores in collaboration with American investigators (evidence level 3)[31] and later developed their own risk algorithm (evidence level 4).[40]

NEW BIOMARKERS: LIPIDS

There is increasing evidence that other lipid measures beyond traditional lipids are important determinants for CVD risk.[41-44] Such factors include analysis of apolipoprotein levels and lipoprotein subclasses, indices of lipoprotein-associated oxidation. Investigation of these biomarkers will provide the opportunity to evaluate whether advanced biomarker testing of lipid measures are predictive of CVD events.

Several large prospective studies have demonstrated that apolipoprotein B (apoB) measurements are equivalent or superior to cholesterol-based indices with respect to risk of coronary artery disease (CAD). For example, in subjects without known CVD, the Quebec Cardiovascular Study found that apoB was the strongest predictor of CVD risk in more than 2000 men followed for 5.5 years even after adjustment for conventional lipid measures.[45] Similar results were reported from AMORIS[46] and ARIC.[47] ApoB levels were also found to be superior to LDL cholesterol in identifying CVD risk for women,[48] in patients with prior myocardial infarction,[49] and those with diabetes.[50] It appears that the apoB measurements are at least as good as LDL cholesterol in terms of predicting risk of CVD events.

Comparisons have been obtained from observational cohorts that have included relatively asymptomatic individuals and from an era when treatment of dyslipidemia was relatively uncommon.[47,51] Specific cut points for lipid and apolipoprotein levels have been proposed as having similar effects on risk,[52] but the actual experience concerning the cardiovascular event predictive capabilities for levels of each of the lipid analytes is not known, especially in the modern era, when medications to treat dyslipidemia are commonly used. Similarly, apoA-I levels appear to discriminate better than HDL-cholesterol individuals with angiographically documented CAD from controls.[53] Thus, the use of the apoB/apoA-I ratio as a new risk factor for CVD and a target for lipid-lowering therapy has been proposed.[54]

Table 2
Evidence and vascular risk estimation

Evidence Level	Risk Factors	Outcomes	Risk Estimation Comparison	Calibration
1 (low)	Measured some, self report for others	Determined not adjudicated	Previously published risk score (categorical variables)	Not evaluated
2	Measured all	Adjudicated	Previously published risk score (categorical variables)	Not evaluated
3	Measured all	Adjudicated	Previously published risk score (continuous variables)	Not evaluated
4	Measured all	Adjudicated	Own Multifactor risk Score (continuous variables)	Usually not applicable
5 (high)	Measured all	Adjudicated	Own Multifactor risk Score (continuous variables)	Externally validated Assessed calibration

Beyond the measurement of traditional lipids and apolipoproteins, there is great interest having more information concerning the predictive utility of LDL and HDL particle number, measurements that are obtained by nuclear magnetic resonance spectroscopy.[55,56] Analyses from Framingham and other observational cohorts for asymptomatic individuals have shown that LDL particle number is highly associated with the development of CVD events, and its effect is at least commensurate with the experience obtained for LDL cholesterol.[57] Increased levels in lipoprotein(a) have also been shown to be predictive of greater risk for CHD, and the evidence for this biomarker has been more convincing in white populations.[58–60]

NEW BIOMARKERS: PROINFLAMMATORY MEASURES

Arterial wall inflammation is a critical antecedent for atherosclerotic events.[61] Vascular disease risk factors such as smoking, sedentary state, excessive alcohol consumption, and central obesity are associated with higher levels of inflammatory markers.[62] High-sensitivity C-reactive protein (hsCRP) is an acute-phase protein that is synthesized and secreted by hepatocytes in response to inflammatory cytokines (eg, interleukin-1 and -6). Inflammatory biomarkers appear to improve CVD risk prediction beyond that achieved by analysis of traditional risk factors in both healthy subjects and patients with acute coronary syndromes,[34] and data from Framingham and the Reynolds Risk Score investigations generally show that hsCRP measurements provide added value for vascular disease prediction.[63–65]

Lipoprotein-associated phospholipase A_2 (Lp-PLA$_2$) is another circulating inflammatory marker that appears to predict future adverse CVD events.[66,67] The effects of Lp-PLA$_2$ appear to differ from the effects observed for hsCRP, and there is utility in measuring both biomarkers.[68,69] Lp-PLA$_2$ is synthesized by inflammatory cells, binds directly to the apoB moiety of LDL, and is preferentially distributed into the small, dense LDL particles. Most of Lp-PLA$_2$ in plasma is on LDL particles, and the molecule hydrolyzes oxidized phospholipids in LDL to form 2 proinflammatory molecules (lysophosphatidylcholine and oxidized nonesterified fatty acids). These bioactive lipid mediators elicit several inflammatory responses that may account for the endothelial dysfunction associated with oxidized LDL in lesion-prone vasculature. A meta-analysis of 14 eligible studies (N = 20,549 patients) demonstrated that elevated levels of either Lp-PLA$_2$ plasma activity (n = 5 studies) or an immunoassay that measured the plasma concentration (n = 9 studies) were both associated with increased risk of CVD events (adjusted odds ratio of 1.60).[70] Levels of hsCRP and Lp-PLA$_2$ levels do not correlate with each other. Moreover, they appear to have independent and additive value in predicting risk for stroke and CAD,[68,71] highlighting the importance of a multi-marker approach to determine vascular disease risk.

ADVANCED BIOMARKERS: LIPOPROTEIN-ASSOCIATED OXIDATION

One proposed unifying mechanism whereby disparate risk factors lead to vascular disease is believed to be by promotion of oxidative stress, which occurs when the production of cellular oxidants exceeds the capacity of cellular antioxidant defense mechanisms. According to the oxidation hypothesis of atherosclerosis, LDL in its native form is not atherogenic, but LDL that has been oxidatively modified is avidly taken up by activated macrophages leading to the formation of foam cells, a key landmark of atherosclerosis.[72,73] Modification of plasma LDL can occur via lipid peroxidation by free radicals[74] or via protein modification by specific oxidant enzymes such as catalase and myeloperoxidase.[75] Whereas interactions of excess reactive oxygen species result in the generation of oxidatively modified LDL (oxLDL), interactions of excess reactive nitrogen species lead to the formation of nytrotyrosine-modified LDL. The contribution of both these forms of damaged LDL will be evaluated in the study participants.

Increased oxidant stress may be a determinant of future CVD events, and biomarkers such as oxLDL and nitrotyrosinated protein have been measured as indicators of oxidant stress.[76–78] High levels of oxLDL have been reported in patients with coronary stenosis (1.9-fold).[79] In more than 3000 older individuals, persons with a low Framingham score had lower oxLDL levels than participants with higher scores.[80]

Myeloperoxidase (MPO) is an enzyme secreted by activated neutrophils and monocyte-derived macrophages. MPO promotes the formation of free radicals that can enhance the generation of oxidized LDL, and thus contributes to the progression of atherosclerotic disease. Several studies have reported that elevated MPO levels at hospital admission are associated with increased risk of recurrent ischemic events in follow-up studies of up to 2 years.[81,82] In fact, in the EPIC Norfolk Prospective Population Study of apparently healthy individuals, high MPO levels are associated with increased risk for CAD during the 8-year follow-up period.[83] In addition, other related biomarkers under investigation include high-sensitivity troponin I, N-terminal pro brain natriuretic protein (ProBNP), and cellular adhesion molecules.[42,84,85]

FUTURE OF CORONARY HEART DISEASE PREDICTION

The prediction of CHD has helped to guide clinical decisions for persons free of clinical CVD at baseline. It is especially helpful in identifying middle-aged individuals who should be treated aggressively with management of cholesterol and blood pressure. As blood pressure and lipid treatment strategies become more widespread, more efficacious, and achievable at lower cost, it makes sense to try to prevent total cardiovascular events. For the preceding reasons it is likely that first CVD events (including total CHD, peripheral arterial disease, cerebrovascular disease, and cardiac failure) may become the clinical outcome of greatest interest and significance in the future.[21,86] Some investigations, especially large cardiovascular registries, have also been involved with the prediction of next cardiovascular events and bedside risk estimation of 6-month mortality in patients surviving admission for an acute coronary syndromes.[87,88]

Coronary disease risk can be estimated by several methods, and recent reports have shown that simple prediction tools can potentially be self-administered. For example, analyses undertaken by Mainous and colleagues[89] for participants in the Atherosclerosis Risk in Communities Study showed that the variables age, diabetes, hypertension, hypercholesterolemia, smoking, physical activity, and family history were predictive of initial CHD events in men, and similar results were available for women. Similarly, Gaziano and colleagues[90] used data from the National Health and Nutrition Examination Survey and showed that a simple set of variables, including age, systolic blood pressure, smoking status, body mass index, reported diabetes status, and current treatment of hypertension were predictive of CHD risk. It has been suggested that such approaches may be useful in developing parts of the world, where lower cost estimates of CHD risk would be particularly useful.

Imaging information related to atherosclerotic burden can be particularly helpful to predict risk of CHD events, but the cost of such procedures is relatively large compared with the low cost of health risk screening.[91] Atherosclerotic imaging may be particularly successful when coupled with reclassification that first identifies persons at intermediate risk by low-cost screening methods and then followed up with an imaging test of an arterial bed (coronary arteries, aorta, or carotid) to reclassify risk, depending on the results of the imaging test. Reclassification strategies may have their greatest utility as a follow-up to sensitive, lower cost, but not highly specific screening strategies such as CHD risk algorithms that are currently in place. Such strategies have not been worked out up to this time and are likely to be considered in the next round of recommendations for screening and follow-up for cardiovascular risk, where risk algorithms are already in place and the ability to undertake atherosclerotic imaging or other specialized laboratory testing is available. Genetic information can potentially be used to develop an estimate of CHD risk, and some investigators have undertaken analyses using this approach.[92] It is likely that this method will achieve greater efficacy when the genetic information is coupled with clinically useful information such as blood pressure and lipid levels.

SUMMARY

Observational studies have provided the richest source of information to develop CHD risk estimation. Most risk estimation has been derived from an era when aggressive treatment of risk factors was not common. Treatment of risk factors with lipid and blood pressure medications will complicate risk estimation in the future. Follow-up intervals of 5 to 15 years are typical for development of CHD risk-estimating equations, and a 10-year interval is commonly used for reporting. Performance criteria for risk estimation include discrimination, calibration, and reclassification. These methods provide information concerning the usefulness of the prediction equation to separate future cases from noncases, allows evaluation on how well the risk-estimating equation might work in other regions, and can help to provide a context for the evaluation of novel risk factors.

REFERENCES

1. Walker SH, Duncan DB. Estimation of the probability of an event as a function of several independent variables. Biometrika 1967;54:167–79.
2. Truett J, Cornfield J, Kannel WB. A multivariate analysis of risk of coronary heart disease in Framingham. J Chronic Dis 1967;20:511–24.
3. Wilson PW, D'Agostino RB, Levy D, et al. Prediction of coronary heart disease using risk factor categories. Circulation 1998;97:1837–47.
4. Schlesselman JJ. Case-control studies. 1 edition. New York: Oxford; 1982.
5. Chobanian AV, Bakris GL, Black HR, et al. The Seventh report of the Joint National Committee on prevention, detection, evaluation, and treatment of

high blood pressure: the JNC 7 report. JAMA 2003; 289:2560–72.

6. Lipid Research Clinics Population Studies. Data book: volume 1. The Prevalence Study 1980 (NIH Publ 80-1527). 1st edition. Bethesda (MD): NIH; 1990.

7. Lipid Research Clinics Program. Manual of laboratory operation. 1st edition. Bethesda (MD): NIH; 1974.

8. Rifkind BM, Segal P. Lipid Research Clinics Program reference values for hyperlipidemia and hypolipidemia. JAMA 1983;250:1869–72.

9. Warnick GR, Myers GL, Cooper GR, et al. Impact of the third cholesterol report from the adult treatment panel of the national cholesterol education program on the clinical laboratory. Clin Chem 2002;48:11–7.

10. McNamara JR, Leary ET, Ceriotti F, et al. Point: status of lipid and lipoprotein standardization. Clin Chem 1997;43:1306–10.

11. Myers GL, Cooper GR, Sampson EJ. Traditional lipoprotein profile: clinical utility, performance requirement, and standardization. Atherosclerosis 1994; 108(Suppl):S157–69.

12. Cooper GR, Myers GL, Smith J, et al. Blood lipid measurements: variations and practical utility. JAMA 1992;267:1652–60.

13. Cooper GR, Smith SJ, Myers GL, et al. Estimating and minimizing effects of biologic sources of variation by relative range when measuring the mean of serum lipids and lipoproteins. Clin Chem 1994;40:227–32.

14. National Diabetes Data Group. Classification and diagnosis of diabetes mellitus and other categories of glucose intolerance. Diabetes 1979;28:1039–57.

15. Report of the Expert Committee on the diagnosis and classification of diabetes mellitus. Diabetes Care 1997;20:1183–97.

16. Assmann G, Cullen P, Schulte H. Simple scoring scheme for calculating the risk of acute coronary events based on the 10-year follow-up of the Prospective Cardiovascular Munster (PROCAM) study. Circulation 2002;105:310–5.

17. Conroy RM, Pyorala K, Fitzgerald AP, et al. Estimation of ten-year risk of fatal cardiovascular disease in Europe: the SCORE project. Eur Heart J 2003; 24:987–1003.

18. Wolf PA, D'Agostino RB, Belanger AJ, et al. Probability of stroke: a risk profile from the Framingham Study. Stroke 1991;3:312–8.

19. Murabito JM, D'Agostino RB, Silbershatz H, et al. Intermittent claudication: a risk profile from the Framingham Heart Study. Circulation 1997;96:44–9.

20. Butler J, Kalogeropoulos A, Georgiopoulou V, et al. Incident heart failure prediction in the elderly: the health ABC heart failure score. Circ Heart Fail 2008;1:125–33.

21. Anderson KM, Odell PM, Wilson PWF, et al. Cardiovascular disease risk profiles. Am Heart J 1991;121: 293–8.

22. Kannel WB, Castelli WP, Gordon T, et al. Serum cholesterol, lipoproteins, and the risk of coronary heart disease: the Framingham Study. Ann Intern Med 1971;74:1–12.

23. Wilson PWF, Castelli WP, Kannel WB. Coronary risk prediction in adults: the Framingham Heart Study. Am J Cardiol 1987;59(G):91–4.

24. Anderson KM, Wilson PWF, Odell PM, et al. An updated coronary risk profile. A statement for health professionals. Circulation 1991;83:357–63.

25. Joint National Committee. The fifth report of the Joint National Committee on detection, evaluation, and treatment of high blood pressure (JNC V). Arch Intern Med 1993;153:154–83.

26. D'Agostino RB Sr, Grundy S, Sullivan LM, et al. Validation of the Framingham coronary heart disease prediction scores: results of a multiple ethnic groups investigation. JAMA 2001;286:180–7.

27. Grundy SM, D'Agostino Sr RB, Mosca L, et al. Cardiovascular risk assessment based on US cohort studies: findings from a National Heart, Lung, and Blood institute workshop. Circulation 2001;104:491–6.

28. Cox DR. Regression models and life tables. J R Stat Soc (B) 1972;34:187–220.

29. Pencina MJ, D'Agostino RB. Overall C as a measure of discrimination in survival analysis: model specific population value and confidence interval estimation. Stat Med 2004;23:2109–23.

30. D'Agostino RB Sr, Nam BH. Evaluation of the performance of survival analysis models: discrimination and calibration measures. Handbook of statistics, vol 23: advances in survival analysis. 1st edition. Amsterdam (Netherlands): Elsevier; 2004. p. 1–26.

31. Liu J, Hong Y, D'Agostino RB Sr, et al. Predictive value for the Chinese population of the Framingham CHD risk assessment tool compared with the Chinese Multi-Provincial Cohort Study. JAMA 2004; 291:2591–9.

32. Diamond GA, Hirsch M, Forrester JS, et al. Application of information theory to clinical diagnostic testing. The electrocardiographic stress test. Circulation 1981;63:915–21.

33. Wilson PW, Nam BH, Pencina M, et al. C-reactive protein and risk of cardiovascular disease in men and women from the Framingham heart study. Arch Intern Med 2005;165:2473–8.

34. Cook NR, Buring JE, Ridker PM. The effect of including C-reactive protein in cardiovascular risk prediction models for women. Ann Intern Med 2006;145:21–9.

35. Pepe MS, Thompson ML. Combining diagnostic test results to increase accuracy. Biostatistics 2000;1: 123–40.

36. Pepe MS, Janes H, Longton G, et al. Limitations of the odds ratio in gauging the performance of a diagnostic, prognostic, or screening marker. Am J Epidemiol 2004;159:882–90.

37. Pencina MJ, D'Agostino RB Sr, D'Agostino RB Jr, et al. Evaluating the added predictive ability of a new marker: from area under the ROC curve to re-classification and beyond. Stat Med 2008;27:157–72.

38. Stevens RJ, Kothari V, Adler AI, et al. The UKPDS risk engine: a model for the risk of coronary heart disease in Type II diabetes (UKPDS 56). Clin Sci (Lond) 2001;101:671–9.

39. Ferrario M, Chiodini P, Chambless LE, et al. Prediction of coronary events in a low incidence population. Assessing accuracy of the CUORE Cohort Study prediction equation. Int J Epidemiol 2005;34:413–21.

40. Wu Y, Liu X, Li X, et al. Estimation of 10-year risk of fatal and nonfatal ischemic cardiovascular diseases in Chinese adults. Circulation 2006;114:2217–25.

41. de Lemos JA, Morrow DA. Brain natriuretic peptide measurement in acute coronary syndromes: ready for clinical application? Circulation 2002;106:2868–70.

42. Blankenberg S, Zeller T, Saarela O, et al. Contribution of 30 Biomarkers to 10-Year cardiovascular risk estimation in 2 population cohorts: the MONICA, Risk, Genetics, Archiving, and Monograph (MORGAM) Biomarker Project. Circulation 2010;121:2388–97.

43. Folsom AR, Chambless LE, Ballantyne CM, et al. An assessment of incremental coronary risk prediction using C-reactive protein and other novel risk markers: the atherosclerosis risk in communities study. Arch Intern Med 2006;166:1368–73.

44. Thompson SG, Kienast J, Pyke SD, et al. Hemostatic factors and the risk of myocardial infarction or sudden death in patients with angina pectoris. European Concerted Action on Thrombosis and Disabilities Angina Pectoris Study Group. N Engl J Med 1995;332:635–41.

45. Lamarche B, Tchernof A, Moorjani S, et al. Small, dense low-density lipoprotein particles as a predictor of the risk of ischemic heart disease in men. Prospective results from the Quebec Cardiovascular Study. Circulation 1997;95:69–75.

46. Walldius G, Jungner I, Holme I, et al. High apolipoprotein B, low apolipoprotein A-I, and improvement in the prediction of fatal myocardial infarction (AMORIS study): a prospective study. Lancet 2001;358:2026–33.

47. Sharrett AR, Ballantyne CM, Coady SA, et al. Coronary heart disease prediction from lipoprotein cholesterol levels, triglycerides, lipoprotein(a), apolipoproteins A-I and B, and HDL density subfractions: the Atherosclerosis Risk in Communities (ARIC) Study. Circulation 2001;104:1108–13.

48. Shai I, Rimm EB, Hankinson SE, et al. Multivariate assessment of lipid parameters as predictors of coronary heart disease among postmenopausal women: potential implications for clinical guidelines. Circulation 2004;110:2824–30.

49. Moss AJ, Goldstein RE, Marder VJ, et al. Thrombogenic factors and recurrent coronary events. Circulation 1999;99:2517–22.

50. Jiang R, Schulze MB, Li T, et al. Non-HDL cholesterol and apolipoprotein B predict cardiovascular disease events among men with type 2 diabetes. Diabetes Care 2004;27:1991–7.

51. Ingelsson E, Schaefer EJ, Contois JH, et al. Clinical utility of different lipid measures for prediction of coronary heart disease in men and women. JAMA 2007;298:776–85.

52. Brunzell JD, Davidson M, Furberg CD, et al. Lipoprotein management in patients with cardiometabolic risk: consensus conference report from the American Diabetes Association and the American College of Cardiology Foundation. J Am Coll Cardiol 2008;51:1512–24.

53. Maciejko JJ, Holmes DR, Kottke BA, et al. Apolipoprotein A-I as a marker of angiographically assessed coronary artery disease. N Engl J Med 1983;309:385–9.

54. van Lennep JE, Westerveld HT, van Lennep HW, et al. Apolipoprotein concentrations during treatment and recurrent coronary artery disease events. Arterioscler Thromb Vasc Biol 2000;20:2408–13.

55. Jeyarajah EJ, Cromwell WC, Otvos JD. Lipoprotein particle analysis by nuclear magnetic resonance spectroscopy. Clin Lab Med 2006;26:847–70.

56. Festa A, Williams K, Hanley AJ, et al. Nuclear magnetic resonance lipoprotein abnormalities in prediabetic subjects in the Insulin Resistance Atherosclerosis Study. Circulation 2005;111:3465–72.

57. Cromwell W, Otvos JD, Keyes MJ, et al. LDL particle number and risk of future cardiovascular disease in the Framingham Offspring Study—implications for LDL management. J Clin Lipidol 2007;1:583–92.

58. Bostom AG, Cupples LA, Jenner JL, et al. Elevated plasma lipoprotein (a) and coronary heart disease in men aged 55 years and younger: a prospective study. JAMA 1996;276:544–8.

59. Scanu AM. Lipoprotein(a) and the atherothrombotic process: mechanistic insights and clinical implications. Curr Atheroscler Rep 2003;5:106–13.

60. Tsimikas S, Brilakis ES, Miller ER, et al. Oxidized phospholipids, Lp(a) lipoprotein, and coronary artery disease. N Engl J Med 2005;353:46–57.

61. Pearson TA, Mensah GA, Alexander RW, et al. Markers of inflammation and cardiovascular disease: application to clinical and public health practice: a statement for healthcare professionals from the Centers for Disease Control and Prevention and the American Heart Association. Circulation 2003;107:499–511.

62. Ridker PM, Brown NJ, Vaughan DE, et al. Established and emerging plasma biomarkers in the

prediction of first atherothrombotic events. Circulation 2004;109:IV6–19.

63. Wilson PWF, Pencina M, Jacques P, et al. C-Reactive protein and reclassification of cardiovascular risk in the Framingham Heart Study. Circ Cardiovasc Qual Outcomes 2008;1:92–7.

64. Ridker PM, Paynter NP, Rifai N, et al. C-reactive protein and parental history improve global cardiovascular risk prediction: the Reynolds Risk Score for men. Circulation 2008;118:2243–51, 4p.

65. Ridker PM, Buring JE, Rifai N, et al. Development and validation of improved algorithms for the assessment of global cardiovascular risk in women: the Reynolds Risk Score. JAMA 2007;297:611–9.

66. Oei HH, van der Meer IM, Hofman A, et al. Lipoprotein-associated phospholipase A2 activity is associated with risk of coronary heart disease and ischemic stroke: the Rotterdam Study. Circulation 2005;111:570–5.

67. Zalewski A, Macphee C. Role of lipoprotein-associated phospholipase A2 in atherosclerosis: biology, epidemiology, and possible therapeutic target. Arterioscler Thromb Vasc Biol 2005;25:923–31.

68. Ballantyne CM, Hoogeveen RC, Bang H, et al. Lipoprotein-associated phospholipase A2, high-sensitivity C-reactive protein, and risk for incident coronary heart disease in middle-aged men and women in the Atherosclerosis Risk in Communities (ARIC) study. Circulation 2004;109:837–42.

69. Sabatine MS, Morrow DA, O'Donoghue M, et al. Prognostic utility of lipoprotein-associated phospholipase A2 for cardiovascular outcomes in patients with stable coronary artery disease. Arterioscler Thromb Vasc Biol 2007;27:2463–9.

70. Garza CA, Montori VM, McConnell JP, et al. Association between lipoprotein-associated phospholipase A2 and cardiovascular disease: a systematic review. Mayo Clin Proc 2007;82:159–65.

71. Ballantyne CM, Hoogeveen RC, Bang H, et al. Lipoprotein-associated phospholipase A2, high-sensitivity C-reactive protein, and risk for incident ischemic stroke in middle-aged men and women in the Atherosclerosis Risk in Communities (ARIC) Study. Arch Intern Med 2005;165:2479–84.

72. Steinberg D, Parthasarathy S, Carew TE, et al. Beyond cholesterol: modifications of low-density lipoproteins that increase its atherogenicity. N Engl J Med 1989;320:915–24.

73. Glass CK, Witztum JL. Atherosclerosis. The road ahead. Cell 2001;104:503–16.

74. McCord JM. Oxygen-derived free radicals in postischemic tissue injury. N Engl J Med 1985;312:159–63.

75. Podrez EA, Schmitt D, Hoff HF, et al. Myeloperoxidase-generated reactive nitrogen species convert LDL into an atherogenic form in vitro. J Clin Invest 1999;103:1547–60.

76. Holvoet P, Harris TB, Tracy RP, et al. Association of high coronary heart disease risk status with circulating oxidized LDL in the well-functioning elderly: findings from the Health, Aging, and Body Composition Study. Arterioscler Thromb Vasc Biol 2003;23:1444–8.

77. Holvoet P, Vanhaecke J, Janssens S, et al. Oxidized LDL and malondialdehyde-modified LDL in patients with acute coronary syndromes and stable coronary artery disease. Circulation 1998;98:1487–94.

78. Holvoet P, Theilmeier G, Shivalkar B, et al. LDL hypercholesterolemia is associated with accumulation of oxidized LDL, atherosclerotic plaque growth, and compensatory vessel enlargement in coronary arteries of miniature pigs. Arterioscler Thromb Vasc Biol 1998;18:415–22.

79. Ehara S, Ueda M, Naruko T, et al. Elevated levels of oxidized low density lipoprotein show a positive relationship with the severity of acute coronary syndromes. Circulation 2001;103:1955–60.

80. Holvoet P, Kritchevsky SB, Tracy RP, et al. The metabolic syndrome, circulating oxidized LDL, and risk of myocardial infarction in well-functioning elderly people in the health, aging, and body composition cohort. Diabetes 2004;53:1068–73.

81. Morrow DA, Braunwald E. Future of biomarkers in acute coronary syndromes: moving toward a multimarker strategy. Circulation 2003;108:250–2.

82. Morrow DA, Sabatine MS, Brennan ML, et al. Concurrent evaluation of novel cardiac biomarkers in acute coronary syndrome: myeloperoxidase and soluble CD40 ligand and the risk of recurrent ischaemic events in TACTICS-TIMI 18. Eur Heart J 2008;29:1096–102.

83. Meuwese MC, Stroes ES, Hazen SL, et al. Serum myeloperoxidase levels are associated with the future risk of coronary artery disease in apparently healthy individuals: the EPIC-Norfolk Prospective Population Study. J Am Coll Cardiol 2007;50:159–65.

84. Omland T, de Lemos JA, Sabatine MS, et al. A sensitive cardiac troponin T assay in stable coronary artery disease. N Engl J Med 2009;361:2538–47.

85. Januzzi JL Jr, Bamberg F, Lee H, et al. High-sensitivity troponin T concentrations in acute chest pain patients evaluated with cardiac computed tomography. Circulation 2010;121:1227–34.

86. D'Agostino RB Sr, Vasan RS, Pencina MJ, et al. General cardiovascular risk profile for use in primary care: the Framingham Heart Study. Circulation 2008;117:743–53.

87. Califf RM, Armstrong PW, Carver JR, et al. 27th Bethesda Conference: matching the intensity of risk factor management with the hazard for coronary disease events. Task Force 5. Stratification of patients into high, medium and low risk subgroups

for purposes of risk factor management. J Am Coll Cardiol 1996;27:1007–19.

88. Eagle KA, Lim MJ, Dabbous OH, et al. A validated prediction model for all forms of acute coronary syndrome: estimating the risk of 6-month postdischarge death in an international registry. JAMA 2004;291:2727–33.

89. Mainous AG III, Koopman RJ, Diaz VA, et al. A coronary heart disease risk score based on patient-reported information. Am J Cardiol 2007;99:1236–41.

90. Gaziano TA, Young CR, Fitzmaurice G, et al. Laboratory-based versus nonlaboratory-based method for assessment of cardiovascular disease risk: the NHANES I Follow-up Study cohort. Lancet 2008; 371:923–31.

91. Detrano R, Guerci AD, Carr JJ, et al. Coronary calcium as a predictor of coronary events in four racial or ethnic groups. N Engl J Med 2008;358: 1336–45.

92. Humphries SE, Yiannakouris N, Talmud PJ. Cardiovascular disease risk prediction using genetic information (gene scores): is it really informative? Curr Opin Lipidol 2008;19:128–32.

93. Expert Panel on Detection, Evaluation, and Treatment of High Blood Cholesterol In Adults. Executive Summary of The Third Report of The National Cholesterol Education Program (NCEP) Expert Panel on detection, evaluation, and treatment of high blood cholesterol in adults (Adult Treatment Panel III). JAMA 2001;285:2486–97.

Interventions for Cardiovascular Disease Prevention

Rajeev Gupta, MD, PhD[a,b,*], Prakash Deedwania, MD[c]

KEYWORDS

- Cardiovascular disease • Prevention • Policy initiative

It is now established that noncommunicable diseases (NCDs), especially cardiovascular diseases (CVD), are major causes of death and disability worldwide, also in low- and middle-income countries.[1] The World Health Organization (WHO) estimates that chronic NCDs are responsible for about 70% of all deaths worldwide of which CVD is the major component.[2] According to the US Institute of Medicine report, there is a large heterogeneity in CVD mortality in different regions of the world (**Fig. 1**). The highest age-adjusted mortality is observed in middle-income countries of eastern Europe, central Asia, and low-income countries in Asia and Africa. Mortality rates are lowest in the high-income countries of North America and western Europe.[3] Mortality has declined significantly in high-income countries, whereas it is increasing in low- and middle-income countries.[4] In low-income developing countries, the increase in coronary heart disease (CHD) and stroke is largely an urban phenomenon and a rapid increase in rural populations has been reported only recently.[5]

Risk factors for CVD have been extensively studied in developed countries. Multiple prospective studies have reported that smoking, high low-density lipoprotein (LDL) cholesterol, low high-density lipoprotein (HDL) cholesterol, hypertension, and type 2 diabetes are major proximate risk factors.[6] All these factors are caused by abnormal lifestyles characterized by sedentary habits, overnutrition, and stress. Only limited prospective studies exist in low-income countries. The international case-control INTERHEART study reported that standard risk factors such as smoking, abnormal lipids, hypertension, diabetes, high waist/hip ratio, sedentary lifestyle, psychosocial stress, and lack of consumption of fruits and vegetables explained more than 90% of acute myocardial infarction events in populations of 52 countries including those of low-income countries.[7] Similar conclusions were reached in limited prospective studies in these countries, urban-rural comparisons in risk factors, and smaller case-control studies.[1,5] The INTERSTROKE study reported that 10 common risk factors explained more than 90% incident hemorrhagic and thrombotic strokes.[8] The risk factors are similar to those in the INTERHEART study but the population-attributable risks are different with greater importance of hypertension and lesser importance of diabetes and lipids (**Table 1**).

Population-based studies in high-income countries have reported that major risk factors such as smoking and hypertension are declining.[9] Management and control of hypertension and hypercholesterolemia are increasing.[10] Reviews of epidemiologic studies in low- and middle-income countries suggest that all the major risk

Conflicts of interest: The author is a member of the Indian Cardiovascular Research and Advocacy Group at St John's Research Institute, St John's Medical College, Bangalore and financially supported by center for excellence grant (BAA HV0912 650066553) from National Heart Lung and Blood Institute under the Global Health Initiative of National Institutes of Health, USA. There are no other financial conflicts of interest relevant to this article.

a Department of Medicine, Fortis Escorts Hospital, JLN Marg, Jaipur 302017, India
b Department of Medicine, Rajasthan University of Health Sciences, Jaipur 302023, India
c Division of Cardiology, Department of Medicine, Veterans Affairs Central California Health Care System/ University of California, San Francisco, Fresno Program, 2615 East Clinton Avenue, Fresno, CA 93703, USA
* Corresponding author. Department of Medicine, Fortis Escorts Hospital, JLN Marg, Jaipur 302017, India.
E-mail address: rajeevg@satyam.net.in

Cardiol Clin 29 (2011) 15–34
doi:10.1016/j.ccl.2010.10.005
0733-8651/11/$ — see front matter © 2011 Published by Elsevier Inc.

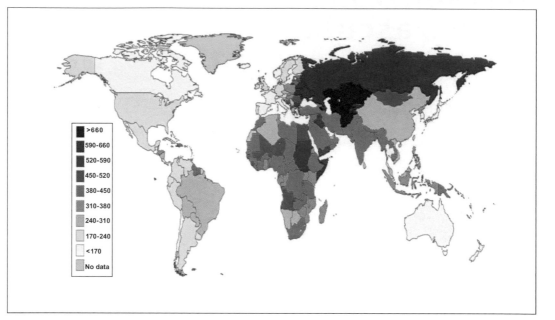

Fig. 1. Cardiovascular mortality patterns vary in different countries. There is substantial variation in age-adjusted mortality with the highest rates in central Asia, eastern and central Europe, and some countries in Africa, and the lowest rates in western Europe and northern America. (*From* Fuster V, Kelly BB, and Board for Global Health. Promoting cardiovascular health in developing world: a critical challenge to achieve global health. Washington DC: Institute of Medicine. 2010. Reprinted with permission from the National Academies Press, Copyright 2010, National Academy of Sciences.)

factors are increasing. Tobacco production, marketing, and consumption have increased significantly in the last 30 years.[11] Smoking is increasing among young people (aged 20–35 years) according to national health surveys in China and India.[12,13] Studies have reported increasing obesity as well as truncal obesity,[14] increasing sedentary lifestyles,[1] and psychosocial stress.[15] The prevalence of hypertension has increased in both urban and rural subjects and is presently 25% to 40% in urban adults and 10% to 15% among rural adults in different parts of

Table 1
Population-attributable risks (%) of various cardiovascular risk factors for CHD and stroke in INTERHEART and INTERSTROKE studies

Risk Factor	INTERHEART (Acute Myocardial Infarction)	INTERSTROKE (Thrombotic or Hemorrhagic Strokes)
Apolipoprotein A/B ratio	49.2	24.9
Hypertension	17.9 (history)	34.6
Smoking	35.7	18.9
Diabetes history	9.9	5.0
High waist/hip ratio	20.1	26.5
Psychosocial stress	32.5	9.8
No regular physical activity	12.2	28.5
Diet/diet score	13.7	18.8
Lack of alcohol intake	6.7	3.8
Cardiac causes	—	6.7

Data from Yusuf S, Hawken S, Ounpuu S, et al. Effect of potentially modifiable risk factors associated with myocardial infarction in 52 countries (the INTERHEART study): case control study. Lancet 2004;364:937–52; and O'Donnel MJ, Xavier D, Liu L, et al. Risk factors for ischaemic and intracerebral haemorrhagic stroke in 22 countries (the INTERSTROKE study): a case-control study. Lancet 2010;376:112–23.

the world.[16] Lipids levels are increasing and serial studies in low-income countries have reported escalating mean levels of total, LDL and non-HDL cholesterol and triglycerides and declining HDL cholesterol.[17,18] Although there are large regional variations in the prevalence of diabetes, it has more than quadrupled among adults in the last 20 years from about 1% to 3% to 10% to 20% in urban areas and 3% to 5% in rural areas in countries of east, west, and south Asia.[19] Diabetes is present in more than half of all adults in south Pacific countries.[20] There is a real epidemic of cardiovascular risk factors and CVD in all parts of the world and this needs an immediate focus on preventive strategies.

PREVENTION STRATEGIES

Progression of CVD is a continuum, and prevention extends across all stages of the disease as shown in **Fig. 2**. The propensity to develop risk factors is either genetic or begins in the early antenatal and postnatal period; risk behaviors start in early adolescence and young adulthood; risk factors commence in young to middle ages; and, depending on the accumulation of risks, the disease manifests in middle age in low-income countries and at older age in high-income countries.[6] The prevention continuum extends across all phases of disease. Social determinants of CVD such as social organization, early life events, life course, social gradient and hierarchy, unemployment, work environment, transport,

social support and cohesion, food, poverty and social exclusion, and low literacy levels influence individual health behaviors and influence primordial, primary as well as secondary prevention.[21] Primary prevention is focused on control of risk factors using both population-based and clinic-based control strategies while secondary prevention strategies involve acute and long-term disease management, including lifestyle changes, revascularization, and pharmacotherapy.

The decline in mortality from CVD in high-income countries is due mainly to a population-wide decrease in risk factors, better risk factor management, and better disease management strategies.[22]

Primordial prevention is focused on decreasing the risk factor load in the population using strategies for increasing awareness and access through education regarding smoking and tobacco cessation, dietary modulation (low fat and high fruit and vegetable intake), and increased physical activity.[23] It also involves addressing the social determinants of health through improvement in daily living conditions; fair distribution of power, money, and resources; and continuous upgrading of knowledge, monitoring, and skills.[24]

Primary prevention is directed toward control of CVD risk factors such as smoking, hypertension, high LDL cholesterol, low HDL cholesterol, metabolic syndrome, and diabetes so that the onset of manifest CVD is avoided or delayed.[23] Secondary prevention involves lifestyle changes, risk factor control, and pharmacologic strategies

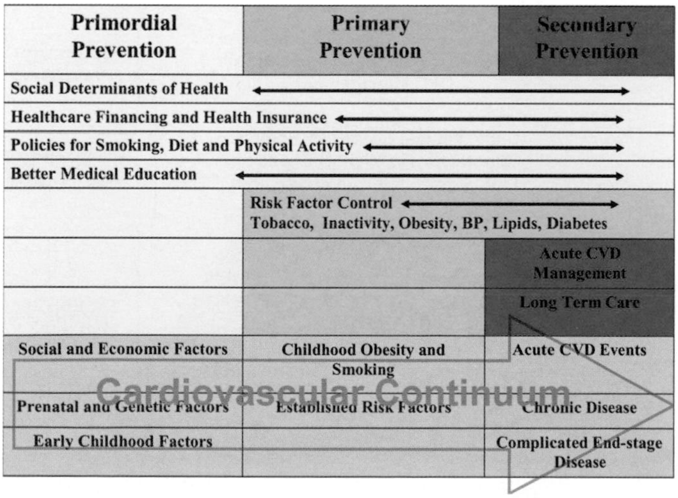

Primordial Prevention	Primary Prevention	Secondary Prevention
Social Determinants of Health ←		→
Healthcare Financing and Health Insurance ←		→
Policies for Smoking, Diet and Physical Activity ←		→
Better Medical Education ←		→
	Risk Factor Control ← Tobacco, Inactivity, Obesity, BP, Lipids, Diabetes	→
		Acute CVD Management
		Long Term Care
Social and Economic Factors	Childhood Obesity and Smoking	Acute CVD Events
Prenatal and Genetic Factors	Established Risk Factors	Chronic Disease
Early Childhood Factors		Complicated End-stage Disease

Cardiovascular Continuum

Fig. 2. The continuum of primordial, primary and secondary levels of prevention extends across the spectrum of cardiovascular disease. Components of primordial prevention (social determinants; healthcare financing and insurance; policies for smoking, diet, and physical activity; and better medical education), primary prevention (primordial prevention factors along with risk factor control) and secondary prevention (acute disease management and long-term therapies) overlap with the CVD progression.

in patients with established CVD (CHD, stroke, and others); tertiary prevention is use of advanced techniques such as coronary interventions and bypass surgery in addition to secondary prevention strategies in patients with established disease.[25] Prevention can also be seen as a pyramid with the greatest focus on tackling social determinants of health and policies directed toward smoking control, promotion of healthy diet, and enhancement of physical activity (**Fig. 3**). These issues along with better health insurance and public health care financing are also important. In developing countries, the medical curriculum has to be extensively revised to focus on CVD. Conventional primary and secondary prevention, which involve control of risk factors and better disease management, also contribute to decline of CVD mortality.[1,5]

Primordial Prevention

Population strategies focus on adoption of healthier lifestyles, which should be adopted as norms for the entire population. There are behavioral and environmental changes applicable especially to high-risk populations (eg, urban or migrant groups) including changes in eating patterns, drinking, smoking, physical activity, and psychosocial factors.[24,26] The risk factors can be prevented by the following primordial prevention strategies:

- Smoking control by a variety of measures such as governmental restrictions on smoking in the workplace and public places, ban on advertising and sponsorship by tobacco companies, enhanced community education programs, and physician-supervised counseling on smoking cessation.
- Generalized and truncal obesity can be avoided by enhanced physical activity and dietary calorie restriction.
- Prevention and control of hypertension can be achieved by reduction of salt, alcohol, and calorie intake, exercise, stress management, and greater intake of calcium, potassium, magnesium, and fiber.
- Prevention and control of hypercholesterolemia and decrease in LDL cholesterol levels can be achieved by reduced intake of saturated fat, meat, and dairy products, and greater intake of polyunsaturated fats and fiber.
- Low HDL cholesterol can be influenced by greater intake of monounsaturated fats, fruits and vegetables, and exercise.
- The incidence of metabolic syndrome and insulin resistance can be reduced by regular physical activity and weight reduction.
- Diabetes can be prevented in high-risk groups by enhanced physical activity and dietary control.

Primordial prevention calls for changing the socioeconomic status of the society. Higher social, economic, educational, and cultural status correlates inversely with smoking, abnormal food patterns, and lack of exercise.[27] To accomplish

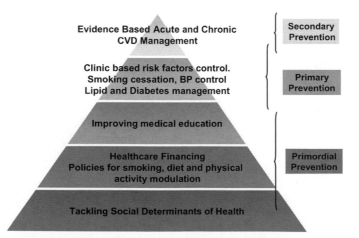

Fig. 3. Cardiovascular prevention pyramid. The greatest benefit and CVD reduction is achieved by primordial prevention measures, which involve tackling the social determinants; public health financing; population policies for smoking cessation, promotion of healthy diet, and physical activity; and changes in medical education curriculum focused on preventive care. Clinic-based primary prevention strategies—which involve control of blood pressure, lipids, and diabetes—are also important. Acute CVD event care and long-term CVD management with secondary and tertiary prevention therapies also contribute to reduction of CVD mortality.

these changes, the WHO recommends the following changes in attitudes, behaviors and social values.[23]

- Encouragement of positive health behavior, prevention of adopting risk behavior, elimination of established risk behaviors, and promotion of the concept of health as a social value.
- Inclusion of established principles and practices of health and general education in a public health program; healthy behavior should be made socially acceptable and should be encouraged.
- Encouragement of CVD health-promoting education in schools; special target groups are children, adolescents, family unit, the underprivileged, and high-risk groups.
- Close collaboration between health personnel and media representatives so that mass media play a major role in health education programs.

Primordial prevention begins in childhood when health risk behaviors begin. Parents, teachers, and peer groups are important in imparting health education to children. Public broadcasting systems, television, and newspapers play an important role in dissemination of health-related information among populations. Suitable strategies to impart information to these print and electronic media should be developed locally.

Primary Prevention

Public education primordial prevention strategies are also applicable in primary prevention, but this strategy depends more on the high-risk approach. Specific high-risk populations are those who smoke or have a family history of CVD, a sedentary lifestyle, or generalized or truncal obesity, and individuals with hypertension, hypercholesterolemia, other dyslipidemia, diabetes, or the metabolic syndrome.[24] Identification of high-risk individuals is also possible using these conditions, as well as risk scoring algorithms such as the Framingham Risk Score, QRISK-1 or QRISK-2, or the WHO risk chart.[28] The effectiveness of the high-risk approach depends directly on practicing physicians and other health care workers. To integrate prevention and treatment at the primary care level, greater emphasis on prevention must be part of the daily practice of medicine. This requires that physicians take an active interest in prevention, that patients are willing to accept and act on preventive advice, and that governments and insurance should be supportive of preventive

treatment. The British Quality Outcomes Framework (QOF) initiative is a good example of better risk factor management at the primary care level that has translated into lower disease incidence.[29]

Guidelines are required for screening and should ordinarily include measurement of height, weight, waist, aerobic fitness, systolic and diastolic blood pressure, total cholesterol, LDL and HDL cholesterol, and blood glucose. Patients should be questioned regarding tobacco use and diet. The updated American Heart Association primary prevention guidelines[30] are useful (**Table 2**). These guidelines are based on compelling scientific evidence that demonstrates that interventions extend overall survival, improve quality of life, and reduce the incidence of acute cardiovascular events. The interventions are smoking cessation, increased physical activity, weight management, blood pressure control, and lipid management. Both population-based and clinic-based approaches are useful.

Secondary Prevention

In patients with established cardiovascular disease (CHD or stroke) the lifestyle changes and risk factor control outlined earlier are essential. The revised American Heart Association guidelines[31] for secondary prevention are useful in this regard (**Table 3**). The interventions include smoking cessation, physical activity, weight management, blood pressure control, lipid management, glycemia management, and pharmacotherapy using antiplatelet drugs, β-blockers, statins, and angiotensin-converting enzyme (ACE) inhibitors. These interventions extend overall survival, improve quality of life, decrease the need for interventional procedures such as coronary angioplasty and bypass surgery, and reduce the incidence of subsequent myocardial infarction.[25]

PREVENTIVE INTERVENTIONS ARE EFFECTIVE

Control of risk factors has led to a 50% to 80% decline in the incidence of CVD in high-income countries.[9] In contrast, in the absence of proper preventive approaches the risk factors are increasing in low- and middle-income countries.[1,5] Of the two approaches to primary prevention, the population approach is used to address the behavioral risk factors at the community level and its success depends on surveillance, population-wide education, partnerships with community organizations, assurance of health services, environmental change, and policy and legislative initiatives. This approach addresses

Table 2
Primary prevention of cardiovascular diseases

Risk Intervention and Goals	Recommendations
Smoking Goal: complete cessation; no exposure to environmental tobacco smoke	• Ask about tobacco use status at every visit • In a clear, strong, and personalized manner, advise to quit
BP control Goal: <140/90 mm Hg; <130/85 mm Hg if renal insufficiency or heart failure is present; <130/80 mm Hg if diabetes is present	• Promote healthy lifestyle modification • Advocate weight reduction; reduction of sodium intake; consumption of fruits, vegetables, and low-fat dairy products; moderation of alcohol intake; and physical activity in persons with BP of >130 mm Hg systolic or 80 mm Hg diastolic. • For persons with renal insufficiency or heart failure, initiate drug therapy if BP is >130 mm Hg systolic or 85 mm Hg diastolic (>80 mm Hg diastolic for patients with diabetes) • Initiate drug therapy for those with BP >140/90 mm Hg if 6 to 12 months of lifestyle modification is not effective • Add BP medications, individualized to patient requirements and characteristics
Dietary intake Goal: an overall healthy eating pattern	• Advocate consumption of a variety of fruits, vegetables, grains, low-fat or nonfat dairy products, fish, legumes, poultry, and lean meats • Match energy intake with energy needs and make appropriate changes to achieve weight loss when indicated • Modify food choices to reduce saturated and trans fats (<10% of calories) by substituting grains and unsaturated fatty acids from fish, vegetables, legumes, and nuts • Limit salt intake to <6 g/d • Limit alcohol intake (<2 drinks/d in men, <1 drink/d in women)
Blood lipid management • Primary goal: LDL-C <160 mg/dL if 1 risk factor is present; LDL-C <130 mg/dL if 2 risk factors are present and 10-y CHD risk is <20%; or LDL-C <100 mg/dL if >2 risk factors are present and 10-y CHD risk is >20% or if patient has diabetes • Secondary goals (if LDL-C is at goal range): if triglycerides are >200 mg/dL, then use non-HDL-C as a secondary goal: non-HDL-C <190 mg/dL for 1 risk factor; <160 mg/dL for 2 risk factors and 10-y CHD risk <20%; non-HDL-C <130 mg/dL for patients with diabetes or for >2 risk factors and 10-y CHD risk >20% • Other targets for therapy: triglycerides <150 mg/dL; HDL-C >40 mg/dL in men and >50 mg/dL in women	• If LDL-C is higher than goal range, initiate additional therapeutic lifestyle changes consisting of dietary modifications to lower LDL-C: <7% of calories from saturated fat, cholesterol <200 mg/d, and, if further LDL-C lowering is required, dietary options (plant stanols/sterols not to exceed 2 g/d and/or increased viscous [soluble] fiber [10–25 g/d]), and additional emphasis on weight reduction and physical activity • If LDL-C is higher than goal range, rule out secondary causes (liver function test, thyroid-stimulating hormone level, urinalysis). After 12 weeks of therapeutic lifestyle change, consider LDL-lowering drug therapy, usually a statin but also consider bile acid–binding resin or niacin. If LDL-C goal not achieved, consider combination therapy (statin/resin/niacin) • After LDL-C goal has been reached, consider triglyceride level: if 150–199 mg/dL, treat with therapeutic lifestyle changes. If 200–499 mg/dL, treat increased non-HDL-C with therapeutic lifestyle changes and, if necessary, consider higher doses of statin or adding niacin or fibrate. If >500 mg/dL, treat with fibrate or niacin to reduce risk of pancreatitis • If HDL-C is <40 mg/dL in men and <50 mg/dL in women, initiate or intensify therapeutic lifestyle changes. For higher-risk patients, consider drugs that raise HDL-C (eg, niacin, fibrates, statins)

(continued on next page)

Table 2
(continued)

Risk Intervention and Goals	Recommendations
Physical activity Goal: at least 30 min of moderate-intensity physical activity on most or all days of the week	• If cardiovascular, respiratory, metabolic, orthopedic, or neurologic disorders are suspected, or if patient is middle-aged or older and is sedentary, consult physician before initiating vigorous exercise program • Moderate-intensity activities (40%–60% of maximum capacity) are equivalent to a brisk walk (15–20 min per mile). Additional benefits are gained from vigorous-intensity activity (60% of maximum capacity) for 20–40 min on 3–5 d/wk • Recommend resistance training with 8–10 different exercises, 1–2 sets per exercise, and 10–15 repetitions at moderate intensity >2 d/wk. Flexibility training and an increase in daily lifestyle activities should complement this regimen
Weight management Goal: achieve and maintain desirable weight (body mass index 18.5–24.9 kg/m^2). When body mass index is <25 kg/m^2, waist circumference >40 inches in men, >35 inches in women	• Initiate weight-management program through caloric restriction and increased caloric expenditure as appropriate • For overweight/obese persons, reduce body weight by 10% in first year of therapy
Diabetes management Goals: normal fasting plasma glucose (<110 mg/dL) and near-normal HbA$_{1c}$ (<7%).	• Initiate appropriate hypoglycemic therapy to achieve near-normal fasting plasma glucose or as indicated by near-normal HbA$_{1c}$ • First step is diet and exercise; second-step therapy is usually oral hypoglycemic drugs: sulfonylureas and/or metformin with ancillary use of acarbose and thiazolidinediones; third-step therapy is insulin • Treat other risk factors more aggressively (eg, change BP goal to <130/80 mm Hg and LDL-C goal to <100 mg/dL)
Chronic atrial fibrillation Goals: normal sinus rhythm or, if chronic atrial fibrillation is present, anticoagulation with INR 2.0–3.0 (target 2.5)	• Irregular pulse should be verified by an electrocardiogram • Conversion of appropriate individuals to normal sinus rhythm • For patients in chronic or intermittent atrial fibrillation, use warfarin anticoagulants to INR 2.0–3.0 (target 2.5) • Aspirin (325 mg/d) or aspirin/clopidogrel combination can be used as an alternative in those with certain contraindications to oral anticoagulation

Abbreviations: HbA$_{1c}$, glycosylated hemoglobin; HDL-C, high-density lipoprotein cholesterol; INR, internationalized normalized ratio; LDL, low-density lipoprotein cholesterol.

Data from Pearson TA, Blair SN, Daniels SR, et al. AHA guidelines for primary prevention of cardiovascular disease and stroke: 2002 update. Circulation 2002;106:388–91.

a selected list of modifiable risk factors such as diet, smoking and tobacco use, sedentary lifestyle, and availability of screening and diagnostic services. The high-risk approach should assess risk factors to determine individual risk. Medical interventions are often required. Evidence-based interventions for primary prevention can be remembered as the ABCs of preventive cardiology (**Box 1**). Secondary prevention strategies, on the other hand, comprise mainly medical interventions in addition to therapeutic lifestyle changes. A comprehensive approach that focuses on a policy-based approach for prevention of cardiovascular disease in all parts of the world, especially in low- and middle-income countries, is suggested.

A large body of scientific evidence supports the concept that policy changes at the government level are the quickest way to improve population health, including chronic diseases.[9,32] North Karelia, Finland, was the first population-level observatory where government-led policy changes

Table 3
Recommended secondary prevention guidelines

Goals	Intervention Recommendation
Smoking	
• Complete cessation • No exposure to environmental tobacco smoke	• Ask about tobacco use status at every visit and advise to quit; assist by counseling and developing a plan for quitting • Urge avoidance of exposure to environmental tobacco smoke at work and home
BP Control	
• <140/90 mm Hg or • <130/80 mm Hg if patient has CHD, diabetes or chronic kidney disease	• Initiate or maintain lifestyle modification: weight control, increased physical activity, alcohol moderation, sodium reduction, and emphasis on increased consumption of fresh fruits, vegetables, and low-fat dairy products • For patients with BP ≥140/90 mm Hg (or ≥130/80 mm Hg for individuals with chronic kidney disease or diabetes) as tolerated, add blood pressure medication, treating initially with β-blockers and/or ACE inhibitors, with addition of other drugs such as thiazides as needed to achieve target blood pressure
Lipid Management	
• Assess fasting lipid profile in all patients during hospitalization for those with an acute cardiovascular or coronary event • Initiate lipid-lowering medication (statins) before discharge according to the following schedule: • LDL-C <100 mg/dL preferably <70 mg/dL: if lower, to reduce by 30% of baseline • If triglycerides are ≥200 mg/dL, non-HDL-C should be <130 mg/dL	• Start dietary therapy; reduce intake of saturated fats (to <7% of total calories), trans-fatty acids, and cholesterol (to <200 mg/d) • Promote daily physical activity and weight management • Start statins in all patients • Encourage increased consumption of omega-3 fatty acids in the form of fish or in capsule form (1 g/d) for risk reduction. For treatment of increased triglycerides, higher doses are usually necessary for risk reduction • Therapeutic options to reduce non-HDL-C are: More intense LDL-C–lowering therapy (increasing statin dose), or Niacin (after LDL-C–lowering therapy), or Fibrate therapy (after LDL-C–lowering therapy)
Physical Activity	
For all patients: • Encourage 30–60 min of moderate-intensity aerobic activity, such as brisk walking, on most, and preferably all, days of the week • An increase in daily lifestyle activities (eg, walking breaks at work, gardening, household work)	• For all patients, assess risk with a physical activity history and clinical status to guide prescription • 30 min, 7 d/wk (minimum 5 d/wk) • Encourage resistance training 2 d/wk • Moderation needed for high-risk patients (eg, recent acute coronary syndrome or revascularization, heart failure)
Weight Management	
• Body mass index 18.5–24.9 kg/m^2 • Waist circumference: men <36 inches, women <31 inches	• Assess body mass index and waist circumference on each visit and consistently encourage weight maintenance/reduction through an appropriate balance of physical activity, caloric intake, and behavioral programs • If waist circumference is ≥31 inches in women and ≥36 inches in men, initiate lifestyle changes and consider treatment strategies for metabolic syndrome as indicated • The initial goal of weight loss therapy should be to reduce body weight by approximately 10% from baseline; further weight loss can be attempted through further assessment

(continued on next page)

Table 3 *(continued)*	
Goals	**Intervention Recommendation**
Diabetes Management	
• HbA$_{1c}$ <7%	• Initiate lifestyle and pharmacotherapy to achieve near-normal HbA$_{1c}$ • Begin vigorous modification of other risk factors (eg, physical activity, weight management, BP control, and cholesterol management as recommended earlier) • Coordinate diabetes care with patient's primary care physician or endocrinologist
Antiplatelet Agents/Anticoagulants	
• Start aspirin 75–162 mg/d and continue indefinitely in all patients unless contraindicated • Start and continue clopidogrel 75 mg/d in combination with aspirin for up to 12 months in patients after acute coronary syndrome or percutaneous coronary intervention with stent placement; in patients with a drug-eluting stent continue dual therapy indefinitely • Manage warfarin to INR of 2.0 to 3.0 for paroxysmal or chronic atrial fibrillation or flutter, and in patients after myocardial infarction when clinically indicated (eg, atrial fibrillation, left ventricular thrombus)	
Renin-Angiotensin-Aldosterone System Blockers	
ACE inhibitors: • Start and continue indefinitely in all patients with left ventricular ejection fraction ≤40% and in those with hypertension, diabetes, or chronic kidney disease, unless contraindicated • Among lower-risk patients with normal left ventricular ejection fraction in whom cardiovascular risk factors are well controlled and revascularization has been performed, use of ACE inhibitors may be considered optional Angiotensin receptor blockers: • Use in patients who are intolerant of ACE inhibitors and have heart failure or have had a myocardial infarction with left ventricular ejection fraction ≤40% • Consider use in combination with ACE inhibitors in systolic-dysfunction heart failure Aldosterone blockade: • Use in patients after myocardial infarction, without significant renal dysfunction or hyperkalemia, who are already receiving therapeutic doses of an ACE inhibitor and β-blocker, have a left ventricular ejection fraction ≤40%, and have either diabetes or heart failure	
β-Blockers	
• Start and continue indefinitely in all patients who have had myocardial infarction, acute coronary syndrome, or left ventricular dysfunction with or without heart failure symptoms, unless contraindicated • Consider chronic therapy for all other patients with coronary or other vascular disease or diabetes unless contraindicated	

Abbreviations: ACE, angiotensin-converting enzyme; BP, blood pressure.
  Data from Smith Jr SC, Allen J, Blair SN, et al. AHA/ACC guidelines for secondary prevention for patients with coronary and other atherosclerotic vascular disease: 2006 update. Circulation 2006;113:2363–72.

(dietary fat control, smoking policies) coupled with population-based educational intervention reduced CVD mortality by 60% to 80% over 20 years.[33] Similar observations have been reported by countries in Europe, North America, and Japan where dietary and smoking policies were put into practice leading to reduced smoking and cholesterol levels.[22,34] A slightly different policy was adopted in the United States where aggressive population-level risk factor control coupled with

appropriate pharmacotherapy led to better control of hypertension and hypercholesterolemia, and reduction of CVD.[9,10]

The decline in CVD mortality in high-income European and North American countries has followed 2 phases.[34] The first phase from 1970 to 1990 was due to population-based measures for risk factor control initiated by changes in policies on smoking, substitution of vegetable oils for animal fats, and promotion of physical activity.

Box 1
The ABCs of preventive cardiology

A Aspirin

B Blood pressure

C Cholesterol control

D Diabetes control

E Exercise regularly

F Food modulation and smoking/tobacco cessation

G Girth control (weight and truncal obesity)

H High alcohol intake control

I Irregular pulse

The second phase of decline from 1990 to date is ascribed to better management of risk factors and treatment of acute CVD syndromes, and short-term as well as long-term use of evidence-based pharmacotherapies. Public health care financing and strengthening of primary, secondary, and tertiary care is important.[24] Influence of policy changes on CVD mortality in different countries is summarized in **Table 4**.[34–39] In countries where population-based tobacco control policies, salt and fat control strategies, and focused control of multiple CVD risk factors (mainly hypertension and hypercholesterolemia) by physicians have been actively pursued, there has been a significant decline in CVD incidence varying from 50% to 90% over a 20- to 30-year period. In middle-income countries of eastern Europe where such initiatives were delayed, there has been a lesser decline (20%–40%). In low-income countries such as China and India, however, no significant policy initiatives exist and there is evidence of increases in CVD prevalence and mortality.

POLICY AND CLINICAL INITIATIVES

The major challenge for governments, health care systems, and clinicians is to develop cost-effective strategies to respond to the threat from CVD with the aim of delaying and eliminating premature onset and reducing mortality and morbidity.[40] Prevention and control of all types of CVD including CHD is a 3-pronged process as highlighted earlier.[23] Primordial strategy involves prevention of risk factors using population-based approaches, primary prevention is control of risk factors using lifestyle changes along with pharmacologic therapies, and secondary prevention is use of aggressive lifestyle and pharmacologic

therapies in patients with known CVD/CHD. All 3 approaches are complementary and policies as well as clinical interventions influence all. We suggest a comprehensive policy and clinical intervention plan that would enhance primordial, primary and secondary preventive strategies (**Table 5**).

Primordial Prevention

These strategies are focused on the population-wide reduction of multiple cardiovascular risk factors. Rose developed the concept of CVD risk as a continuum in a population and showed that all pathophysiologic factors were continuously distributed in a population.[41] He opined that high-risk and sick individuals simply represented the extreme end of the statistical distribution. From this hypothesis evolved the concept of population-wide control of risk factors. This would shift the mean levels of risk factors (eg, cholesterol, systolic blood pressure) in the standard normal curve to the left and decrease the number of high-risk individuals. The principal concepts of the Rose hypotheses were continuity of risk and its population impact; more disease in subjects at low risk as compared to less numbers in people with high risk; prediction of cases using population mean of risk factors; difference in causes of CVD among population and individuals; societal characteristics that influence risk; and implications on policy, research, and population action.[42] The policy and clinical actions for primordial prevention are summarized in the remainder of this section.

Improving socioeconomic environment and literacy

The social issues involved in the occurrence of premature CVD and other NCDs are multiple and include the social gradient, stress, early life events, social exclusion, improper working conditions, lack of social support, addictions including tobacco and alcohol, food scarcity or excess and uneven distribution, lack of proper transport, illiteracy and low educational status.[21,43] There are macrolevel factors (governance failure, geopolitics, natural resources decline, economic policies, population growth, demographic trap, and so forth) and microlevel factors (cultural barriers, poverty trap, lack of innovation and savings, absence of trade/business, technological reversal, adverse productivity shock, gender bias, adolescence-related, and so forth).[43] Sen[44] highlights health as a developmental issue and focuses on individual empowerment using literacy as a tool for better health. Multiple national programs exist in all countries to improve the socioeconomic status of the population ranging from literacy improvement, employment generation,

Table 4
Policy changes in Europe, North America, and other countries that led to decline in CVD mortality

Country	Political Agenda		Risk Factor Prevention			Better Risk Factor and Disease Management				Decline in CVD Mortality	
	Strengthening of Health Care Systems for Acute and Chronic CVD Care	Public Health Care Financing and Insurance	Tobacco Control Policies	Food-modification Initiatives	Physical Activity Promotion	Chronic Diseases/ CVD-focused Physician Education	Aggressive Population-based Pharmacologic Risk Factor Control	CVD-focused Primary Care	CVD-focused Secondary/ Tertiary Care	Period Evaluated	Percent Change
Western Europe[34]	++++	++++	+++	++	++	++++	++	+++	+++	1970–2000	(–) 40%–45%
Finland[33]	++++	++++	+++	++	+++	++++	++	+++	+++	1972–2007	(–) 75%–80%
Germany[35]	++++	++++	+++	++	+++	++++	++	+++	+++	1980–2000	(–) 39%–50%
Spain[34]	++++	++++	+++	+++	+++	++++	++	+++	+++	1970–2000	(–) 48%–50%
England[36]	++++	++++	+++	++	++	++++	+++	++++	+++	1984–2004	(–) 48%–52%
Australia[37]	++++	++++	+++	++	++	++++	+++	++++	+++	1968–2000	(–) 83%
United States[38]	+++	++	++	++	++	++++	++++	+++	++++	1970–2000	(–) 60%
Russia[34]	++	+++	++	+	+	+++	++	++	+++	1970–2000	(–) 10%
Eastern Europe[34]	++	++	++	++	++	+++	++	++	++	1985–2000	(–) 16%
China[39]	+	+++	+	++	++	++	+	+	++	1985–2004	(+) 27%–50%
India[5]	+	+	++	0	0	+	0	0	+++	No data	–

Scale of 0 to 4+.

Table 5
Policy and clinical agenda for CVD prevention and control in low- and middle-income countries

Policy Domain	Existing Policies or Programs in Most Low-income Countries	Unmet Actionable Needs
Socioeconomic and education	National literacy missions, right to education act, employment guarantee act, and so forth	Strengthen policy initiatives Linking these to health Interministerial collaboration
National CVD control program	National CVD and diabetes control programs National health programs	Scaling up and integration with National Rural health Mission and National Urban Health Mission
Health care financing	State-level initiatives for families designated below poverty line Multiple public and private insurance providers	Health insurance for CVD including for risk factor management, acute care, and secondary prevention Integration and social marketing of existing initiatives
Medical education and training of health care workers	Largely profession driven, cure-centric continuing medical education events	Structured, public health, preventive approach A formal preventive cardiology education and certifications
Tobacco control	FCTC and tobacco control legislations	Strengthen implementation of FCTC guidelines and legislation
Healthy diet	Minimal organized efforts	Focus on control of saturated fats, trans fats, salt, and alcohol Industry initiatives for alternative strategies
Improved physical activity	Minimal organized efforts	Better urban planning with interministerial collaboration Worksite and school-based interventions
Aggressive primary prevention and preventive health care delivery	Existing network of primary health centers, district hospitals, and teaching hospitals in public sector A larger number of private care providers, mostly unorganized, and a smaller more organized corporate sector in urban areas	Needs orientation to CVD and diabetes care Needs quality control and standardization
Evidence-based acute and chronic CVD care	Minimal and fractured	Better acute care Chronic care delivery improvement and use of evidence-based therapies

and social security. These policies are directed to the specific social issue or population group but not in the context of disease prevention or control. Improving literacy reduces unhealthy behaviors (eg, smoking) and increases awareness of risk factors. It also promotes adherence to lifestyle and pharmacotherapies for primary and secondary prevention.[45] Both general literacy and health literacy should be part of CVD control programs.[45,46] Interministerial collaboration is essential for policy implementation on CVD prevention and control, and constitution of national commissions of macroeconomics and health is needed as advocated by the United Nations. These

should encompass ministries of health, finance, planning, technical education, human development, urban development, youth affairs, sports, women and child development, agriculture, food and civil supplies, industry, commerce, and transport.

National CVD health programs

A major public health initiative is development and implementation of a focused national CVD control program. Multiple examples of such initiatives exist in high-income countries. Multisectoral and multifactorial CVD control initiatives were implemented in European countries in the mid-1960s and early 1970s. The US-based National High

Blood Pressure Control Program and National Cholesterol Education Programs are examples of focused and successful prevention programs. In contrast, the existing national health programs in most low-income countries are directed towards communicable diseases and maternal and child health. For example, in India, although a national program for control of CVDs and diabetes has been initiated as a pilot, it has not been scaled up because of paucity of funds.[32] In China also only ad hoc programs exist for CVD control.[47] We believe that these should be a public health priority and the program must be spread widely; the scope and funding must be substantially increased. A political will to initiate and sustain these programs is needed.

Health care financing and universal health insurance

An important area for CVD control is health care financing by governments. There is an inverse relationship between health care financing by the government and disease burden. The countries with the largest expenditure on health (excluding the United States) have more healthy people. It is possible to reduce the mortality and burden of CVD by population-wide fiscal policies.[45] Financing is needed for implementation of programs not only to control tobacco, alcohol, and dietary fat but also to improve urban design and provide better education within the existing national programs. Health insurance for acute and chronic diseases is virtually nonexistent in many low-income countries.[48] In the US millions suffer ill health due to lack of health insurance and preventive care.[49] In India more than 80% of the population pays out of pocket for health-related expenses, and every year almost 30 million individuals are pushed into poverty as a result of catastrophic health care expenditure.[50]

Changing medical education curriculum

Primordial and primary prevention of chronic NCDs, especially CVD and CHD, is not a major component of medical school curricula in most low-income countries. Continuing medical education for general physicians, general practitioners, and others about advances in cardiovascular and other forms of therapy should be mandatory.[32,51] Physicians should be encouraged to use global risk-assessment tools such as the Framingham Risk Score.[52] They have to be aware of the guidelines. Although there is evidence that most clinicians manage their patients according to the guidelines, the uptake of preventive efforts is limited. Establishment of systems to address the multilevel contexts that influence the development and maintenance of prevention-related health behaviors is important. Hospitals and health care systems should be encouraged to develop and provide preventive cardiology services and systems for the community.[53] There should be training and certification for preventive CHD specialists who can train the practitioners and paramedics in strategies of prevention and health promotion. Training of health care workers and allied health professionals for systematic or opportunistic screening is important. This would lead to early diagnosis of risk factors and their management. There is also a need for creation of a cadre of NCD health care workers not only for screening but also for monitoring of individuals and ensuring compliance. These workers should also be trained to educate the populace in the early diagnosis of acute CVD events and to ensure referral.[32]

Tobacco control

An important policy action for CVD prevention and control is enforcement of strict antitobacco laws. It is now well recognized that smoking in any form and the use of nonsmoked tobacco are equally dangerous to health, especially cardiovascular health. Smoking and tobacco use is rampant in rural communities and in urban areas with low socioeconomic status in most low-income countries.[11–13] Comprehensive legislation on tobacco control and adoption of the WHO Framework Convention on Tobacco Control (FCTC) by various governments is an important step in this direction.[54] Studies from Europe and North America have reported that strict enforcement of FCTC has resulted in reduced admissions for CHD as well as decreased mortality.[55] Laws need to be amended to comply with the provisions of the FCTC. There is a considerable gap in policy and its application all over the world. The government needs to approve antismoking laws and educate the public through organized programs with media support and strictly enforce the tobacco control legislation.

Healthy diet, salt, and alcohol

Diet is a very controversial area and the current evidence-based practices adopted by western countries should be evaluated before these are implemented elsewhere is the world. For low-income countries, WHO has concluded that as a society moves up the socioeconomic scale substantial changes occur in diet.[56] These include greater consumption of calories, fats, saturated fats, trans fats, salt, refined carbohydrates and sugars, and decreased intake of high-fiber foods, legumes, and vegetables. A healthy diet should be the opposite.

WHO guidelines[56] promote (1) increased intake of fruits and vegetables (at least 500 g per day), legumes, and whole grain foods; (2) reduced intake of fried foods, processed foods, soft drinks containing calories, and other unhealthy foods; (3) limitation of the daily intake of total fat to 25% to 35% of calories, and saturated fat <7% of calories, by limiting the use of butter, full-fat dairy products, trans fats, and tropical oils (palm oil and coconut oil) and increased intake of monounsaturated fats up to 20%; (4) reduction of the dietary glycemic load by cutting down on carbohydrates, especially refined carbohydrates; (5) reduction of the intake of salt to less than 2.5 g sodium or less than 6 g of salt (1 teaspoon of salt) per day; and (6) moderate consumption of nuts, lean meat, fish, and alcohol. Government policies are important to translate knowledge into practice.[57]

For years the food and nutrition policies of the governments in low-income countries have focused on the problem of undernutrition. The dual epidemic of under- and overnutrition needs a different response. The focus should be on a balanced healthy diet that tackles the problems of both rather than overweight/obesity alone. The following steps can have major immediate effects: (1) promotion of healthy nutrition in the general population by implementation of guidelines on chronic diseases, diabetes, and obesity; (2) creation of culturally sensitive health educational material; (3) subsidies for producing and distributing healthy foods and fruits; (4) penal taxation on unhealthy saturated and hydrogenated fats and subsidies on vegetable oils; (5) food labeling including portion size, calories, total fat, saturated fat, trans fat, protein, carbohydrates, sodium, sugar, and fiber; (6) availability of healthy foods in schools and work sites; and (7) reduction of salt content in processed food.

Many high income countries have implemented food content labeling specifically for fats, saturated fats, trans-fats and salt.[58] The consequences of such initiatives have to be prospectively assessed. Presently there is no evidence of the efficacy of such efforts as shown by increasing rates of obesity in all high-income countries.[9] Salt is important in the genesis and perpetuation of hypertension and has a direct correlation with CVD.[59] Diets in most tropical countries have a very high salt content, typically 10 to 12 g of salt intake per day. A lower intake of 5 to 6 g of salt per day is suggested by international guidelines.[30,31] Recommendations regarding alcohol intake for CVD prevention are confusing. The overall harm of alcohol due to high blood pressure, liver disease, accidents, and injuries is much more than its protective effects on CVD.[60] As a policy alcohol use should be discouraged in the community as well as for the individual.

Physical activity promotion

Regular physical activity is extremely important for CVD prevention.[30] The recommended physical activity is 30 to 45 minutes of moderate-intensity activity such as brisk walking every day.[61] Evidence from Europe and North America reports a beneficial effect of population-based initiatives on increasing physical activity with a public health perspective. Occupational physical activity and creating special time for employees has been the focus of WHO.[62] There are examples of multiple comprehensive work site health promotion programs that focus on improvement of physical activity.[63] These work site intervention programs change health-related behaviors with reduced tobacco use and increased physical activity.[64] The habit of active participation in physical activity programs, games, and sports begins in early childhood and continues into adulthood; therefore, physical education should be given greater emphasis in schools and colleges.[65] Yoga can be part of the physical activity of school children; regular participation not only improves physical capacity but also improves adherence to other strategies for improving health.[66] Individual level promotion of physical activity is also important. However, initiation and persistence with the habit of increased physical activity requires strong motivation and discipline.

Urban planning is important for public health and can improve human well-being, emphasize needs assessment and service delivery, manage complex social systems, focus at the population level, and rely on community-based participatory methods.[67,68] For CVD prevention, the construction and use of foot paths and cycle paths should be encouraged.[69] A uniform urban development policy is needed that should be guided not only by aesthetics but also by the health needs of the population. Traditionally, planning should involve community needs for transportation, housing, commercial/office buildings, natural resource use, environmental protection, and health care infrastructure.

Primary Prevention

This strategy focuses on control of risk factors (**Table 2**). Although the number of CVD risks is high, interventions focused on the major risk factors (smoking, high BP, high LDL cholesterol, low HDL cholesterol, and diabetes) have shown to lead to a substantial decline in the incidence of CVD.[9] Primary prevention strategies should focus on improving health care delivery and target-oriented control of risk factors.[30]

Health care delivery for primary prevention

In countries with fractured health care systems, such as most low-income countries and the US, the primary care delivery mechanisms and primary prevention services are chaotic.[49] For proper delivery of chronic health care, the medical infrastructure needs to be structured like a pyramid. In this pyramid, the maximum emphasis has to be at the primary level, that is, at the level of first contact, which should be easily accessible (both physically and in terms of affordability) to everyone. Each successive rung needs to be equipped to perform more complex tasks for more complex conditions. This has to be followed up with a referral system along this pyramid. Such a system minimizes waste (in the form of trivial or self-limiting illnesses being treated at district- or state-level hospitals) and enhances accessibility as observed in many western European countries.[29] In most low-income countries, such a system is in operation on paper but in reality this system is woefully inadequate.[53] As a policy, preventive health care and chronic disease surveillance should be delivered by primary care physicians or trained community health workers.[70]

Risk factor control

Aggressive primary prevention is critical to preventing CVD in those who are in the high-risk category with the 4 key objectives: (1) avoidance of all tobacco products and passive exposure to tobacco, (2) control of dyslipidemia, (3) control of blood pressure, and (4) control of blood glucose and diabetes through intense lifestyle modification and medication if necessary.

A key recommendation of the American Heart Association Primary Prevention Guidelines (**Table 2**) is that CVD risk should be assessed in all individuals through careful history, physical examination, and selected laboratory testing.[30] Risk factors such as tobacco use, poor diet, alcohol intake, lack of physical activity, and family history of CHD should be routinely evaluated at every visit. Physical parameters such as blood pressure, pulse, height, weight, body mass index, and waist circumference should be measured regularly. Physiological parameters such as lipid profile and fasting blood glucose levels should be measured in all adults 20 years of age or older. The CVD risk assessment should not be time-consuming or expensive and should be amenable to performance outside of health care facilities. This assessment should be performed once every 5 years in healthy individuals and more frequently in high-risk persons.

The next step in risk factor assessment is calculation of a global risk score in persons aged 40 years and older.[28] One benefit of this approach is the identification of those who are at high risk not because of a single markedly elevated risk factor but rather because of the presence of several modestly elevated risk factors. Several global risk factor assessment tools are available, but the revised Framingham risk factor assessment tool[52] is the most used worldwide.

Traditionally, risk estimation has been used to inform the patient of the importance of changes in risk behaviors or the need for treatment. The use of this information may differ from patient to patient and among health care providers and insurers. Increasingly, health care providers have used risk stratification to better reserve aggressive interventions for those at the highest risk. Interventions to lower LDL cholesterol are illustrative.[70] Clinical trials with statins have convincingly demonstrated benefits in every stratum of individual, varying from low-risk persons to the situation of high-risk secondary prevention. The rationale moves from efficacy to cost-effectiveness. The JUPITER trial, therefore, added C-reactive protein measurement as a risk marker, and results showed that in this subgroup of high-risk primary prevention rosuvastatin was particularly effective.[71] Similar arguments are provided for blood pressure control and use of aspirin in high-risk asymptomatic persons.

A novel approach in primary prevention is the use of multiple pharmacological agents for primary prevention, the polypill concept.[72] Because increasing age is the most important CVD risk factor, Wald and Law proposed that a combination of three antihypertensive agents (at half dose) with a statin, aspirin and folic acid could reduce the incidence of CVD by more than 80% if given to the whole population aged more than 55 years. No formal outcome trials are available, but a study reported that such a combination effectively reduced CVD risk factors in mild- to moderate-risk individuals.[73] The demonstrated calculated risk reduction was about 60% instead of the 80% suggested by Wald and Law. Several trials are ongoing to assess the efficacy of such an approach for primary prevention, and until these results are available, this combination is not recommended.[74]

Community worker—based models for chronic disease risk factor control have been tried in many settings with variable results.[75] This strategy is useful for management of infections, pregnancy-related outcomes and malnutrition.[76] Use of practitioners of alternative systems of medicine could be important for chronic disease risk factor management. Individual focused care should identify high-risk individuals using proper algorithms[28] and control the risk factors using lifestyle changes and pharmacotherapy.

Secondary Prevention

Acute cardiovascular disease management and appropriate long-term medical care are crucial in preventing CVD-related mortality. A substantial reduction in CVD-related mortality in high-income countries is the result of better acute coronary care and long-term management.[9,25,34] In contrast, availability of care and its standard is variable in low-income countries. Better quality CVD care systems and manpower need to be developed in these countries.

Acute cardiovascular care

In high-income countries a large network of public or privately funded advanced CVD care centers exist. Although in certain high-income countries such care is not uniformly accessible, in most countries of North America, Europe, and Australasia availability and accessibility of such care has reduced CVD mortality substantially.[9] Publicly funded primary and secondary health care systems for acute CVD care need to be developed in low- and middle-income countries. In many low- and middle-income countries, management practices for acute coronary syndromes are driven by guidelines and are optimal.[77] Accessibility and availability issues should be resolved.

Secondary prevention therapies

Guidelines recommend that lifestyle changes, aspirin, beta-blockers, ACE inhibitors, and statins should be used in all patients with symptomatic CVD (**Table 3**).[31] Secondary prevention thus comprises medical interventions and therapeutic lifestyle changes that aim to reduce complications, recurrent events, and disease progression in patients with established CVD. Many high-risk patients without established CVD may also be appropriate candidates for secondary prevention strategies such as those with diabetes, left ventricular hypertrophy, symptomatic carotid atherosclerosis, peripheral vascular disease, aortic aneurismal disease, and chronic renal

---

Table 6
Barriers to Adherence to Evidence-Based Therapies for Chronic Diseases

Health Systems Related	Health Care Provider Level	Individual Patient Level
• Low perceived need by health care bureaucrats and managers	• Lack of proper education and motivation	• Lack of motivation and commitment
• Government policies for tobacco/food	• Absent continuing medical education programs	• Failure to realize seriousness of problem
• Lack of "heart friendly" infrastructure	• Lack of continuity of care	• Older age
• Resource constraints and cost of equipment and drugs, especially for NCDs	• Fixed clinician perceptions	• Female gender
	• Overburdened with number of patients	• Low SES
• Lack of advocacy/ lobbying	• Lack of understanding of patient needs	• Social isolation, especially in the elderly
• Poor access and availability of medical manpower and medicines	• Costs	• Finance-related factors and costs
• Media apathy and conflicting messages	• Neglecting to involve patients in choices	• Significant co-morbid conditions
• No insurance cover for OPD management	• Prescribing complex regimens	• Failure to sustain lifestyle changes
• Use of non-standardized formulary and frequent changes	• Failure to explain benefits and side effects	• Lack of quality information
• Undergraduate medical education not focused on NCDs	• Lack of focus on lifestyle changes	• No insurance cover
• Overburdened health care system with communicable diseases	• Overtreatment	• Distance and geographic factors
	• Low clinician referrals	• Confusing messages from multiple stake-holders

insufficiency.[25] Treatment of elevated lipoproteins reduces CVD events by approximately 30% to 40% and overall mortality by 20% in high-risk patients. A similar reduction is achieved for treatment of high blood pressure in very high-risk patients and those with co-morbidities. There was low use of secondary prevention therapies in Europe and North America in the late 1990s but the situation has improved as a result of policy focus on better management.[78] In low- and middle-income countries, studies have reported that there is a rapid decline as patients move from tertiary to secondary and primary care and there is low use of various evidence-based medicines, especially statins and β-blockers.[79] This is caused by barriers to proper management at health care systems, health care providers, and at the patient level as shown in **Table 6**. All these need to be addressed if the compliance to long-term CVD preventive therapy is to be enhanced.

SUMMARY

The epidemic of CVD worldwide and especially in low- and middle-income countries needs an urgent policy and clinical response for its control. It is no longer a disease of the rich or the well educated. Strategies that have been successful in upper- to middle-income countries are available and need to be implemented.[80] Most of the achievements are attributable to social change involving culture, housing, and food. **Table 5** prioritizes the agenda for governments and physicians. Political and bureaucratic will and policies for improving the human development index should be implemented. Initiation of a national cardiovascular disease control program is important. The medical curricula need to be extensively revised to incorporate these diseases into the mainstream. Financing mechanisms have to be developed for supporting health care infrastructure at primary and secondary levels and for public-funded health insurance and overall strengthening of health systems.[81] Suitable policies and clinical initiatives should replace clinical inertia for tobacco control, dietary fat control, and better physical activity. Both primary prevention for target-oriented control of CVD risk factors and pharmacotherapy-based secondary prevention should be practiced. The ABCs of preventive cardiology should be remembered by all (**Box 1**). Facilities for the management of CVD risk factors in primary care and acute and chronic disease management in secondary care are needed. Implementation of these policies can delay the occurrence of acute cardiovascular events by at least 10 years,

reduce the mortality burden by at least 25% to 30%, decrease use of tertiary care, save money, and reduce the inexorable march of CVDs in the world.

REFERENCES

1. Gersh B, Mayosi B, Sliwa K, et al. The epidemic of cardiovascular diseases in the developing world: global implications. Eur Heart J 2010;31:642–8.
2. World Health Organization. Preventing chronic diseases: a vital agenda. Geneva: World Health Organization; 2005.
3. Fuster V, Kelly BB, Board for Global Health. Promoting cardiovascular health in the developing world: a critical challenge to achieve global health. Washington: Institute of Medicine; 2010. Available at: http://www.iom.edu/Reports/2010/Promoting-Cardiovascular-Health-in-the-Developing-World-A-Critical-Challenge-to-Achieve-Global-Health.aspx. Accessed 12 September 2010.
4. Yusuf S, Reddy S, Ounpuu S, et al. Global burden of cardiovascular diseases: part I: general considerations, the epidemiologic transition, risk factors, and impact of urbanization. Circulation 2001;104: 2746–53.
5. Gupta R, Joshi PP, Mohan V, et al. Epidemiology and causation of coronary heart disease and stroke in India. Heart 2008;94:16–26.
6. Burke GL, Bell RA. Global trends in cardiovascular disease. In: Wong ND, Black HR, Gardin JM, editors. Preventive cardiology. 2nd edition. New York: McGraw-Hill; 2005. p. 22–43.
7. Yusuf S, Hawken S, Ounpuu S, et al. Effect of potentially modifiable risk factors associated with myocardial infarction in 52 countries (the INTERHEART study): case control study. Lancet 2004;364: 937–52.
8. O'Donnel MJ, Xavier D, Liu L, et al. Risk factors for ischaemic and intracerebral haemorrhagic stroke in 22 countries (the INTERSTROKE study): a case-control study. Lancet 2010;376:112–23.
9. Leupker RV. Decline in incident coronary heart disease. Why are rates falling? Circulation 2008; 117:592–3.
10. Kaplan NM, Opie LH. Controversies in hypertension. Lancet 2006;367:168–76.
11. Jha P, Ranson MK, Ngyuyen SK, et al. Estimates of global and regional smoking prevalence in 1995 by age and sex. Am J Public Health 2002;92:1002–6.
12. Jha P, Jacob B, Gajalakshmi V, et al. A nationally representative case-control study of smoking and death in India. N Engl J Med 2008;358:1137–47.
13. Gu D, Kelly TN, Wu X, et al. Mortality attributable to smoking in China. N Engl J Med 2009;360:150–9.
14. Monteiro CA, Moura EC, Conde WL, et al. Socioeconomic status and obesity in adult population of

developing countries: a review. Bull World Health Organ 2004;82:940–6.

15. Kearney PM, Whelton M, Reynolds K, et al. Global burden of hypertension: analysis of worldwide data. Lancet 2005;365:217–23.

16. Suchday S, Kapur S, Ewart CK, et al. Urban stress and health in developing countries: development and validation of a neighbourhood stress index for India. Behav Med 2006;32:77–86.

17. Gaziano T. Cardiovascular disease in the developing world and its cost-effective management. Circulation 2005;112:3547–53.

18. Gupta R, Guptha S, Agrawal A, et al. Secular trends in cholesterol lipoproteins and triglycerides and prevalence of dyslipidemias in an urban Indian population. Lipids Health Dis 2008;7:40.

19. Gupta R, Kumar P. Global diabetes landscape - type 2 diabetes mellitus in South Asia: epidemiology, risk factors and control. Insulin 2008;3:78–94.

20. Coughlan A, McCarty DJ, Jorgensen LN, et al. The epidemic of NIDDM in Asian and Pacific island populations: prevalence and risk factors. Horm Metab Res 1997;29:323–31.

21. Marmot M, Wilkinson RG. Social determinants of health. Oxford: Oxford University Press; 1999.

22. Tunstall-Pedoe H, editor. MONICA monograph and multimedia sourcebook. Geneva: World Health Organization; 2003.

23. World Health Organization. Prevention of cardiovascular disease. Guidelines for risk assessment and management of cardiovascular risk. Geneva: World Health Organization; 2007.

24. World Health Organization, Commission on Social Determinants of Health. Closing the gap in a generation: health equity through action on the social determinants of health. Geneva: World Health Organization; 2009.

25. Brook RD, Greenland P. Secondary prevention. In: Wong ND, Black HR, Gardin JM, editors. Preventive cardiology. 2nd edition. New York: McGraw-Hill; 2000. p. 515–42.

26. Deedwania PC, Gupta R. Prevention of coronary heart disease in Asian populations. In: Wong ND, Black HR, Gardin JM, editors. Preventive cardiology. New York: McGraw-Hill; 2000. p. 503–16.

27. Bambra C, Gibson M, Sowden A, et al. Tracking the wider social determinants of health and health inequities: evidence from systematic reviews. J Epidemiol Community Health 2010;64:284–91.

28. Brindle P, Beswick A, Fahey T, et al. Accuracy and impact of risk assessment in the primary prevention of cardiovascular disease: a systematic review. Heart 2006;92:1752–9.

29. Dunbar JA. The quality and outcomes framework reduces disparities in health outcomes for cardiovascular disease. J Epidemiol Community Health 2010;64:841–2.

30. Pearson TA, Blair SN, Daniels SR, et al. AHA guidelines for primary prevention of cardiovascular disease and stroke: 2002 update. Circulation 2002; 106:388–91.

31. Smith SC Jr, Allen J, Blair SN, et al. AHA/ACC guidelines for secondary prevention for patients with coronary and other atherosclerotic vascular disease: 2006 update. Circulation 2006;113: 2363–72.

32. Reddy KS, Shah B, Varghese C, et al. Responding to the threat of chronic diseases in India. Lancet 2005;336:1744–9.

33. Vartiainen E, Laatikainen T, Peltonen M, et al. Thirty five year trends in cardiovascular risk factors in Finland. Int J Epidemiol 2010;39:504–18.

34. Kesteloot H, Sans S, Kromhout D. Dynamics of cardiovascular and all-cause mortality in Western and Eastern Europe between 1970 and 2000. Eur Heart J 2006;27:107–13.

35. Muller-Riemenschneider F, Andersohn F, Willich SN. Trends in age-standardised and age-specific mortality from ischaemic heart disease in Germany. Clin Res Cardiol 2010;99:511–8.

36. Allender S, Scarborough P, O'Flaherty M, et al. Patterns of coronary heart disease mortality over the 20th century in England and Wales: possible plateaus in the rate of decline. BMC Public Health 2008;8:148.

37. Taylor R, Dobson A, Mirzaei M. Contribution of changes in risk factors to the decline of coronary heart disease mortality in Australia over three decades. Eur J Cardiovasc Prev Rehabil 2006;13: 760–8.

38. Ford ES, Ajani UA, Croft JB, et al. Explaining the decrease in US deaths from coronary disease, 1980–2000. N Engl J Med 2007;356:2388–98.

39. Cheng J, Zhao D, Zeng Z, et al. The impact of demographic and risk factor changes on coronary heart disease deaths in Beijing, 1999–2010. BMC Public Health 2009;9:30.

40. Reddy KS. Cardiovascular disease in non-Western countries. N Engl J Med 2004;350:2438–40.

41. Rose G. Rose's Strategy of Preventive Medicine. Oxford: Oxford University Press; 2008.

42. Khaw KT, Marmot M. The Rose concept and applications: commentary. In: Rose G, editor. Rose's Strategy of Preventive Medicine. Oxford: Oxford University Press; 2008. p. 3–31.

43. Gupta R, Kumar P. Social evils, poverty, and health. Indian J Med Res 2007;126:279–88.

44. Sen A. Development as freedom. New York: Alfred A Knopf; 1999.

45. Gaziano T, Reddy KS, Paccaud F, et al. Cardiovascular disease. In: Jamison DT, Breman JG, Measham AR, Alleyne G, Cleason M, Evans DB, Jha P, Mills A, Musgrove P, editors. Disease control priorities in developing countries. 2nd edition. New

York: Oxford University Press and World Bank; 2006. p. 645–62.

46. DeWatt DA, Berkman ND, Sheridan T, et al. Literacy and health outcomes: a systematic review of the literature. J Gen Intern Med 2004;19: 1228–39.

47. Sun J, Wang Y, Chen X, et al. An integrated intervention program to control diabetes in overweight Chinese women and men with type 2 diabetes. Asia Pac J Clin Nutr 2008;17:514–24.

48. Chen MH. Asia Pacific agrees health financing plan. Lancet 2010;375:1426.

49. Brown JR, O'Connor GT. Coronary heart disease and prevention in the United States. N Engl J Med 2010;362:2150–3.

50. Van Doorslaer E, O'Donnell O, Rannan-Eliya R, et al. Effect of payments for health care on poverty estimates in 11 countries in Asia: an analysis of household survey data. Lancet 2006;368:1357–64.

51. Nishtar S. Prevention of coronary heart disease in South Asia. Lancet 2002;360:1015–8.

52. D'Agostino RB, Vasan RS, Pencina MJ, et al. General cardiovascular risk profile for use in primary care: the Framingham Heart Study. Circulation 2008; 117:743 53.

53. Beaglehole R, Ebrahim S, Reddy S, Voûte J, Leeder S; Chronic Diseases Action Group. Prevention of chronic diseases: a call to action. Lancet 2007;370:2152–7.

54. World Health Organization. WHO Framework Convention on Tobacco Control. Available at: http://www.who.int/fctc/text_download/en/index.html. Accessed 10 May 2010.

55. Mackay DF, Irfan MO, Haw S, Pell JP. Meta-analysis of the effect of comprehensive smoke-free legislation on acute coronary events. Heart 2010;96: 1525–30.

56. World Health Organization. Diet, nutrition and prevention of chronic diseases. Geneva: World Health Organization; 2002.

57. Lawrence M. Do food regulatory systems protect public health? Public Health Nutr 2009;12:2247–9.

58. Mozaffarian D, Katan MB, Ascherio A, et al. Trans fatty acids and cardiovascular disease. N Engl J Med 2006;3554:1601–13.

59. Strazzullo P, D'Elia L, Kandala NB, et al. Salt intake, stroke, and cardiovascular disease: meta-analysis of prospective studies. BMJ 2009;338:b4567.

60. Costanzo S, Di Castelnuovo A, Donati MB, et al. Alcohol consumption and mortality in patients with cardiovascular disease: a meta-analysis. J Am Coll Cardiol 2010;55:1339–47.

61. Pate RR, Pratt M, Blair SN, et al. Physical activity and public health: a recommendation from the Centers for Disease Control and Prevention and the American College of Sports Medicine. JAMA 1995;273: 402–7.

62. Conn V, Hafdahl A, Cooper P, et al. Meta-analysis of workplace physical activity interventions. Am J Prev Med 2009;37:330–9.

63. Abraham C, Graham Rowe E. Are worksite interventions effective in increasing physical activity? A systematic review and meta-analysis. Health Psychol Rev 2009;3:108–44.

64. Prabhakaran D, Jeemon P, Goenka S, et al. Impact of a worksite intervention program on cardiovascular risk factors: a demonstration project in an Indian industrial population. J Am Coll Cardiol 2009;53: 1718–28.

65. Katz DL. School based interventions for health promotion and weight control: not just waiting on the world to change. Annu Rev Public Health 2009; 30:253–72.

66. Enas EA, Singh VN, Munjal YP, et al. Recommendations of the second Indo-US health summit on prevention and control of cardiovascular disease among Asian Indians. Indian Heart J 2009;61:265–74.

67. Kochtitzky CS, Frumkin H, Rodriguez R, et al. Urban planning and public health at CDC. MMWR Morb Mortal Wkly Rep 2006;50(Suppl 2):34–8.

68. Brownson RC, Kelly CM, Eyler AA, et al. Environmental and policy approaches for promoting physical activity in the United States: a research agenda. J Phys Act Health 2008;5:488–503.

69. Frumkin H. Urban sprawl and public health. Public Health Rep 2002;117:201–17.

70. Wilson MA, Pearson TA. Primary prevention. In: Wong ND, Black HR, Gardin JM, editors. Preventive cardiology. 2nd Ed. New York: McGraw-Hill; 2005. p. 493–514.

71. Ridker PM, Danielson E, Fonseca FAH, et al. Rosuvastatin to prevent vascular events in men and women with elevated C-reactive protein. N Engl J Med 2008;359:2195–207.

72. Wald NJ, Law MR. A strategy to reduce cardiovascular disease by more than 80%. BMJ 2003;326: 1419–22.

73. The Indian Polycap Study (TIPS), Yusuf S, Pais P, Afzal R, et al. Effects of a polypill (Polycap) on risk factors in middle aged individuals without cardiovascular disease (TIPS): a phase II, double blind, randomized trial. Lancet 2009;373:1341–51.

74. Reddy KS. The preventive polypill: much promise, insufficient evidence. N Engl J Med 2007;356:212.

75. Vishwanathan M, Kraschnewski J, Nishikawa B, et al. Outcomes of community health worker interventions. Evid Rep Technol Assess 2009;181:1–144.

76. Arifeen SE, Hoque DM, Akter T, et al. Effects of the integrated management of childhood illness strategy on childhood mortality and nutrition in a rural area in Bangladesh: a cluster randomised trial. Lancet 2009;374:393–403.

77. Xavier D, Pais P, Devereaux PJ, et al. Treatment and outcomes of acute coronary syndromes in India

(CREATE): a prospective analysis of registry data. Lancet 2008;371:1435—42.

78. Kotseva K, Wood D, De Backer G, et al. Cardiovascular prevention guidelines in daily practice: a comparison of EUROASPIRE I, II and III surveys in eight European countries. Lancet 2009;373: 929—40.

79. Sharma KK, Gupta R, Agrawal A, et al. Low use of statins and other coronary secondary prevention therapies in primary and secondary care in India. Vasc Health Risk Manag 2009;5:1004—13.

80. Khoury MJ, Gwinn M, Ioannidis PA. The emergence of translational epidemiology: from scientific discovery to population health impact. Am J Epidemiol 2010;172:517—24.

81. Sundewall J, Swanson RC, Betigeri A, et al. Health systems strengthening: current and future activities. Lancet 2010. DOI:10.1016/S0140-6736(10)60679-4.

Women and Heart Disease

L. Veronica Lee, MD[a], JoAnne M. Foody, MD[b],*

KEYWORDS

• Coronary artery disease • Women • Risk factors
• Hypertension • Hyperlipidemia

The overall death rate from cardiovascular disease (CVD) has declined and exceeded the American Heart Association (AHA) goal of a 25% decline in CVD and stroke, but the observed reduction has been significantly less for women. In women cardiovascular events such as hypertensive heart disease, myocardial infarction (MI), and stroke is 245 per 1000; ten times the death rate for breast cancer.[1] In fact, in the United States heart disease causes more than one-third of all deaths and most of these occur in women (52.8% [459,096] in 2004), not men. Although the presentation of heart disease is "delayed" in women at an older age than men, and women are considered "protected," heart disease is not a disease of younger men and the elderly. CVD is the leading cause of death in women older than 65 years, but it is the second leading cause of death in women aged 45 to 64 and the third leading cause in younger women aged 25 to 44 years, an age group that is often considered to be unlikely to have significant heart disease.[2] Unfortunately, women remain unaware of CVD risk, as established by a survey conducted by the AHA that found only 57% of women were cognizant that heart disease was a significant cause of death for women. Women and health care professionals alike continue to view death from heart disease as a threat primarily to middle-aged men.[3]

The disparity between genders in the incidence of CVD may be the result of significant differences in both cardiovascular risk factors and presentation. Risk factor modification has been shown to have a different impact on cardiovascular risk for men and women. A recent analysis of NHANES (National Health and Nutrition Examination Survey) data attributed 47% of cardiovascular death reduction that has been demonstrated over the past 2 decades to a combination of acute therapies such as revascularization and both primary and secondary prevention.[4] At least 44% of the decrease demonstrated was the result of risk factor reduction. In this article, recent data of unique sex-specific characteristics of both risk for and presentation of CVD, and the current understanding of how clinical outcome can be improved by targeting specific risk factors to reduce the overall risk of CVD in women, are reviewed.

CARDIOVASCULAR DISEASE RISK FACTORS

The impact of traditional risk factors, although the same, is different on men and women. There is an increase in the incidence of significant risk factors in women that may explain the high rate of CVD that has been observed. With the exception of tobacco use, women have a higher prevalence of all traditional risk factors than men. One-third of women older than 20 years have hypertension, almost half have a total cholesterol of 200 mg/dL or greater, approximately one-quarter have prediabetes mellitus, nearly one-fifth are cigarette smokers, greater than one-third are obese (body mass index [BMI; calculated as the weight in kilograms divided by height in meters squared,

The authors have nothing to disclose.
[a] Clinical Research and Development, Building 500-2, Lantheus Medical Imaging, 331 Treble Cove Road, North Billerica, MA 01821, USA
[b] Division of Cardiology, Brigham and Women's Hospital, Harvard Medical School, 75 Francis Street, Boston, MA 02155, USA
* Corresponding author.
E-mail address: jfoody@partners.org

Cardiol Clin 29 (2011) 35–45
doi:10.1016/j.ccl.2010.11.002
0733-8651/11/$ — see front matter © 2011 Elsevier Inc. All rights reserved.

ie, kg/m^2] ≥30), and more than two-thirds when surveyed report a sedentary lifestyle.[2] Of concern, all of these risk factors are increasing with the exception of smoking cigarettes, as the obesity epidemic propagates globally.

HYPERTENSION

The most common traditional cardiovascular risk factor for women is hypertension. By age 75 years, 85% of women in the United States have hypertension based on the JNC VII (Seventh Report of the Joint National Committee on Prevention, Detection, Evaluation, and Treatment of High Blood Pressure) definition of a blood pressure goal of less than 140/90 mm Hg. However, women have a lower blood pressure than men for most of their life until menopause, which suggests that a lower target blood pressure is indicated for women than men. There is not a threshold blood pressure at which heart disease and stroke risk begins, but there is a linear relationship that demonstrates increased risk even in men and women with prehypertensive or "normal" blood pressure.[5] As a result, the AHA Prevention Guidelines recommend the importance of maintaining an optimal systolic blood pressure (SBP) of less than 120 mm Hg for women.

As women transition to menopause they begin to develop systolic hypertension at an increasing rate. Men who develop hypertension early tend to develop diastolic hypertension, rarely seen in women. Risk factors for the development of hypertension before menopause in women include polycystic ovary disease, renal artery stenosis, oral contraceptive use, and pregnancy. Dietary supplementation with folate in women has been shown to decrease the occurrence of new-onset hypertension.[6] Systolic hypertension becomes more common in older men, although the rate of new-onset hypertension is more rapid in women than men once women reach menopause. Other hemodynamic measures are also different between men and women, with a wider pulse pressure, higher cardiac output, and lower systemic vascular resistance being more common in women.[7]

The mechanism of developing hypertension after menopause has been shown to be the result of menopause itself and independent of both age and BMI, although these are known risk factors for hypertension in both genders.[8] The absence of estrogen after menopause is believed to contribute to postmenopausal hypertension by vasoconstriction of the vascular bed through both renin-angiotensin-aldosterone and sodium-sensitive pathways.[9,10]

Putative treatable contributors to the development of postmenopausal hypertension include folate deficiency, sleep apnea, and the loss of the nocturnal dip (10 mm Hg dip in SBP during sleep) in blood pressure. The nocturnal dip has been associated with an increase in cardiovascular events, and has been shown to be lost in postmenopausal women and restored with hormonal therapy.[11]

Blood pressure reduction benefit in women was assessed in a meta-analysis of 7 trials. Although women received benefits from drug therapy, because of a lower event rate it was less pronounced than in men.[12] The SYMPHONY trial demonstrated that while being treated for acute coronary syndromes women were given on average more medications than men; however, women were less likely to reach a target blood pressure above what would now be considered optimal.[13] At present, many antihypertensives are available to choose from and although the response to medications for blood pressure lowering appears to be similar between men and women, women tend to have more treatment-related side effects. Because routine use of antihypertensives is necessary for adequate and stable control, the higher incidence of side effects becomes a significant factor in determining patient compliance. In addition, the need on average for more than 2 medications to achieve a target blood pressure of less than 140/90 mm Hg, let alone optimal blood pressure control, increases the risk of compounding side effects.

There is a significant risk of maternal and fetal mortality in women with chronic or new-onset hypertension in pregnancy. In addition, hypertensive pregnant women are at an increased risk of thromboembolism, hemorrhage, eclampsia, premature delivery, and abruptio placentae. In addition, a woman who has a hypertensive pregnancy is at an increased risk for the development of long-term hypertension and a residual increased risk for CVD. At present there are limited data regarding therapy for hypertensive pregnancies, and it is often withheld until a diastolic blood pressure greater than 105 mm Hg or SBP of greater than 160 mm Hg is reached. Medications that are currently recommended in pregnancy include hydralazine, labetalol, methyldopa, nicardipine, and nifedipine.

DYSLIPIDEMIA

A significant independent risk factor for coronary artery disease (CAD) in both men and women is increased concentrations of low-density lipoprotein cholesterol (LDL-C) and reduced levels of high-density lipoprotein cholesterol (HDL-C). CAD risk is dependent on lipid and lipoprotein concentrations that vary not only with age, diet, genetics, and physical activity in both men and women but also the ovarian function of women. Total cholesterol increases more slowly in women than men until the sixth decade, at which time the levels increase at a more rapid rate in women until they surpass that in age-matched men. Women have a lower cardiovascular risk than men at any given concentration of total cholesterol. Supporting this, the Framingham study demonstrated that total cholesterol levels greater than 295 mg/dL were associated with a reduced rate of MI in women of 60% more than that of men.[14]

HIGH-DENSITY LIPOPROTEIN CHOLESTEROL

Until puberty, boys have higher concentrations than girls of HDL-C. However, as puberty begins HDL-C levels, while staying the same in girls, begin to decline in boys. In young men HDL-C remains stable whereas HDL-C in young women starts to slowly increase until they are about 20% greater than men by menopause. Postmenopause levels of HDL-C begin to decline by a total of 3.5 mg/dL, a level that still remains higher than that of men in advanced age.[15] The Framingham investigators found that for every 10 mg/dL increase in HDL-C the risk of CAD was decreased by 40% to 50% in women, a more pronounced benefit than in men. The effect of the increases in HDL-C counterbalances the atherogenic effect of LDL-C twice over. Even at modestly reduced levels of HDL-C between 35 and 50 mg/dL, higher rates of CAD and CAD-related mortality have been found. As a result, the current American College of Cardiology recommendations are for a higher target HDL-C in women.[16]

LOW-DENSITY LIPOPROTEIN CHOLESTEROL

From birth, women have lower LDL-C level than men until rapid increases begin in the middle of the fifth decade as a result of menopause, exceeding that of age-matched men whose LDL-C levels remain stable.[16] LDL-C concentration of 130 mg/dL or greater is an independent risk factor for HDL-C for both men and women. However, until recently there has been controversy regarding the part that LDL-C plays in the risk of CAD in women because of the limited prospective studies evaluating this and the cardioprotective effects of relatively elevated HDL-C. It is known that a poor prognosis is associated with very high concentrations of LDL-C in both genders, but is unclear at lower LDL-C levels in women. A primary

prevention study in Japanese men and women aged 40 to 70 years, the MEGA study, was a randomized open-label study in patients with total cholesterol of 5.7 to 7.0 mmol/L receiving either dietary counseling or 10 to 20 mg/d of pravastatin.[17] Of the 5356 subjects enrolled, 68.4% were women, and the incidence of CAD in women was 2 to 3 times less than that of the men. The composite of CAD-related events of angina, revascularization, MI, or sudden death was 26% lower in women on statin therapy (19.1% lower cholesterol) than dietary control (4.9% lower cholesterol) (P value not significant and similar to findings in men). Older women at least 60 years old received a greater benefit than women who were younger.

The JUPITER study evaluated 15,548 men 50 years or older and women 60 years or older in a primary prevention study of patients with elevated high-sensitivity C-reactive protein of greater than 2.0 mg/L and LDL-C levels of 130 mg/dL or less, randomized to treatment with rosuvastatin 20 mg (38.5% women) or placebo (37.9% women) daily.[18] A significant reduction in the composite end point of MI, stroke, arterial revascularization, hospitalization for unstable angina, or cardiovascular mortality was found with a mean follow-up of 1.9 years (rosuvastatin 0.77 vs placebo 1.36 per 100 person-years hazard ratio [HR] 0.56, 95% confidence interval [CI] 0.46–0.69; P<.00001) and was adequately powered for subset analysis of women showing a reduction in HR of 46% compared with 42% of men. However, because of the age criteria, benefit was only assessed in the older and postmenopausal women enrolled, leaving open for debate the utility in younger women. As a result guidelines support the use of statins in women with cardiovascular risk, but the best time to initiate therapy is not clearly defined. Younger women with isolated LDL-C and risk factors such as early menopause, diabetes, and family history should be evaluated for medical therapy in addition to counseling for both lifestyle and dietary modification.

TRIGLYCERIDES

Until middle age, triglycerides increase at a slower rate in women than in men, then men's levels decline while women's continue to increase until age 70 years, until reaching comparable levels to men. Triglyceride concentrations are independent predictors of CVD even when adjusted for other comorbidities and risk factors. Elevated triglyceride levels are common in women who are older and postmenopausal, and are likely the result of the concomitant presence of insulin resistance, metabolic syndrome, obesity, and atherogenic lipoproteins.

DIABETES MELLITUS

One of the most important risk factors for heart disease in women is diabetes mellitus, irrespective of age. Diabetes triples the incidence of heart disease in women and doubles the risk for MI when compared with nondiabetic women, and the described gender-specific delay of the age of onset of heart disease in women as a whole is lost in diabetic women. Diabetic men, on the other hand, are only twice as likely to develop heart disease as nondiabetic men. The higher risk of heart disease seen in diabetic women is likely related at least in part to the common association with multiple other known traditional risk factors such as hypertension, obesity, and smoking. Frequently, diabetic women have a constellation of risk factors associated with the metabolic syndrome, including an increased BMI, low HDL-C levels, impaired glucose tolerance, and elevated triglyceride concentrations. Diabetic women as a whole have higher lipoprotein levels as compared with nondiabetic women, and these levels are markedly higher than those observed in either diabetic or nondiabetic men.[19]

Control of other traditional risk factors in diabetic women and men was assessed in a recent study, which found that SBP was less controlled in diabetic women compared with men (46.6% vs 41.2%) as was LDL-C (28.3% vs 22.4%), although the medical regimens were not significantly different and were of similar intensity.[20] Therefore, the clustering of additional traditional risk factors may explain part of the increase in event rate seen in diabetic women. This inference is supported by a recent study that followed risk factors over years and their association to the development of heart disease. The highest HR was found during the first 10 years in women for diabetes (5.38) and smoking (3.84). Subsequent follow-up showed a decline in the HR, reaching a nadir at longer than 20 years of follow-up (diabetes 1.71, smoking 1.60). Of note, BMI had a greater significance in men during the first 10 years, but other traditional risk factors did not demonstrate a significant change in HR over time.[21]

SMOKING

In the United States there has been a 50% decline in smoking since 1965 in people older than 18 years and as of 2005, 23.9% of men and 18.1% of women continue to smoke cigarettes.[22]

Mortality is earlier in cigarette smokers than nonsmokers, and women who smoke die earlier than their male counterparts (14.5 vs 13.2 years, respectively). There is a dose-dependent association between smoking cigarettes and the incidence of MI in women who smoke beyond the age of 44 years. Women who smoke 1 to 5 cigarettes daily have an increased incidence of MI of 2.5, which increases further in women who smoke 40 cigarettes daily to 74.6.[23] There is an increase in other cardiovascular events such as stroke, aortic aneurysm, and peripheral artery disease. Cigarette smoking is recognized to cause endothelial dysfunction, increase the risk of restenosis in cardiovascular stents, elevate blood pressure, and alter cholesterol levels. Although overall smoking rates have declined in the United States, this reflects a more rapid decline in the numbers of men than women who smoke. Concerning is the higher prevalence of cigarette smoking in young women than in young men who are 17 years or younger. This discrepancy may be the result of the reasons for starting and continuing to smoke cigarettes being very different between women and men, and consequently smoking is a distinguishing behavioral risk factor. There is a role of social and psychological support and views of self that is demonstrated in the increased likelihood of young Caucasian women as compared with African American women to be able to stop smoking and at an earlier age.

OBESITY AND VISCERAL ADIPOSITY

During the 26-year follow-up of participants in The Framingham study for the development of CAD, obesity was determined to be an independent risk for women. Middle-aged women were found to have increased rates of the development of CAD with only mild to moderate increase in weight.[24] The Nurses' Health Study demonstrated an increase in relative risk of 1.8 to 3.3 in women with a BMI of 45 to 49 and greater than 29, respectively.[25,26] In the United States 33.2% of women older than 20 years had elevated BMIs of 25 or higher, which suggests from the findings above that they are all at an increased risk of developing CAD.[2] BMI does not result in a true percentage of body fat, which would be more precise in its determination of risk. The accuracy of BMI is dependent on such factors as age, gender, and muscle mass, which was not controlled for in the aforementioned assessment.

The waist-hip ratio (WHR) in both men and women may be a more important assessment of CAD risk than absolute weight measurements because it takes into account the distribution of body fat. Truncal obesity (considered the male, android, or apple pattern) instead of weight gain at the hips (considered the female, pear pattern) in women is associated with a greater increase in CAD and, interestingly, is associated with higher LDL-C and lower HDL-C levels. The INTERHEART Study investigated the relationship of both WHR and BMI to acute MI in a case-control study of 27,098 participants (12,461 cases, 14,637 controls) in 52 countries and multiple racial and ethnic groups. WHR, as well as both waist and hip circumferences, were associated with an increased risk of MI even after adjustment for other risk factors ($P<.0001$). When comparing the top 2 quintiles for WHR and BMI, the respective population-attributable risks of MI were 24.3% (95% CI 22.5–26.2) compared with only 7·7% (6.0–10.0), suggesting that WHR may be more significantly associated than BMI with the risk of MI in many racial and ethnic groups.[27] The clustering of metabolic abnormalities related to insulin resistance is present in patients with abdominal obesity, especially visceral obesity. Imaging studies have been used to assess the impact of the regional fat distribution in the body, and have shown that increases in visceral fat are related to metabolic disturbances associated with the metabolic syndrome such as glucose intolerance, insulin resistance, hyperinsulinemia, small, dense LDL-C particles, low HDL-C levels, hypertriglyceridemia, and elevated apolipoprotein B (apoB) concentrations. Després and colleagues[28] has suggested that visceral obesity is a marker of a dysmetabolic state that may result in the development of metabolic syndrome. As such, an elevated triglyceride level in the presence of an increased waist circumference may add to the determination of the presence of increased visceral fat.

The PROCEED Cohort was a prospective study in Germany and the United States of 10,816 subjects with BMI scores of 20 to 35, evaluated using waist circumference as a discriminator for health care cost in overweight and obese subjects. The investigators found that irrespective of BMI, the annual health care costs were higher in individuals with increased waist circumference (increase by16%–18% in Germany, 20%–30% in United States), suggesting that public health initiatives to increase awareness of this risk may be cost-effective.[29]

SLEEP APNEA

Sleep apnea is an independent risk factor for CAD, stroke, and arrhythmia, and is estimated to be present in 9% of middle-aged men and only 4% of women according to epidemiologic clinically-based studies. It is known that the prevalence is higher in groups such as those with hypertension, chronic renal disease, morbid obesity, the elderly, and a history of CAD or stroke.[30,31] However, it is most likely underdiagnosed in women who tend to have a smaller neck and therefore pharynx to obstruct, and a higher incidence of obesity and hypothyroidism. The gender-specific presentation may also result in underdiagnosis by health professionals who are unaware of these differences. Similarly to the "atypical" presentation in women of CAD, women with sleep apnea present with symptoms of fatigue,[32] and more sleep disturbances such as staying and falling asleep.[33] The Wisconsin Sleep Cohort Study demonstrated that women were more likely to report daytime sleepiness even in the absence of or only mild sleep apnea. It is essential that women patients are asked about sleep habits, daytime sleepiness, fatigue, and snoring to improve diagnosis and treatment of women with sleep apnea.

The effect of sleep apnea on cardiovascular morbidity and mortality was assessed during a 10-year follow-up of 392 men and women with CAD referred for cardiac catheterization. No relationship was found with subsequent death or MI, but a significant elevation in the risk of stroke was found. Subjects with an apnea-hypopnea index (number of apneas and hypopneas per hour of sleep) of 5 to 15 had an increased risk of 2.44 (95% CI 1.08–5.52) and in those with an apnea-hypopnea index of 15 or greater, risk was increased 3.56-fold (95% CI 1.56–8.16) compared with patients without sleep apnea ($P = .011$ trend).[34] This and other studies have shown a higher risk associated with the presence of sleep apnea in men as compared with women for stroke, heart failure, and CAD.[35] This finding may result from the potential difference in mechanism between women and men because the pattern of hypopnea and apnea occurs mainly in rapid eye movement (REM) sleep in women and in non-REM sleep in men.[36,37]

PHYSICAL INACTIVITY

Physical inactivity has been demonstrated to be as much of a risk factor as smoking in the development of CAD.[38,39] Women as a whole have a more sedentary lifestyle and do less regular vigorous exercise than men. There has been a slight increase in physical activity in women by 8.6% from 2001 to 2005, with 46.7% of women in 2005 doing at least 30 minutes on most days of physical activity.[40] Even modest increases in physical activity in women with a sedentary

Table 1
ABCDEs for CVD prevention in nonpregnant women

A	Angiotensin-converting enzyme inhibitors	Women post-MI, CHF, LV systolic dysfunction, LVH, nephropathy, CVD, and/or diabetes or hypertension. Similar recommendations to men. Avoid in pregnancy. Increased incidence of side effects compared with men (cough, angioedema)
	Angiotensin II receptor blockers	Women with diabetes, nephropathy, hypertension, or LVH. If ACE-I intolerant post-MI, CHF, LV systolic dysfunction. Similar recommendations to men. Avoid in pregnancy
	Antianginals	Women with known inducible ischemia and nitrate responsive chest pain without significant CAD. Include: nitrates, calcium channel blockers, β-blockers
	Anticoagulants: warfarin, heparin, GP IIb/IIIa platelet receptor inhibitor	Warfarin: women with atrial fibrillation, LV aneurysm or LV thrombus Heparin (UF or LMWH): reduce weight dosing similar indications as for men GP IIb/IIIa receptor inhibitor: women at high risk (troponin-positive NSTEMI), may have increased risk of bleeding. Not for troponin-negative NSTEMI
	Antiplatelet: ASA, clopidogrel	For women at risk of stroke, or >65 y without contraindications. Women with known CVD or at high risk. Clopidogrel in same patients if ASA intolerant or in women after stent for CVD
B	β-Blockers	Women post-MI, at high risk of MI, inducible ischemia, symptomatic tachycardias, CHF, hypertension
	BP control	Women with low CVD risk <140/90 mm Hg Women at high risk for CVD, DM, nephropathy <130/80 mm Hg Therapy should be risk directed (eg, β-blockers post-MI) otherwise consider: ACE-I, calcium channel blockers, thiazide diuretics. Second tier: ARBs and β-blockers Consider secondary causes of HTN (renal artery stenosis), sleep apnea, lifestyle modification: low sodium, high potassium (unless kidney disease) diet, folic acid supplementation, exercise, stress management, smoking cessation
C	Calcium channel blockers	
	Cigarette Smoking	Smoke-out date, counseling, buproprion, nicotine patch, varenicline. Weight gain associated with cessation normalizes within 1 year if related to smoking cessation
	Cholesterol	Good: HDL >50 mg/dL, increase exercise, 3 oz red wine a day, weight loss exercise, fish or flax seed oil, niacin, fibrates Bad: LDL <100 mg/dL for high risk consider lowering to <70 mg/dL, diet, weight loss, exercise, HMG CoA reductase inhibitors, niacin, fibrates, increased fiber in diet, avoid *trans* fatty acids (hydrogenated or partially hydrogenated oils) Ugly: Triglycerides <150 mg/dL, improve glycemic control, improve diet (less processed food), weight loss, exercise

D	Depression and anxiety	Women should be screened and treated for depression and anxiety because both can increase the risk of CVD and make risk factors harder to treat
	Diabetes	Impaired fasting glucose (110–124 mg/dL): lifestyle change, weight loss, exercise. Diabetes: improve glycemic control with lifestyle change, medications with goal Hb A1c <6.5%. Lowest risk at Hb A1c <6%
	Diet and weight management, sleep apnea	Emphasis on lifestyle change, portion control, and a diet high in fiber, fruits, and vegetables, whole grains, low in sodium, low in saturated fat and cholesterol; avoid processed foods, BMI <25, waist hip ratio ≤0.8% body fat of <25% (most accurate measure). Screen women for sleep apnea if snoring, sleep disturbance, hypertension, fatigue, weight gain, atypical chest pain, arrhythmia, CVD, or stroke. Not all patients are overweight
	Diuretics, direct renin inhibitors	Caution in women with symptoms of dehydration, dryness, and incontinence. Excellent at lower dose as adjunctive therapy for hypertension. Direct renin inhibitors have few side effects in women, but clinical outcome trial data are pending
E	Ejection fraction	ACE-I (ARB if intolerant) and β-blocker for all women with CHF or decreased LV systolic function. Aldosterone antagonist if severe CHF and low risk of hyperkalemia. Digoxin with caution. High-risk women ICD using guidelines as in men
	Exercise	Aerobic exercise at least 30 min daily on most days. For women doing little to no exercise initiate a walking regimen with goals using a pedometer. For weight loss may need to increase to an hour. Resistance training with lighter weights and frequent repetitions. Address limitations to physical exercise with physical therapy. Cardiac rehabilitation for women post-MI, revascularization, CHF, chronic angina
	Ego and self-esteem	Women as primary caregivers often put their needs last and this social view has to be addressed when prescribing therapy and treatment

Abbreviations: ACE-I, angiotensin-converting enzyme inhibitor; ARB, angiotensin II receptor blocker; ASA, acetylsalicylic acid; BMI, body mass index; CAD, coronary artery disease; CHF, congenital heart failure; CVD, cardiovascular disease; GP, glycoprotein; Hb A1c, hemoglobin A1c; HDL, high-density lipoprotein; HMG-CoA, 3-hydroxy-3-methylglutaryl-coenzyme A; HTN, hypertension; ICD, implantable cardioverter defibrillator; LDL, low-density lipoprotein; LMWH, low molecular weight heparin; LV, left ventricular; LVH, left ventricular hypertrophy; MI, myocardial infarction; NSTEMI, non-ST segment elevation myocardial infarction; UF, unfractionated.

lifestyle that lead to small increases in fitness have been demonstrated to produce valuable reductions in blood glucose levels, blood pressure, improved lipid profiles, and weight loss.[41,42] The AHA has developed the GROW program to encourage exercise in the workplace to encourage awareness that exercise is a key element to any prevention program.

Little is known about the best types of physical activity to encourage reductions in cardiovascular risk. A recent study suggests that there were significant benefits in right ventricular systolic function by echocardiography, blood pressure, and waist circumference in 50 middle-aged abdominally obese women when doing bicycling as opposed to walking over a 6-month period.[43] This finding suggests that there may be incremental benefit to encouraging additional more vigorous and varied physical activity in women once an initial pattern of routine exercise is tolerated and established.

PREVENTION

The Framingham Risk Score has been used clinically, as well as by insurance companies to determine risk an individual patient's eligibility for certain types of cardiovascular testing such as stress tests. However, it has been shown to significantly underestimate risk in women because of the exclusion of significant risk factors in women such as insulin resistance, obesity, and family history. In response, the new American Cardiology Guidelines for Women recommend that all women are at risk of CAD who have any risk factors for CAD, and should be treated as a population at risk. These guidelines go beyond previously established target goals for lipids in the NCEP ATP III and hypertension in the JNC VII, establishing more aggressive lower levels as optimal to reduce risk. Optimal risk for women as defined by the guidelines require a woman to have a Framingham risk score of less than 10%, no other cardiovascular risk factors, and to be leading a healthy lifestyle. Not only women with CAD at high risk but also any woman with a history of peripheral vascular disease, aortic aneurysm, chronic kidney disease, stroke, diabetes, and 10-year global risk of 20% or greater by Framingham score are considered at high risk and as suitable for secondary prevention. All other women are considered to be at risk, highlighting that the preponderance of all adult women are at risk of CAD and have risk factors that need to be attended to by the public health care system.[21] **Table 1** summarizes the goals for preventive care for nonpregnant women.

Once an initial assessment of each woman patient is performed, an individually tailored program to target the key risk factors for each patient needs to be implemented with serial follow-up and management to attain and maintain established goals. A preventive plan should include lifestyle modification, and when required preventive therapy and additional diagnostic assessments. The risk factors for stroke are similar to those for CAD and potential causes of stroke assessed for, such as atrial fibrillation. In addition, many of the same risk factors for CAD have also been associated with an increased risk of developing cancer.

HORMONE REPLACEMENT THERAPY

Clinical trials studying the reduction of cardiovascular risk associated with the treatment of menopause with hormone replacement therapy (HRT) did not demonstrate a reduction in risk of CAD, but potentially harmful effects. In a randomized control trial of 16,605 healthy postmenopausal women, the Women's Health Initiative (WHI), women received either placebo or a combined therapy containing both estrogen and progesterone. An increased risk of breast cancer (HR 1.26), pulmonary embolism (HR 2.13), stroke (HR 1.41), and cardiovascular events (HR 1.29) in part of the study caused it to be stopped early.[44,45] A meta-analysis of 22 randomized trials (n = 4124) found similar results in women treated with hormonal therapy compared with placebo with an increase in cardiovascular events (HR 1.39; 95% CI 0.48–3.95).[46] The Heart and Estrogen/progestin Replacement Study (HERS), a multicenter, randomized, double-blind, placebo-controlled trial in 2763 postmenopausal women, was the first to study the cardioprotective effect of estrogen.[47] In women receiving HRT there was a 52% increased risk of cardiovascular events in the first year. After a 6.8-year follow-up no benefit of CVD was detected.[48] Reduction in cardiac mortality, MI, or CAD progression, even with a more favorable LDL-C and HDL-C profile, has not been demonstrated in additional studies: the Estrogen in the Prevention of Reinfarction Trial (ESPRIT) (n = 1017, 2-year therapy), the Estrogen Replacement and Atherosclerosis (ERA) trial (n = 309, 3.2-year follow-up), and the Women's Angiographic Vitamin and Estrogen (WAVE) trial (n = 423).[49,50] Similar studies to evaluate the benefit of secondary stroke prevention using estrogen therapy have not been able to show benefit.[51,52]

These findings are in opposition to the pathophysiologic and epidemiologic data that find a benefit with estrogen replacement therapy. Effects on lipid profile are well established, with increases in HDL-C and reductions in LDL-C. The progression of carotid intimal thickness is slowed, and improvement in diastolic measurements of heart function by echocardiogram has been shown with HRT.[53,54] In addition, return of the restorative nocturnal dip during 24-hour blood pressure monitoring has been demonstrated in menopausal women treated with hormonal therapy.[55]

At present it remains unclear whether different combinations of hormonal therapy, distinct methods of delivery, or their use in younger versus older postmenopausal women would result in a beneficial effect on cardiovascular outcomes. Given the abundance of clinical trial data, currently available HRT administered long-term for the prevention of CVD cannot be supported. Decisions to continue or to initiate HRT whether or not CAD is present must be made on an individual basis assessing the risks against the non-CAD benefits of HRT.[56] The Kronos Early Estrogen Prevention Study (KEEPS) will further inform our clinical decision making in this area once it is completed.

SUMMARY

The most common cause of death in women remains CAD. Despite tremendous improvements in the reduction of risk, diagnosis and treatment of CVD remains gender-specific. There is a significant burden of risk in women, which may explain some of the differences observed. To reduce the higher mortality seen in women during the first MI, more aggressive and earlier screening and treatment of underlying risk factors is required to reduce the CAD epidemic in women.

REFERENCES

1. National Center for Health Statistics. Center for Disease Control and Prevention. Compressed mortality file: underlying cause of death 1979–2004. Atlanta (GA). Centers for Disease Control and Prevention. Available at: http://wonder.cdc.gov/mortSQL.html. Accessed October 1, 2010.
2. Rosamond W, Flegal K, Furie K, et al. Heart disease and stroke statistics—2008 update: a report from the American Heart Association Statistics Committee and Stroke Statistics Subcommittee. Circulation 2008;117:e1–121.
3. Lewis SJ. Cardiovascular disease in postmenopausal women: myths and reality. Am J Cardiol 2002;89:5E.
4. Ford ES, Ajani UA, Croft JB, et al. Explaining the decrease in U.S. deaths from coronary disease, 1980-2000. N Engl J Med 2007;356:2388–98.
5. Vasan RS, Larson MG, Leip EP, et al. Impact of High-normal blood pressure on the risk of cardiovascular disease. N Engl J Med 2001;345:1291–7.
6. Forman JP, Rimm EB, Stampfer MJ, et al. Folate intake and the risk of incident hypertension among US women. JAMA 2005;293(3):320–9.
7. Safar ME, Smulyan H. Hypertension in women. Am J Hypertens 2004;17(1):82–7.
8. Zanchetti A, Facchetti R, Cesana GC, et al. Menopause-related blood pressure increase and its relationship to age and body mass index: the SIMONA epidemiological study. J Hypertens 2005;23:2269–76.
9. Ramírez-Expósito MJ, Martínez-Martos JM. Hypertension, RAS, and gender: what is the role of aminopeptidases? Heart Fail Rev 2008;13(3):355–65.
10. Schulman IH, Raij L. Salt sensitivity and hypertension after menopause: role of nitric oxide and angiotensin II. Am J Nephrol 2006;26:170–80.
11. Butkevich A, Abraham C, Phillips RA. Hormone replacement therapy and 24-hour blood pressure profile of postmenopausal women. Am J Hypertens 2000;13:1039–41.
12. Gueyffier F, Boutitie F, Boissel JP. Effect of antihypertensive drug treatment on cardiovascular outcomes in women and men. A meta-analysis of individual patient data from randomized, controlled trials. The INDANA Investigators. Ann Intern Med 1997; 126(10):761–7.
13. Frazier CG, Shah SH, Armstrong PW. Prevalence and management of hypertension in acute coronary syndrome patients varies by sex: observations from the sibrafiban versus aspirin to yield maximum protection from ischemic heart events postacute coronary syndromes (SYMPHONY) randomized clinical trials. Am Heart J 2005;150(6):1260–7.
14. Kannel WB. The Framingham study: historical insight on the impact of cardiovascular risk factors in men versus women. J Gend Specif Med 2002;5:27.
15. Bittner V. Lipoprotein abnormalities related to women's health. Am J Cardiol 2002;90:77i.
16. Mosca L, Banka CL, Benjamin EJ. Evidence-based guidelines for cardiovascular disease prevention in women: 2007 update. Circulation 2007;115:1–20.
17. Mizuno K, Nakaya N, Ohashi Y, et al. Usefulness of pravastatin in primary prevention of cardiovascular events in women: analysis of the Management of Elevated cholesterol in the primary prevention Group of Adult Japanese (MEGA Study). Circulation 2008;117:494–502.
18. Ridker P, Danielson E, Fonseca FA, et al. Rosuvastatin to prevent vascular events in men and women with elevated C-reactive protein. N Engl J Med 2008;359:2195–207.
19. Walden CE, Knopp RH, Wahl PW, et al. Sex differences in the effect of diabetes mellitus on lipoprotein triglyceride and cholesterol concentrations. N Engl J Med 1984;311:953.

20. Ferrare A, Mangione CM, Kim C. Sex disparities in control and treatment of modifiable cardiovascular disease risk factors among patients with diabetes. Diabetes Care 2008;31:69–74.

21. Berry JD, Dyer A, Carnethon M, et al. Association of traditional risk factors with cardiovascular death across 0 to 10, 10 to 20, and >20 year follow-up in men and women. Am J Cardiol 2008;101(1):89–94.

22. National Center for Health Statistics. Health, United States, 2007: with chartbook on trends in the health of Americans. Hyattsville (MD): National Center for Health Statistics; 2007. Available at: http://www.cdc.gov/nchs/hus.htm. Accessed October 1, 2010.

23. US Department of Health and Human Services. The health consequences of smoking: a report of the surgeon general. Atlanta, GA: US Department of Health and Human Services, Public Health Service, Centers for Disease Control and Prevention, National Center for Chronic Disease Prevention and Health Promotion, Office on Smoking and Health; 2004. Available at: www.cdc.gov/tobacco/sgr/sgr_2004/index.htm. Accessed October 1, 2010.

24. Mosca L, Grundy SM, Judelson D, et al. Guide to preventive cardiology for women. AHA/ACC Scientific Statement Consensus panel statement. Circulation 1999;99:2480.

25. Barrett-Connor E. Heart disease in women. Fertil Steril 1994;62(6 Suppl 2):127S.

26. Kritz-Silverstein D, Barrett-Connor E. Long-term postmenopausal hormone use, obesity, and fat distribution in older women. JAMA 1996;275:46.

27. Commerford P, Lang CC, Rumboldt Z, et al. Obesity and the risk of myocardial infarction in 27 000 participants from 52 countries: a case-control study. Lancet 2005;366(9497):1640–9.

28. Després P, Lemieux I, Bergeron, et al. Abdominal obesity and the metabolic syndrome. contribution to global cardiometabolic risk. Arterioscler Thromb Vasc Biol 2008;28:1039.

29. Pendergast K, Wolf A, Sherrill B, et al. Impact of waist circumference difference on health-care cost among overweight and obese subjects: the PROCEED Cohort. Value Health 2010;13(4):402–10.

30. Al Lawati NM, Patel SR, Ayas NT. Epidemiology, risk factors, and consequences of obstructive sleep apnea and short sleep duration. Prog Cardiovasc Dis 2009;51(4):285–93.

31. Young T. Analytic epidemiology studies of sleep disordered breathing—what explains the gender difference in sleep disordered breathing. Sleep 1993;16(Suppl 8):S1–2.

32. Chervin RD. Sleepiness, fatigue, tiredness, and lack of energy in obstructive sleep apnea. Chest 2000;118(2):372–9.

33. Baldwin CM, Griffith KA, Nieto FJ, et al. The association of sleep-disordered breathing and sleep symptoms with quality of life in the Sleep Heart Health Study. Sleep 2001;24(1):96–105.

34. Valham F, Moore T, Rabben T, et al. Increased risk of stroke in patients with coronary artery disease and sleep apnea: a 10-year follow-up. Circulation 2008;118:955–60.

35. Gottlieb DJ, Ywnokyan G, Newman AB, et al. Prospective study of obstructive sleep apnea and incident coronary heart disease and heart failure. Circulation 2010;122:352–60.

36. Ware JC, McBrayer RH, Scott JA. Influence of sex and age on duration and frequency of sleep apnea events. Sleep 2000;23(2):165–70.

37. O'Connor C, Thornley KS, Hanly PJ. Gender differences in the polysomnographic features of obstructive sleep apnea. Am J Respir Crit Care Med 2000;161:1465–72.

38. Dubbert PM, Carithers T, Sumner AE, et al. Obesity, physical inactivity, and risk for cardiovascular disease. Am J Med Sci 2002;324:116.

39. Lawler JM, Hu Z, Green JS, et al. Combination of estrogen replacement and exercise protects against HDL oxidation in post-menopausal women. Int J Sports Med 2002;23:477.

40. CDC. 2001 and 2005 BRFSS summary data quality reports. CDC; 2002 and 2006. Available at: http://ftp.cdc.gov/pub/data/brfss/2001summarydataqualityreport.pdf. and http://ftp.cdc.gov/pub/data/brfss/2005summarydataqualityreport.pdf. Accessed October 1, 2010.

41. Miller TD, Fletcher GF. Exercise and coronary artery disease prevention. Cardiologia 1998;43:43.

42. Grundy SM, Bazzarre T, Cleeman J, et al. Prevention Conference V: Beyond secondary prevention: identifying the high-risk patient for primary prevention: medical office assessment: Writing Group I. Circulation 2000;101:E3.

43. Eriksson M, Udden J, Hemmingsson E, et al. Impact of physical activity and body composition on heart function and morphology in middle-aged, abdominally obese women. Clin Physiol Funct Imaging 2010;30(5):354–9.

44. Rossouw JE, Anderson GL, Prentice RL, et al. Risks and benefits of estrogen plus progestin in healthy postmenopausal women: principal results from the Women's Health Initiative randomized controlled trial. JAMA 2002;288:321.

45. Hays J, Ockene JK, Brunner RL, et al. Effects of estrogen plus progestin on health-related quality of life. N Engl J Med 2003;348:1839.

46. Hemminki E, McPherson K. Impact of postmenopausal hormone therapy on cardiovascular events and cancer: pooled data from clinical trials. BMJ 1997;315:149.

47. Grady D, Applegate W, Bush T, et al. Heart and Estrogen/progestin Replacement Study (HERS): design,

methods, and baseline characteristics. Control Clin Trials 1998;19:314.

48. Grady D, Herrington D, Bittner V, et al. Cardiovascular disease outcomes during 6.8 years of hormone therapy: heart and estrogen/progestin Replacement Study follow-up (HERS II). JAMA 2002;288:49 [Erratum, JAMA 2002, 288:1064].

49. Cherry N, Gilmour K, Hannaford P. Oestrogen therapy for prevention of reinfarction in postmenopausal women: a randomized placebo controlled trial. Lancet 2002;360:2001.

50. Herrington DM, Howard TD, Hawkins GA, et al. Estrogen-receptor polymorphisms and effects of estrogen replacement on high-density lipoprotein cholesterol in women with coronary disease. N Engl J Med 2002;346:967.

51. Hurn PD, Brass LM. Estrogen and stroke: a balanced analysis. Stroke 2003;34:338.

52. Viscoli CM, Brass LM, Kernan WN, et al. A clinical trial of estrogen-replacement therapy after ischemic stroke. N Engl J Med 2001;345:1243.

53. Dubuisson JT, Wagenknecht LE, D'Agostino RB. Association of hormone replacement therapy and carotid wall thickness in women with and without diabetes. Diabetes Care 1998;21(11): 1790–6.

54. Aldrighi JM, Alecrin IN, Caldas MA, et al. Effects of estradiol on myocardial global performance index in hypertensive postmenopausal women. Gynecol Endocrinol 2004;19(5):282–92.

55. Kaya C, Dincer Cengiz S, Cengiz B, et al. The long-term effects of low-dose 17β-estradiol and dydrogesterone hormone replacement therapy on 24-h ambulatory blood pressure in hypertensive postmenopausal women: a 1-year randomized, prospective study. Climacteric 2006;9(6): 437–45.

56. Mosca L, Collins P, Herrington DM, et al. Hormone replacement therapy and cardiovascular disease: a statement for healthcare professionals from the American Heart Association. Circulation 2001;104: 499.

Primary and Secondary Prevention Strategy for Cardiovascular Disease in Diabetes Mellitus

Sundararajan Srikanth, MD[a], Prakash Deedwania, MD[b],*

KEYWORDS

- Diabetes mellitus • Cardiovascular disease
- Primary prevention

Diabetes is a metabolic and a vascular disease manifested by arterial inflammation and endothelial dysfunction leading to micro- and macrovascular pathology. Type 2 diabetes has reached worldwide epidemic proportions. By the year 2025 the number of individuals with diabetes mellitus in the world is expected to exceed 350 million with a prevalence of 4.4%.[1] Diabetes continues to affect a substantial proportion of the adult population in the United States. From the National Health and Nutrition Enhancement Survey (NHANES) 1999/2000 data,[2] 8.3% of persons aged 20 years or more had either diagnosed or undiagnosed diabetes, and this percentage increased to 19.2% for persons aged 60 years or more in the United States. Men and women were affected similarly by diabetes. In 1999/2000, an additional 6.1% of adults had impaired fasting glucose, increasing to 14.4% for persons aged 60 years or more; men were affected more than women.[3] Overall, an estimated 14.4% of the US population aged 20 years or more and 33.6% of those aged 60 years or more had either diabetes or impaired fasting glucose. In the last decade, type 2 diabetes has also been diagnosed more frequently in children and adolescents concomitant with the increasing prevalence of obesity and decreased physical activity in this population.

Cardiovascular (CV) diseases are the leading cause of morbidity and mortality in the general population. Haffner and colleagues[4] initially reported that patients with type 2 diabetes without a history of myocardial infarction (MI) have the same risk of coronary artery disease (CAD) as those without diabetes with a history of MI. Subsequently the National Cholesterol Education Program stated that diabetes is considered a coronary heart disease (CHD) risk equivalent.[5] The baseline risk of CV disease is multiplied 2- to 4-fold in persons with diabetes mellitus with a higher case fatality rate compared with patients without diabetes.[6] There are a few articles questioning the conclusion that the diabetic state confers CV risk equivalent to that of preexisting CAD. The most recent article based on data from the REACH registry suggests that the CV risk of a person with diabetes without additional risk factors lies in between that of an individual without diabetes and someone with established CV disease.[7] However, the diabetic cohort in the REACH registry had a much greater

a Division of Cardiology, VACCHCS/CMC, UCSF Program at Fresno, Fresno, CA, USA
b Division of Cardiology, Department of Medicine, Veterans Affairs Central California Health Care System/ University of California, San Francisco, Fresno Program, 2615 East Clinton Avenue, Fresno, CA 93703, USA
* Corresponding author. Division of Cardiology, Department of Medicine, Veterans Affairs Central California Health Care System/University of California, San Francisco, Fresno Program, 2615 East Clinton Avenue, Fresno, CA 93703.
E-mail address: deed@fresno.ucsf.edu

Cardiol Clin 29 (2011) 47–70
doi:10.1016/j.ccl.2010.11.004
0733-8651/11/$ – see front matter. Published by Elsevier Inc.

adherence to statin therapy, which explains the lower event rates. Recent data from the Danish population study and the million women study from Europe, both of which were prospective long-term studies in the general population, show that in the diabetic cohort who are not on statin therapy the risk of CV disease is equivalent to that of an individual without diabetes but with known CAD.[8,9] Moreover a recent meta-analysis of individual records from studies in the Emerging Risk Factors Collaboration involving nearly 700,000 individuals reported a doubling of risk for CAD as well as for stroke independent of other conventional risk factors in the presence of diabetes mellitus thus reinforcing the fact that the CV risk in the presence of diabetes approximates that of CV risk in the individual with prior ischemic coronary event.[10]

CV disease accounts for 65% of deaths in persons with type 2 diabetes mellitus. Much of the morbidity and mortality is from atherosclerotic CAD, congestive heart failure and sudden cardiac death. Advances in medical therapy, interventional techniques and surgical techniques have resulted in only modest improvements in mortality from CV disease in men with diabetes and in fact mortality rates during the last decade have risen for women with diabetes and CV disease (**Fig. 1**).[11]

The excess CV mortality and morbidity in the diabetic population reflects the general vascular inflammation that is seen in this disease state. Significant progress has been made in elucidation of the mechanism and consequences of the metabolic perturbations in the diabetic state. The disease is characterized by insulin resistance and is commonly associated with the metabolic syndrome. Sensitivity to insulin is variable in the population at large. Insulin resistance develops as a result of a complex interplay of genetic and environmental factors. Hyperinsulinemia occurs as an adaptive response to increasing insulin resistance.

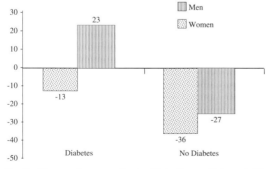

Fig. 1. Change in age-adjusted 8- to 9-year CV mortality in NHANES for 30 years. (*Data from* Gu K, Cowie CC, Harris MI. Diabetes and decline in heart disease mortality in US adults. JAMA 1999;281:1291–7.)

PATHOGENESIS OF TYPE 2 DIABETES MELLITUS

Type 2 diabetes develops when insulin-resistant individuals cannot maintain the degree of excess insulin secretion needed to overcome insulin resistance. The development of the overt diabetic condition is preceded by a prediabetic phase which usually lasts 6 to 8 years (**Fig. 2**). The prediabetic milieu is characterized by hyperinsulinemia, hypertension, and endothelial dysfunction. Insulin resistance and hyperglycemia seem to set the stage for the development of the metabolic syndrome characterized by dyslipidemia, endothelial dysfunction, hypercoagulability, hypertension, and truncal obesity, which is present in approximately 25% of adults in the United States.[12] The metabolic syndrome also known as the insulin resistance syndrome or cardiovascular dysmetabolic syndrome (CDS), is a constellation of metabolic abnormalities that are associated with a higher risk of CV disease and mortality.[13] The metabolic risk factors for CV disease that make up the metabolic syndrome do not directly cause type 2 diabetes but are frequently associated with it (**Table 1**). Multiple prospective observational studies demonstrate a strong association between the metabolic syndrome and the risk for subsequent development of type 2 diabetes.[14] The risk of diabetes seems to increase with increasing components of the metabolic syndrome.[15]

Both type 2 diabetes and CV disease stem from a complex interaction of insulin resistance and visceral obesity. Clearly environmental factors in the form of excess calorie intake contribute significantly to the genesis of type 2 diabetes in addition to genetic tendencies. Visceral adipose tissue acts as an endocrine factory releasing various adipokines with effects on the vascular, hepatic, and muscular tissues (**Fig. 3**). Positive energy balance in the adipose tissue may mediate insulin resistance by lipotoxicity in various tissues. Free fatty acids inhibit insulin-stimulated peripheral glucose uptake while promoting the development of dyslipidemia, characterized by low high-density lipoprotein-cholesterol (HDL-C), high triglycerides, and increased small dense low-density lipoprotein-cholesterol (LDL-C). Other adipokines promote systemic inflammation, and increase oxidant stress promoting thrombosis. These effects interfere with the normal function of the vascular endothelium, and result in reduced nitric oxide bioavailability followed by disruption of the structural integrity of the endothelial monolayer. This break in the integrity of the endothelium allows entry of LDL-C in the media, which on further modification by oxidation and monocyte ingestion leads to the formation of the classic foam cells. Accumulation of foam cells

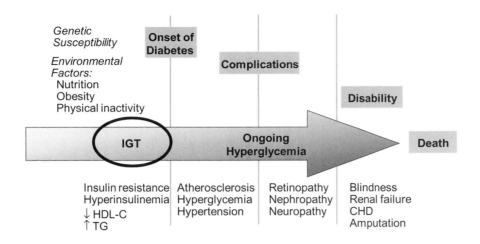

IGT=impaired glucose tolerance; CHD=congestive heart disease

Fig. 2. Natural history of type 2 diabetes disease progression.

leads to the formation of fatty streaks that are classically believed to lead to atherosclerosis.

The approach to management of the patient with diabetes should prioritize the goal of reducing CV morbidity and mortality while also addressing microvascular complications (nephropathy and retinopathy). For this to transpire, interventions should be targeted at the basic pathophysiologic processes that have been identified as risk factors leading to atherosclerosis and CV disease and are manifest more aggressively in the patient with diabetes (**Box 1**). In the following sections, the current literature pertaining to individual risk factor intervention for primary and secondary prevention of CV disease in the patient with diabetes is briefly reviewed. The rationale for a comprehensive risk reduction strategy based on available data is emphasized.

SIGNIFICANCE AND TREATMENT OF INDIVIDUAL RISK FACTORS IN TYPE 2 DIABETES MELLITUS
Dyslipidemia

Hypertriglyceridemia was one of the first metabolic abnormalities recognized to be associated with insulin resistance. The mechanism of hypertriglyceridemia is understood to be caused by differential insulin sensitivity of the tissues in the individual's body. Defects in the ability of insulin to mediate muscle use of glucose and inhibit lipolysis in adipose tissues seem to be the primary

---

Table 1
The International Diabetes Federation diagnostic criteria for the metabolic syndrome (diagnosis is made when 3 or more risk factors are present)

Criterion	Defining Level
Central obesity (waist circumference)	Europid men >94 cm (south Asian >90 cm), Europid and south Asian women >80 cm
Plus any 2 of the following	
Increased triglycerides	$\geq$1.7 mmol/L or on specific treatment for this abnormality
Reduced HDL-C	Men <1.03 mmol/L, women <1.29 mmol/L, or on specific treatment for this abnormality
Hypertension	Systolic BP $\geq$130 mm Hg, or diastolic BP $\geq$85 mm Hg or on specific treatment for this abnormality
Abnormal glycoregulation	Fasting plasma glucose $\geq$5.6 mmol/L, or previously diagnosed type 2 diabetes mellitus

Abbreviation: BP, blood pressure.
Adapted from Alberti KG, Zimmet P, Shaw J. The metabolic syndrome–a new worldwide definition. Lancet 2005;366:1059.

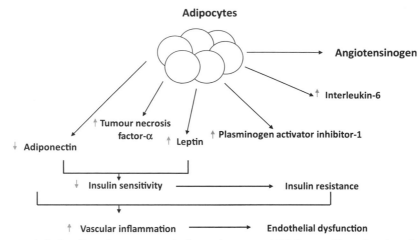

Fig. 3. Adipocyte role in insulin resistance, metabolic syndrome, and CV disease. (*From* Deedwania PC, Volkova N. Current treatment options for the metabolic syndrome. Curr Treat Options Cardiovasc Med 2005;7:63; with permission.)

abnormalities that cause the insulin-resistant state.[16] The resistance at the level of the muscle and adipose tissue leads to persistently higher ambient levels of insulin and free fatty acids. In response to the higher free fatty acid level, the hepatic tissue increases the rate of conversion of free fatty acids to triglycerides. This is accentuated by the normal insulin sensitivity of the hepatic tissues in the face of compensatory hyperinsuline-mia. The appreciation of the difference in the insulin sensitivity of the various tissues has led to better understanding of the abnormalities caused by insulin resistance. Although the classic diabetic dyslipidemia is characterized by high serum triglyc-eride levels, low levels of HDL-C and an increased number of small dense LDL particles, there are additional lipid abnormalities as well.[17,18]

LDL-C is the major cholesterol-rich lipoprotein that mediates the link between serum cholesterol and atherosclerosis. The interaction of LDL-C with monocytes transforms them into the foam cells that are seen in atherosclerotic plaques. This interaction of the monocytes with LDL occurs only when the LDL is modified by acetylation, oxidation, or glycosylation as realized in diabetes mellitus. Moreover the small dense LDL particles that are abundant in diabetes mellitus are particu-larly atherogenic.[19] Thus, quantitative and qualita-tive lipid abnormalities mediate the increased risk of atherosclerosis in diabetes mellitus as shown by the MRFIT and United Kingdom Prospective Diabetes Study (UKPDS)[20,21] data. Evaluation of the importance of various risk factors for CAD in UKPDS shows that LDL-C and HDL-C are the best predictors of CHD (**Table 2**).

In the diabetic population the prevalence of hypertriglyceridemia and low HCL-C levels is approximately twice as high and the prevalence of high LDL-C levels is not different compared with the nondiabetic population.[22] However what-ever the amount of LDL-C in the diabetic indi-vidual, the LDL is atherogenic (type B small dense LDL) and therefore treatment with statins has been found to be highly effective in preventing macrovascular events. Initial data on the benefits of statins in patients with diabetes were obtained from subgroup analyses of the major secondary intervention trials such as the Scandinavian Sim-vastatin Survival Study (4S) and CARE trials.[23,24] In the 4S study, simvastatin led to a 35% decrease in LDL-C resulting in a 42% decrease in the inci-dence of nonfatal MI and CV mortality. A meta-analysis of the CARE (Cholesterol and Recurrent Events) and LIPID (Long-term Intervention with Pravastatin in Ischemic Disease) studies showed a 25% decrease in incidence of major coronary events and revascularizations in the subgroup of patients with diabetes.

Box 1
Cardiac risk factors in type 2 diabetes

Hyperglycemia

Hypertension

Atherogenic dyslipidemia

Increased platelet aggregation

Increased plasminogen activator inhibitor-1

Increased thrombogenicity

Increased fibrinogen level

Increased von Willebrand factor

Decreased tissue plasminogen activator

Table 2
Stepwise selection of risk factors[a] in 2693 diabetics with time to first event as dependent variable: UKPDS CAD (n = 280)

Position in Model	Variable	P value
First	LDL-C	<0.0001
Second	HDL-C	0.0001
Third	Hemoglobin A_{1c}	0.0022
Fourth	Systolic BP	0.0065
Fifth	Smoking	0.056

[a] Adjusted for age and sex.
Data from Turner RC, Millns H, Neil HA, et al. Risk factors for coronary artery disease in non-insulin dependent diabetes mellitus: United Kingdom Prospective Diabetes Study (UKPDS: 23). BMJ 1998;316:823–8.

More recently the benefits of high-dose statins were shown in the Treating to New Targets (TNT) study, which compared atorvastatin 80 mg/d to 10 mg/d in patients with stable CAD.[25] A subanalysis showed that major CV events were reduced by 25% in patients with diabetes receiving high-dose atorvastatin supporting the use of intensive lipid-lowering regimens (**Fig. 4**).

Further post hoc analysis of the TNT study was done to investigate the effect of intensive lipid lowering on future CV events in patients with diabetes, with or without coexisting mild to moderate chronic kidney disease (CKD).[26] Compared with 10 mg of atorvastatin, 80 mg of atorvastatin reduced the relative risk of major CV events by 35% in patients with diabetes and CKD and by 10% in patients with diabetes and normal estimated glomerular filtration rate. The absolute risk reduction in patients with diabetes and CKD was substantial, yielding a number needed to treat of 14 to prevent 1 major CV event in 4.8 years (**Fig. 5**). This result is very encouraging and is in contrast to previous observations in patients with diabetes and end-stage renal disease.

These data from the TNT analysis of the diabetic cohort provide strong support for the prevailing recommendations of reducing LDL-C to levels less than 70 mg/dL as recommended by various guidelines including the American Diabetes Association (ADA). From the TNT data, further reduction of LDL-C with intensive statin therapy provided no safety concerns in patients with diabetes and diabetes along with CKD. It is instructive to look at some of the other secondary prevention trials preceding the TNT trial (**Fig. 6**).

In the diabetic cohort of the 4S study, LDL-C decreased from a mean of 186 mg/dL to 119 mg/dL (36% reduction) on simvastatin with a 55% reduction in CHD. In the diabetic cohort of the LIPID trial, the LDL changed from a mean of 150 mg/dL to 112 mg/dL on pravastatin with a 19% risk reduction in CHD. The CARE cohort started with a mean LDL of 136 mg/dL, which decreased to 98 mg/dL with a 25% risk reduction in CHD on pravastatin. In the Health Protection Study, mean LDL decreased from 127 to 89 mg/dL (30% reduction) with a 21% reduction in CHD events. The results of the post hoc analysis of the diabetic subgroup from TNT

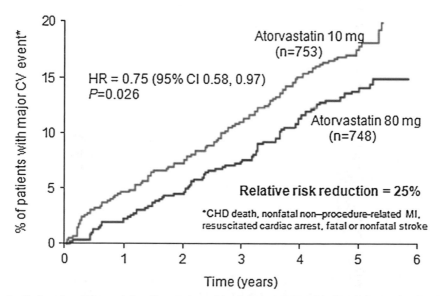

Fig. 4. Time to first major CV event in all patients with diabetes: TNT trial. (*Data from* Shepherd J, Barter P, Carmena R, et al. Effect of lowering LDL cholesterol substantially below currently recommended levels in patients with coronary heart disease and diabetes: the Treating to New Targets (TNT) study. Diabetes Care 2006;29:1220–6.)

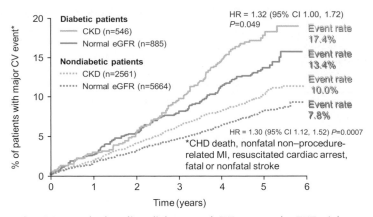

Fig. 5. Time to first major CV event by baseline diabetes and CKD status: the TNT trial.

extend this linear declining trend seen in the CHD event rates with declining LDL-C levels, similar to the results seen in the overall study. End-of-treatment mean LDL-C levels were 98.6 mg/dL with atorvastatin 10 mg and 77.0 mg/dL with atorvastatin 80 mg in the TNT cohort. These data show that by aggressive LDL-C reduction, between the 4S placebo group and the TNT atorvastatin 80 mg group, statin therapy alone was able to achieve a 70% reduction of CHD events. Thus, the target LDL-C for secondary prevention of CHD in the setting of diabetes should be 70 mg/dL. Moreover, aggressive reduction of LDL-C should be sought in this population from the outset.

Although the studies mentioned earlier included only diabetic patients with established CHD, the findings from the Heart Protection Study support the use of lipid-lowering therapy in diabetes without clinically evident atherosclerotic disease.[27] This study, which included almost 4000 people with diabetes without prior CHD, demonstrated a 26% risk reduction of nonfatal MI, CV death, stroke, or revascularizations in the group of subjects treated with simvastatin 40 mg/d (**Fig. 7**).

The Collaborative Atorvastatin Diabetes Study (CARDS), involving patients with type 2 diabetes, was halted 2 years early because patients allocated to atorvastatin had significant reduction (37%) in combined CV end points compared with those receiving placebo (**Fig. 8**).[28] In this primary prevention study, 2838 persons with type 2 diabetes between the ages of 40 and 75 years with no previous history of CHD, stroke, or other major CV events and a documented history of at least 1 of retinopathy, micro-/macroalbuminuria, hypertension or current smoking, LDL equal to or less than 4.14 mmol/L (160 mg/dL), and triglycerides equal to or less than 6.78 mmol/L (600 mg/dL) were randomized to either placebo or atorvastatin 10 mg daily. Patients who received 10 mg daily of atorvastatin had a 37% reduction in major CV events such as acute MI, stroke, angina, and revascularization compared with control patients. This was a landmark trial that was designed specifically to answer the question of primary prevention of micro- and macrovascular disease in the diabetic population. Treatment with atorvastatin resulted in benefit even in individuals with LDL

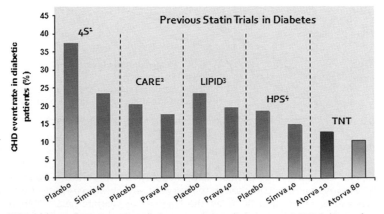

Fig. 6. What does TNT add to what was already known about diabetes and CHD? (*Data from* Refs.[24,27,84,85])

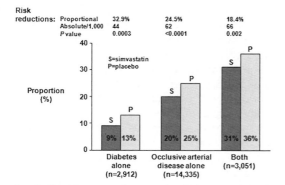

Fig. 7. Health Protection Study diabetes substudy: absolute effects on 5-year rates of first major vascular event. (*Adapted from* Heart Protection Study Collaborative Group. MRC/BHF Heart Protection Study of cholesterol-lowering with simvastatin in 5963 people with diabetes: a randomised placebo-controlled trial. Lancet 2003;361:2005–16; with permission.)

levels lower than 100 mg/dL at the time of initiation of the medication.

Although there is a great deal of evidence supporting the use of statins in diabetics for CV risk reduction, there is less evidence for interventions directed at diabetic dyslipidemia (high triglyceride and low HDL). The fibrate class of lipid-lowering drugs is useful for lowering increased triglyceride or non–HDL-C levels. However, clinical trial data with these drugs have shown mixed results. The Helsinki Heart Study involved 135 patients with type 2 diabetes without concurrent CVD.[29] A 68% relative risk reduction in coronary death and nonfatal MI was seen in association with a 10% reduction in LDL and 26% reduction in triglycerides with gemfibrozil 600 mg twice a day. However, this result did not reach statistical significance because of the small sample size. The FIELD trial randomized 9795 individuals with type 2 diabetes at risk

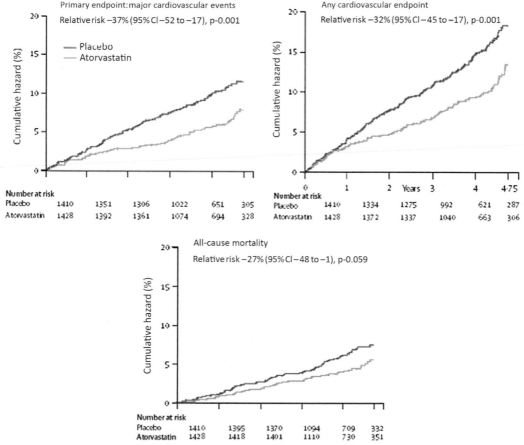

Fig. 8. Collaborative Atorvastatin Diabetes Study (CARDS). Cumulative hazard of primary end point, all-cause mortality, and any cardiovascular end point for heterogeneity. (*Data from* Colhoun HM, Betteridge DJ, Durrington PN, et al. Primary prevention of cardiovascular disease with atorvastatin in type 2 diabetes in the Collaborative Atorvastatin Diabetes Study (CARDS): multicentre randomised placebo-controlled trial. Lancet 2004;364:685–96.)

for CAD to either fenofibrate 200 mg/d or placebo.[30] Statins and other lipid-lowering therapy were allowed any time after randomization. There was no difference in the primary composite end point of CHD death or nonfatal MI. The secondary composite end point of total CV disease events was lower in the fenofibrate group (12.5% vs 13.9%, $P = .035$), primarily because of a reduction in nonfatal and coronary revascularization. Patients in the placebo group were more frequently treated with other lipid-lowering therapy, predominantly statins, during the 5-year follow-up, which may have negated any treatment effect differences between the fenofibrate and placebo groups.

The ACCORD Lipid trial evaluated treatment with fenofibrate compared with placebo among patients with type 2 diabetes treated with an open-label statin medication.[31] Among the 5518 patients randomized into the study, the addition of fenofibrate to statin therapy was not superior to statin therapy alone. Although fenofibrate reduced triglyceride levels, there was only a small difference in mean HDL and no difference between LDL-C between groups, which could help to explain lack of benefit (**Fig. 9**).

However, most subjects in the ACCORD study treated with fenofibrate did not have increased triglyceride or low HDL-C. Those subjects with residual atherogenic dyslipidemia as identified by an increased triglyceride level and low HDL-C had a significant 31% reduction in primary end point (first occurrence of nonfatal MI, nonfatal stroke, or death from CV causes). The risk associated with atherogenic dyslipidemia was 17.3%, which is comparable with the risk in individuals with prior CV disease. This finding is consistent with the results of previous studies using fibric acid derivatives (**Fig. 10**). Thus, although the overall ACCORD lipid trial seems to be negative, subgroup analysis would suggest that there is value to adding fenofibrate to a statin in diabetic individuals with residual risk arising from atherogenic dyslipidemia.

To summarize, the goals of therapy as recommended by the Adult Treatment Panel III (ATP III) of the National Cholesterol Education Program include a LDL-C target of less than 100 mg/dL; serum triglyceride level less than 150 g/dL and HDL-C greater than 40 mg/dL.[32] The panel also recommends a secondary target of therapy in non–HDL-C (total cholesterol minus HDL-C). In diabetic individuals with a triglyceride level greater than or equal to 200 mg/dL, the non–HDL-C goal is 130 mg/dL. The choice of a particular agent depends on the baseline lipid profile. If baseline LDL-C is less than 100 mg/dL, statin therapy should be initiated based on risk factor assessment. A statin is the drug of choice if LDL-C is greater than 100 mg/dL. If triglycerides are equal to or greater than 500 mg/dL, treatment options include fibrates or niacin to lower triglyceride level before initiating LDL-lowering therapy. Although there is no official modification by the National Cholesterol Education Program (NCEP), a recent advisory from the NCEP as well as ADA guidelines suggests that because of the associated high risk of coronary events, the appropriate LDL target for the diabetic population may be 70 mg/dL.[33,34] However, in light of the FIELD and recent ACCORD lipid trials, the role of additional treatment with

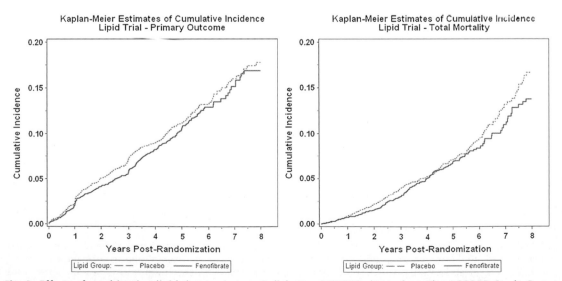

Fig. 9. Effects of combination lipid therapy in type 2 diabetes: ACCORD. (*Data from* The ACCORD Study Group. Effects of combination lipid therapy in type 2 diabetes mellitus. N Engl J Med 2010;362:1563–74.)

Trial (Drug)	Primary Endpoint: Entire Cohort (P-value)	Lipid Subgroup Criterion	Primary Endpoint: Subgroup
HHS (Gemfibrozil)	-34% (0.02)	TG > 200 mg/dl LDL-C/HDL-C > 5.0	-71% (0.005)
BIP (Bezafibrate)	-7.3% (0.24)	TG ≥ 200 mg/dl	-39.5% (0.02)
FIELD (Fenofibrate)	-11% (0.16)	TG ≥ 204 mg/dl HDL-C < 42 mg/dl	-27% (0.005)
ACCORD (Fenofibrate)	-8% (0.32)	TG ≥ 204 mg/dl HDL-C ≤ 34 mg/dl	-31%

Fig. 10. Comparison of ACCORD subgroup results with those from prior fibrate studies. (*Data from* Refs.[29–31,86])

fibrate to further improve the outcome is an open question.

Hypertension

Hypertension is seen in about 60% to 80% of individuals with type 2 diabetes. As with the metabolic syndrome this often predates the manifestation of overt diabetes. There is significant association between the blood pressure and insulin sensitivity.[35,36] The mechanisms believed to mediate hypertension include insulin resistance and diabetic nephropathy. Insulin resistance and concurrent hyperinsulinemia possibly cause sodium retention by the kidneys, stimulate growth of vascular smooth muscle cells and affect endothelial function, vascular reactivity, and blood flow.

Several trials have been published regarding the treatment of hypertension in diabetes mellitus. They have shown beyond reasonable doubt that adequate control of blood pressure can protect against macrovascular and microvascular complications. In the Hypertension in Diabetes Study (a substudy of UKPDS), diabetic subjects were randomized into groups with different blood pressure control targets (**Fig. 11**). After a mean follow-up of more than 8 years there was a relatively greater decrease in diabetes-related mortality by 32%, stroke incidence by 44%, and congestive heart failure incidence by 56% in the aggressively treated group (mean blood pressure 144/82 mm Hg on treatment) compared with the less aggressively treated group (mean blood pressure of 154/87 mm Hg).[37]

The Hypertension Optimal Treatment (HOT) trial showed that targeting diastolic blood pressure to less than 80 mm Hg in patients with diabetes was associated with a 51% reduction of CV mortality in a 4-year period compared with the group with a target diastolic blood pressure of less than 90 mm Hg.[38] If the diabetic subgroup was removed from the analysis, the benefit in the rest of the population did not achieve statistical significance. The ACCORD study randomized a total of 4733 patients with type 2 diabetes mellitus to intensive antihypertensive therapy with a target systolic pressure of less than 120 mm

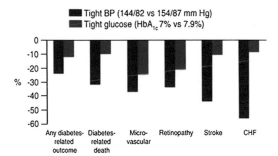

Fig. 11. UKPDS: comparison between tight control of blood pressure and glycemia on risk of diabetes complications. (*Data from* UK Prospective Diabetes Study (UKPDS) Group. Intensive blood-glucose control with sulphonylureas or insulin compared with conventional treatment and risk of complications in patients with type 2 diabetes(UDPDS 33). Lancet 1998;352: 837–53; and UK Prospective Diabetes Study Group. Tight blood pressure control and risk of macrovascular and microvascular complications in type 2 diabetes: UKPDS 38. BMJ 1998;317:703–13.)

Hg or standard therapy for systolic pressure target less than 140 mm Hg. After 1 year, the mean systolic blood pressure was 119.3 mm Hg in the intensive therapy group and 133.5 mm Hg in the standard therapy group. At 1 year there was no difference in the primary composite outcome (nonfatal MI, nonfatal stroke, or death from CV causes). It should perhaps not come as a surprise that there was no improvement in the primary composite outcome because control of blood pressure to a value less than 130 mm Hg systolic has not been shown to improve coronary events in most studies. On the other hand, there is a close correlation between systolic blood pressure and risk of stroke rate down to a lower value of 115 mm Hg. In the ACCORD study, it was shown that decreasing systolic blood pressure down to a mean value of 119.3 mm Hg was associated with decrease in all strokes and nonfatal strokes (**Fig. 12**).[39]

Results from the ADVANCE study are also instructive in the management of hypertension in the patient with diabetes.[40] ADVANCE was a 2 × 2 factorial study, in which 11,140 patients were randomized to either intensive glucose control or standard glucose therapy, and fixed-dose combination of perindopril and indapamide, or placebo. After a 6-week run-in phase with usual glucose control, patients who tolerated and complied with the blood pressure regimen were randomized to either intensive glucose control, or a strategy of standard glucose control. After a mean of 4.3 years of follow-up, 73% of those assigned active treatment and 74% of those assigned to control remained on randomized treatment. Compared with patients assigned to placebo, those who received active therapy had a mean reduction in systolic blood pressure of 5.6 mm Hg (mean systolic blood pressure of 134.7 mm Hg active vs 140.3 mm Hg placebo) and diastolic blood pressure of 2·2 mm Hg (mean diastolic blood pressure 74.8 mm Hg active vs 77 mm Hg placebo). The relative risk of death from CV disease was reduced by 18% ($P = 0.03$) and death from any cause was reduced by 14% ($P = 0.03$) (**Fig. 13**). This benefit was attributed mostly to reduction in microvascular events.

So the natural question that arises is what should be the target blood pressure for therapy in the patient with diabetes? Although guidelines have recommended target blood pressure less than 130/80 mm Hg or 120/75 mm Hg in those with CKD,[41] this target had not been supported by prospective, large-scale, randomized controlled trials specifically designed to evaluate the benefit of targeted therapy to a goal of blood pressure less than 130/80 mm Hg. The ACCORD blood pressure study is the first such trial where treatment directed to a goal of less than 120/80 mm Hg was prospectively evaluated against a blood pressure goal of less than 140/80 mm Hg. Although the findings of the ACCORD trial have not yet been incorporated into guidelines, it seems reasonable in the meanwhile to consider that the target blood pressure for most patients with diabetes should be less than 130/85 mm Hg.

The other important take-home message from UKPDS and other trials is that adequate control of blood pressure generally requires the use of 2 or more antihypertensive agents.[42] As regards the choice of specific antihypertensive agents,

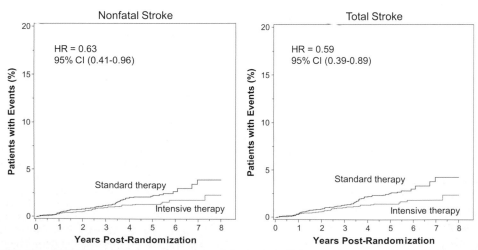

Fig. 12. Effects of intensive blood pressure control in type 2 diabetes: the ACCORD study. (*Data from* The ACCORD Study Group. Effects of intensive blood-pressure control in type 2 diabetes mellitus. N Engl J Med 2010;362:1575–85.)

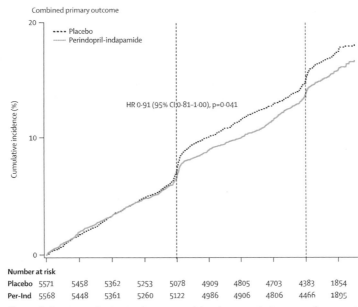

Combined primary outcome

Fig. 13. ADVANCE: effect of therapeutic strategies on combined macro-/microvascular events. (*Data from* Patel A, ADVANCE Collaborative Group, MacMahon S, et al. Effects of a fixed combination of perindopril and indapamide on macrovascular and microvascular outcomes in patients with type 2 diabetes mellitus (the ADVANCE trial): a randomised controlled trial. Lancet 2007;370:829.)

some guidance can be obtained by analysis of various antihypertensive trials. In general, the degree of blood pressure reduction obtained is more important than which agents are used. Moreover, because therapy requires use of multiple antihypertensive medications at the outset, the preferred initial drug is a moot point. Nevertheless angiotensin-converting enzyme inhibitors (ACE-I) have generally been recommended as preferred initial drugs. There are persuasive data from the Heart Outcomes Prevention Evaluation (HOPE) study in support of the use of ACE-I.[43] Approximately 3500 patients with diabetes with at least 1 additional classic CV risk factor were randomized to either placebo or ramipril in the study. Patients with proteinuria, congestive heart failure, recent MI, or stroke were excluded (as these are established indications for ACE-I). The combined outcome of MI, stroke, and CV deaths was significantly lower in the ramipril-treated group.

Although ACE-I remain the cornerstone of therapy for patients with type 1 diabetes and nephropathy, the RENAAL (Reduction of End Points in Non-Insulin-Dependent Diabetes Mellitus with the Angiotensin II Antagonist Losartan) and IDNT (Irbesartan Diabetic Nephropathy Trial) studies support initial therapy with angiotensin receptor blockers (ARBs) in type 2 diabetes. The RENAAL study showed that losartan improves renal outcomes in patients with type 2 diabetes and nephropathy more than that attributable to blood pressure control alone. The

renoprotective effect of losartan corresponded to an average delay of 2 years in the need for dialysis or kidney transplantation. CV outcomes were secondary end points in the RENAAL and IDNT trials, and with the exception of heart failure for losartan, no benefits on CV outcomes were statistically significant. In contrast, the HOPE trial showed that ACE-I, specifically ramipril, had the greatest evidence for prevention of CV outcomes in patients with renal insufficiency, regardless of diabetic status. Because evidence has shown that patients with increased serum creatinine level (≥1.4 mg/dL) are just as likely to die from CV disease as they are to reach end-stage renal disease, it is unclear which should be the focus for treatment for clinicians. Using a strictly evidence-based approach, this question can only be answered by yet another large, long, randomized controlled trial. Given the similarity of actions between ARB and ACE, it is likely there is considerable overlap of both benefits and side effects between the two, although ARB may have a lower incidence of cough and hyperkalemia. Nevertheless, ARBs represent the only evidence-based treatment strategy for patients with type 2 diabetes mellitus and proteinuria, and have been recommended as initial treatment of choice by the National Kidney Foundation.[44] To conclude, pharmacologic therapy to block the renin-angiotensin-system should be mandatory in patients with diabetic nephropathy (which includes patients with microalbuminuria). In the absence of evidence-based data, the selection of the appropriate antihypertensive agent should be tailored to the needs of the patient with careful consideration of both medical and economic factors.

β-Blockers are recommended and provide cardioprotection in patients with established CHD, and therefore when additional therapy is needed, β-blockers should be considered in appropriate patients. The role of calcium channel blocker therapy was clarified by the recently published ACCOMPLISH trial.[45] The diabetic subgroup in this study involving 6946 subjects were randomized to treatment with benazepril plus amlodipine or benazepril plus hydrochlorthiazide. A subgroup of 2842 high-risk patients with diabetes (previous CV or stroke events) was further analyzed. Although the mean blood pressure achieved was similar in both treatment groups, there were clear benefits with the benazepril plus amlodipine combination in CV end points. The difference between the 2 treatment groups showed that contemporary treatment with benazepril and amlodipine was noted to be progressively better in higher-risk groups, that is, individuals with diabetes and high-risk diabetic individuals (**Fig. 14**).

In summary, reduction of increased blood pressure to the target blood pressure should be the primary goal. This point is well demonstrated in the UKPDS study, which showed that in the group with aggressive blood pressure control with either captopril or atenolol, there was no difference in end points, whereas a significant difference was noted between the aggressively treated group and the control group (see **Fig. 11**). It is appropriate to initiate a specific group of antihypertensive drugs based on compelling indications related to the individual patient. Because most hypertensive patients with diabetes require more than 2 antihypertensive agents, it is prudent to start therapy with at least 2 drugs, usually as a combination product to promptly achieve the target blood pressure and reduce risk of CV events. In general one of those drugs in combination should be a renin-angiotensin-system blocking agent. Based on recent data from the ACCOMPLISH trial, it may be reasonable to consider initial therapy with an ACE-I and dihydropyridine calcium channel blocker especially in the high-risk patient with diabetes. Assimilating the findings of the ACCORD and ADVANCE trials, it is likely that JNC 8 will give specific recommendations for the management of blood pressure in the patient with diabetes.

Hyperglycemia

A causal relationship between hyperglycemia and microvascular disease is well established. Studies have also documented benefit of glycemic control by delaying or preventing manifestations of microvascular disease. However, the relationship between hyperglycemia and macrovascular disease has been a subject of constant debate. The largest study

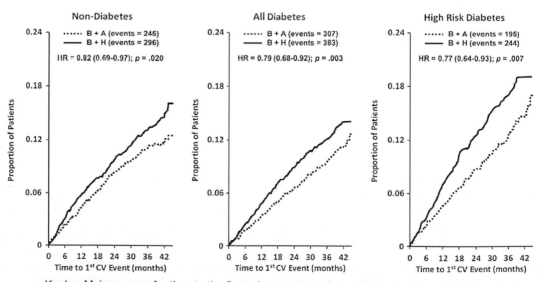

Kaplan-Meier curves for time to the first primary composite end point in patients without diabetes, with diabetes, and with high-risk diabetes (as defined in the text). CV cardiovascular; HR hazard ratio; B+ A benazepril plu amlodipine; B + H benazepril plus hydrochlorothiazide

Fig. 14. Time to first events in major patient subgroups: ACCOMPLISH trial. (*Adapted from* Weber MA, Bakris GL, Jamerson K, et al. Cardiovascular events during differing hypertension therapies in patients with diabetes. J Am Coll Cardiol 2010;56:77–85; with permission.)

addressing this issue is the UKPDS.[46,47] It was a study designed to answer the question whether intensive control of glucose compared with conventional treatment in newly diagnosed type 2 diabetics lowers the risk of complications. After a mean follow-up of more than 10 years of approximately 2500 patients in each group, intensive therapy showed a 12% reduction in any diabetes-related end point and a significant reduction in the microvascular end points (25% reduction; P = .0099). A 16% reduction in MI (P = .052) and nonsignificant reduction in diabetes-related and all-cause mortality was noted in the intensively treated group. Thus, although the value of tight glycemic control for prevention of microvascular disease is undisputable, the UKPDS does not strongly suggest a similar benefit in controlling macrovascular disease.

The EPIC-Norfolk study found a continuous relationship between all-cause mortality and glycosylated hemoglobin, even for values in the nondiabetic range.[48] In this European study, 4662 men aged 45 to 79 years who had had glycosylated hemoglobin measured at the baseline survey in 1995 to 1997 were followed up to December 1999. The main outcome measures were mortality from all causes, CV disease, ischemic heart disease, and other causes. Men with known diabetes had increased mortality from all causes, CV disease, and ischemic disease (relative risks 2.2, 3.3, and 4.2, respectively, P<.001 independent of age and other risk factors) compared with men without known diabetes. The increased risk of death among men with diabetes was largely explained by the HbA_{1c} concentration. HbA_{1c} was continuously related to subsequent all-cause, CV, and ischemic heart disease mortality throughout the population distribution, with lowest rates in those with HbA_{1c} concentrations less than 5%. An increase of 1% in HbA_{1c} was associated with a 28% increase in risk of death independent of age, blood pressure, serum cholesterol level, body mass index (BMI, calculated as weight in kilograms divided by the square of height in meters), and cigarette smoking habit; this effect remained after men with known diabetes, an HbA_{1c} concentration of 7% or more, or history of MI or stroke were excluded. These data argue in favor of the 16% risk reduction for MI in UKPDS being a significant difference.

Postprandial hyperglycemia has also been identified as a potential risk factor for CV disease.[49] The DECODE study was undertaken on the initiative of the European Diabetes Epidemiology Study Group in 1997. Baseline data on glucose concentrations at fasting and 2 hours after the 75-g oral glucose tolerance test from 13 prospective European cohort studies, which included 18,048

men and 7316 women aged 30 years or older were collected. After a mean follow-up period of 7.3 years, mortality increased with increasing 2-hour glucose within each fasting glucose classification. However, for 2-hour glucose classifications of impaired glucose tolerance and diabetes, there was no trend for increasing fasting glucose concentrations, which would suggest that fasting glucose concentrations alone do not identify individuals at increased risk of death associated with hyperglycemia. However, there are no universally accepted guidelines for therapy. The American College of Endocrinology recommends a 2-hour postprandial glucose level of less than 140 mg/dL.

The threshold to which glycemic control needs to be corrected has probably been adequately answered by the recently published data from the ACCORD trial.[50] The goal of the trial was to evaluate intensive glycemic control through currently available means (ie, glycated hemoglobin [HbA_{1c}] <6%), compared with standard glycemic control (ie, HbA_{1c} 7.0–7.9%) among patients with type 2 diabetes mellitus with known CV disease or with additional risk factors for CV disease. At 1 year, HbA_{1c} was 6.4% versus 7.5%, respectively. The glycemic arm of the trial was stopped prematurely because of excess deaths reported in the intensive treatment group. Although there was no identifiable cause for excess death in the intensively treated group in the ACCORD trial, a strategy of lowering HbA_{1c} to a mean of less than 6.5% may not be advisable. These results were somewhat mirrored by the ADVANCE trial, which is the largest trial on diabetes treatments to date.[51] In this trial, 11,140 patients with type 2 diabetes were randomly assigned to undergo either standard glucose control or intensive glucose control with gliclazide and other agents to achieve an HbA_{1c} value of 6.5% or less. At the end of 5 years, the mean HbA_{1c} was 6.5% in the intensive control arm versus 7.3% in the standard therapy arm. The main finding of this study was that gradually implemented intensive glucose control, with a goal of achieving an HbA_{1c} of 6.5% or less, was associated with a significant reduction in some microvascular complications of diabetes, but not macrovascular complications. Intensive glucose control was also associated with a higher incidence of hospitalizations and severe hypoglycemia. A recent presentation by the ADVANCE group indicated that severe hypoglycemia was associated with significant increased risk of CV and all-cause mortality.

The choice of hypoglycemic therapy should be influenced by consideration of multiple factors including BMI, renal function, comorbidities, financial issues, and patient preferences. In general, overweight individuals should preferably be initially started on metformin in the absence of contraindications. The thiazolidinediones (TZDs), which form an important therapeutic drug class, are effective in reducing blood sugar. Their hypoglycemic action is mediated by increasing muscle uptake of glucose, thereby decreasing insulin resistance. They also reduce hepatic glucose production. The primary action of these drugs is mediated via activation of the peroxisome proliferator-activated receptor (PPAR)-γ receptor, a nuclear receptor with a regulatory role in differentiation of cells. This receptor is expressed in adipocytes, vascular tissue, and other cell types. These drugs have been shown to improve endothelial function, reduce intraabdominal adipose tissue, improve pancreatic β cell function and exert antiinflammatory actions that may contribute to antiatherosclerotic effects. However, not all these effects may be class effects. Pioglitazone and rosiglitazone are 2 thiazolidinediones that are currently available.

The prospective pioglitazone clinical trial (PROactive) randomized more than 5000 patients with type 2 diabetes and documented CV disease to pioglitazone or placebo as add-on therapy to other hypoglycemic treatment.[52] Among patients with type 2 diabetes, treatment with pioglitazone was not associated with a reduction in the primary composite event compared with placebo at an average follow-up of 3 years. Although pioglitazone was not associated with a reduction in the primary composite event (coronary and peripheral events), it was associated with a reduction in the secondary composite end point of coronary events (death, MI, or stroke). In addition, there was a reduction in the need to add insulin to glucose-lowering regimens. The incidence of heart failure and heart failure hospitalizations was higher in the pioglitazone group compared with placebo. The tendency of pioglitazone for sodium retention may explain the higher heart failure rates in the pioglitazone group.

Meta-analysis of trials using rosiglitazone in the treatment of diabetes show variable results regards adverse CV outcomes. Concern regarding use of rosiglitazone arose after the meta-analysis by Nissen and colleagues.[53] In this meta-analysis involving 42 trials, a small increase in MI was shown compared with the comparator group (placebo, metformin, sulfonylurea, or insulin). An independent meta-analysis performed by the manufacturers of rosiglitazone (Glaxo-Smith-Kline) showed similar findings. Most studies included in these meta-analyses were not designed to explore CV outcomes, which were not uniformly collected or adjudicated; therefore, MI

and other CV events were noted as adverse events. The RECORD study, however, was designed to evaluate the effect of rosiligtazone on CV events and mortality.[54] Of 4447 patients from Europe and Australasia, 2222 people on metformin were assigned to addition of rosiglitazone (1117) or sulfonylurea (1105), and 2225 patients on a sulfonylurea were assigned to addition of rosiglitazone (1103) or metformin (1122). All-cause mortality, CV mortality, and MI were also similar between the rosiglitazone and active control arms. However, these results need to be considered in the context of the small number of events and greater statin use in the rosiglitazone group. The incidence of heart failure was higher as was the risk of bone fractures in the rosiglitazone arm. An updated meta-analysis by Nissen and Wolski[55] published this year, again reported a significantly increased risk of MI (odds ratio 1.28) but not CV mortality. Exclusion of the RECORD trial from the analysis yielded similar results with a higher estimate of the odds ratio for MI. The 2008 ADA and the European Association for the Study of Diabetes (EASD) consensus algorithm recommended against the use of rosiglitazone, because of concern regarding safety and the availability of alternative therapies, including pioglitazone, that do not have the same concerns.[56] The last word on the usefulness of TZDs in the management of hyperglycemia in patients with diabetes continues to be debated and clinicians should make individualized judgment when considering its use for any particular patient.

Recent publication of a 10-year follow-up of intensive glucose control in type 2 diabetes from the UKPDS study cohort has raised the concept of a legacy effect.[57] In the UKPDS study, 4209 patients with newly diagnosed type 2 diabetes were randomized to either conventional therapy (dietary restriction) or intensive therapy (either sulfonylurea or insulin or, in overweight patients, metformin). In posttrial monitoring, patients returned to community- or hospital-based care with no attempt to maintain their previously randomized therapies. The median follow-up was 17 years, with close to 9 years of posttrial follow-up. Although between-group differences in HbA$_{1c}$ were lost within a year of cessation of assigned treatments, levels of HbA$_{1c}$ continued to decrease in both groups for 5 years reflecting appropriate risk factor management. In the sulfonylurea/insulin group, reduction in risk persisted for microvascular disease and any diabetes-related outcome at 10 years (**Fig. 15**). In addition, reductions were also noted for diabetes-related death, MI, and death from any cause. Furthermore, in the group treated with metformin, significant risk reductions

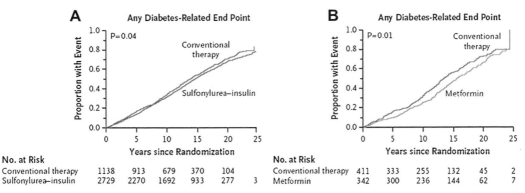

Fig. 15. Ten-year follow-up of intensive glucose control in type 2 diabetes: UKPDS (*A, B*). (*Adapted from* Holman RR, Paul SK, Bethel A, et al. 10-year follow-up of intensive glucose control in type 2 diabetes. N Engl J Med 2008;359:1577–89; with permission.)

persisted for any diabetes-related outcomes, MI, and death from any cause without any effect on microvascular disease. The persistence and emergence of benefits, despite early loss of within-trial differences in HbA_{1c} levels between the intensive therapy group and the conventional therapy group, has been called the legacy effect.

To summarize, although glycemic control does significantly affect the incidence of microvascular complications the effect on macrovascular CV outcomes is less obvious especially in those with prolonged duration of diabetes or preexisting CV disease. In addition, there seems to be a lower threshold value of glycemic control (HbA_{1c} of 6.5%) under which the risk of therapy may outweigh the benefits. Moreover, the strategy and medications used for glycemic control may have an effect on outcomes. Based on the results of the recent trials as noted earlier, the ACC, American Heart Association (AHA), and ADA issued a consensus statement recommending maintenance of A_{1c} levels at or less than 7% for most people with diabetes and recommending that a comprehensive risk factor reduction should be instituted for CV risk reduction in all patients with diabetes.

Increased Thrombotic Tendency

The patient with diabetes has many prothrombotic factors increasing the risk for arterial thrombosis leading to MI or strokes. These include platelet dysfunction, increased fibrinogen levels, increased von Willebrand factor, increased factor VII, increased plasminogen activator inhibitor type-I (PAI-1), and reduced tissue plasminogen activator (TPA) levels. Although various abnormalities in the thrombotic pathway have been described, successful therapeutic interventions

have been proved only with antiplatelet therapy, which is discussed briefly in this section.

The multiple biochemical and functional abnormalities in platelet function in type 1 and type 2 diabetes lead to increased platelet aggregability and adhesiveness. The correction of this increased platelet aggregability and adhesiveness with antiplatelet agents such as aspirin should logically reduce CV events in diabetics. Until recently, there were no prospective studies designed for investigating the therapeutic role of aspirin in the diabetic cohort. Evidence available from small diabetic subgroups in studies on the general population was used to guide recommendations about use of aspirin in patients with diabetes. The Primary Prevention Project is one such study that enrolled 1031 diabetic subjects.[58] In this study efficacy of low-dose aspirin (100 mg/d) in primary prevention of CV events was studied in individuals with one or more of the following risk factors: hypertension, hypercholesterolemia, diabetes, obesity, family history of premature MI, or being elderly. After a mean follow-up of 3.6 years, there was significantly lower frequency of CV deaths and total CV events in the group treated with aspirin. The US Physicians' Health Study (USPHS), was a 5 year primary prevention trial on nearly 23,000 healthy men that included 533 men with diabetes. Among the men with diabetes, 4% of those treated with aspirin (325 mg every other day) had an MI versus 10.1% of those who received placebo (relative risk of 0.39). The Antithrombotic Trialists' (ATT) Collaboration recently published an individual patient-level meta-analysis of the 6 large trials of aspirin for primary prevention in the general population.[59] These trials collectively enrolled more than 95,000 participants, including almost 4000 with diabetes. Overall, the meta-analysis found that aspirin reduced the risk of vascular events by 12%, with the largest reduction being for nonfatal MI. There was little effect on total stroke or CHD death. Some heterogeneity was noted regards differences in aspirin's effects based on sex.

Three of the trials in the meta-analysis focused on the effect of aspirin exclusively among patients with diabetes. The ETDRS trial examined the effect of 650 mg of aspirin daily versus placebo among 3711 patients with type 1 or type 2 diabetes between 18 and 70 years of age with some degree of retinopathy. Patients on aspirin had a lower risk of nonfatal or fatal MI (relative risk 0.85). However, there was a higher but nonsignificant increase in incidence of stroke with aspirin (relative risk 1.18, 99% confidence interval [CI] 0.88–1.58).[60] The POPADAD randomized 1276 adults with type 1 or 2 diabetes more than 40 years old and asymptomatic peripheral vascular disease to aspirin (and/or antioxidant therapy) or placebo.[61] No difference was seen in the 2 composite primary end points (death from CHD or stroke, nonfatal MI or stroke, or amputation above ankle AND death from CHD or stroke). Rates of discontinuation of study medication were high. The Japanese Primary Prevention of Atherosclerosis with Aspirin for Diabetes (JPAD) study was a randomized, open-label trial of aspirin for primary prevention involving 2539 Japanese patients with type 2 diabetes. After an average follow-up of 4.4 years there was no difference in the primary composite end point of fatal or nonfatal ischemic heart disease, fatal or nonfatal stroke, and peripheral arterial disease (hazard ratio 0.8, 95% CI 0.58–1.1). The combined secondary end point of coronary and cerebrovascular mortality was significantly different (hazard ratio 0.1, CI 0.01–0.79). However, on a prespecified subgroup analysis, subjects older than 65 years had significantly lower incidence of the primary end point on aspirin.

Thus, none of the trials mentioned provides definitive results. Based on these and other studies, the US Preventive Services Task Force recently recommended encouraging aspirin use in men aged 45 to 79 years and women aged 55 to 79 years, and not encouraging aspirin use in younger adults regardless of the presence or absence of diabetes.[62,63] Two ongoing studies with combined sample size of more than 15,000 individuals with diabetes will provide additional information on the role of low-dose aspirin for the prevention of CV events. Aspirin and Simvastatin Combination for Cardiovascular Events Prevention Trial in Diabetes (ACCEPT-D) is an open-label Italian primary prevention trial comparing aspirin 100 mg daily to no aspirin among adults more than 50 years old with diabetes who are also on simvastatin.[64] The second trial, A Study of Cardiovascular Events in Diabetes (ASCEND), will also examine the effects of 100 mg aspirin daily versus placebo for primary prevention among men and women more than 40 years of age with either type 1 or type 2 diabetes.[65]

To provide guidelines for management, the ADA, AHA, and ACC recently published an expert consensus document recommending low-dose aspirin (75–162 mg/d) as primary prevention for adults with diabetes who are at increased CVD risk (10 year risk of CVD events more than 10%) and are not at increased risk for bleeding (prior gastrointestinal bleeding, peptic ulcer disease, or concurrent use of medication such as nonsteroidal antiinflammatory drugs or warfarin).[66] The accurate determination of CVD risk should be made using clinical tools such as the UKPDS Risk Engine, ARIC CHD Risk Calculator or ADA Risk Assessment Tool (**Box 2**).

The efficacy of aspirin for secondary prevention of CV events is suggested from a meta-analysis of secondary prevention trials by the Antithrombotic Trialists' Collaboration (ATC). The ATC meta-analysis included 287 trials with total involvement of 212,000 high-risk patients.[67] In more than 4500 patients with diabetes studied in the ATC, the incidence of vascular events was reduced from 23.5% with control treatment to 19.3% with antiplatelet therapy ($P<.01$). Although the overall incidence of vascular events in the diabetic subgroup was much higher, the benefit of antiplatelet therapy in the patients with and without diabetes was comparable. In the HOT study, half of the 1501 patients with diabetes mellitus included in each target group were randomly allocated to receive aspirin. The CV event rate was reduced by 15% and MI by 36% compared with placebo. The relative effects of aspirin were similar in nondiabetic and diabetic subjects.[38]

COMPREHENSIVE CV RISK REDUCTION IN DIABETES MELLITUS
Multiple Risk Factor Intervention

With established diabetes mellitus all modifiable risk factors should be addressed. These include

---

Box 2
Indications for aspirin use for primary prevention in high-risk patients with diabetes

1. Obesity
2. Hypertension
3. Cigarette smoking
4. Family history of CHD
5. Micro- or macroalbuminuria
6. Atherogenic dyslipidemia

hypertension, hyperglycemia, smoking, dyslipidemia, obesity, dietary indiscretion, and physical inactivity. Although studies in the past focused on a single risk factor such as glycemic control or hypertension, there is clear evidence that therapy directed to address the concurrent CV risk factors that frequently coexist in the patient with diabetes is essential to provide comprehensive CV risk reduction. This approach is substantiated by results of multiple randomized controlled trials of intensive glycemic control that have failed to show a definite independent link between glycemic control and CV risk reduction. It is thus apparent that to reduce the associated high risk of CV events, the focus of treatment should be on addressing all of the CV risk factors in patients with diabetes, and should not just be confined to glycemic control as the risk of CV events is additive for various risk factors that are frequently present in patients with diabetes.

Intervention should start with dietary advice and advice regarding physical activity. Early initiation of a moderate exercise program may be the best strategy for reducing the risk of later macrovascular complications. Several studies have shown that higher leisure-time physical activity is associated with reduced total and CVD mortality among patients with diabetes or impaired glucose tolerance. The Look AHEAD trial is a multicenter, randomized clinical trial that evaluates the effectiveness of intentional weight loss in reducing CVD events among patients with type 2 diabetes. Although the study is focused on weight loss, its findings are relevant for multilevel intervention effects on CVD risk factors in diabetes. The Look AHEAD investigators conducted an interim analysis to evaluate changes in risk profile at the end of 1 year.[68] Participants assigned to the intensive lifestyle intervention lost an average 8.6% of their initial weight versus 0.7% in the diabetes support and education group (P<.001). A greater proportion of intensive lifestyle intervention participants had reductions in glycemia, hypertension, and lipids, which resulted in decreased requirement of pharmacologic therapy. Dietary advice should include recommendations regarding optimal fat intake. It is recommended that intake of polyunsaturated fat should be limited to 10% of calorie intake, although there is a lack of evidence to support this. Consumption of fish high in omega-3 fatty acids (1–2 servings/wk), reduced the risk of coronary death and total mortality in epidemiologic studies and randomized clinical trials, and this benefit seems to extend to those with diabetes as well.[69] Several cohort studies have an association between dietary glycemic load and incidence of type 2 diabetes. Prospective cohort studies

have also reported an inverse association between whole grain consumption and risk of diabetes and CHD. Moderate alcohol consumption (1–2 drinks or 10–20 g of alcohol per day) shows a benefit on CHD incidence in the general population. This benefit also extends to the diabetic population.

As noted in the preceding discussion in this article, individual interventions on CV risk factors in patients with diabetes give a 15% to 30% risk reduction. The results of these studies have been scrutinized in detail leading to the establishment of treatment guidelines with specific targets regarding glycemic control, blood pressure, and lipid levels (**Table 3**). Although addressing individual risk factors in the patient with diabetes is a logical extension of the findings from currently available evidence, this has limited potential in achieving the maximal attainable benefit for CV risk reduction. A more appropriate approach would be to address multiple risk factors concurrently with the hope of obtaining a comprehensive risk reduction.

Although such a strategy would require considerable effort on the part of the physician and the patient, available data do suggest a comprehensive risk reduction approach to the management of patients with diabetes is beneficial. The Danish Steno-2 study was the first long-term trial among people with type 2 diabetes to evaluate the effect of an intensified, multi-targeted intervention compared with conventional multifactorial treatment on CVD and its risk factors.[73] At a mean follow-up of 7.8 years, patients receiving the intensive therapy showed a 53% (95% CI 27–76) reduction in risk of CVD. The number needed to treat in the Steno-2 study was 5 (ie, 1 CVD event will be prevented in every 5 patients treated intensively for 7.8 years) (**Fig. 16**).

The ADDITION study is an ongoing international trial, similar to the Steno-2 protocol. The overall aim of the ADDITION study is to evaluate screening methods for prevalent undiagnosed type 2 diabetes, and to develop and evaluate optimized intensive treatment of diabetes and associated risk factors among people 40 to 69 years of age.[74] The ADDITION investigators recently evaluated changes in CVD risk factor profile at the end of 1 year of follow-up among 79 general practices in the southwestern region of the Netherlands. Overall, the 1-year data indicated that the intensive multilevel intervention resulted in a significant reduction in CVD risk factors without worsening health-related quality of life at the end of the first year of follow-up.[75] The data on incident CVD and mortality from this trial are not yet available.

In summary, there is supportive evidence from trials suggesting a benefit of an intensive multifactorial approach for CVD prevention in diabetes. An

Table 3
Goals for risk factor management in diabetes

Risk Factor	Goal of Therapy	Reference[b]
Cigarette smoking	Complete cessation	ADA, AHA
Blood pressure (with proteinuria)	<130/80 mm Hg <125/75 mm Hg	JNC VII, ADA JNC VII, ADA
LDL-C (measured annually) For age >40 y	<70 mg/dL for secondary prevention[a] Without CVD but ≥1 risk factor, LDL goal is <100 If LDL is <100 at baseline, statin based on additional risk factors	ATP III, ADA
For age <40 y	Without CVD, but estimated to have high risk of CVD, LDL-C goal is <100 mg/dL	
Triglycerides 200–499 mg/dL Triglycerides >500 mg/dL	Non–HDL-C <130 mg/dL Fibrate/niacin before LDL lowering Non-HDL <130 mg/dL Target triglycerides <150 mg/dL	ATP III, AHA ADA
HDL-C <40 mg/dL(<50 mg/dL in women)	Increase HDL	ATP III, ADA
Prothrombotic state	Low-dose aspirin therapy (patients with CHD and other high-risk factors including age >40 y)	ADA, AHA
Glucose	Hemoglobin A₁c <7%	ADA, AHA
Overweight and obesity (BMI ≥25 kg/m²)	Lose 5%–7% of body weight	ADA, AHA
Physical inactivity	150 min moderate aerobic exercise or at least 90 min vigorous aerobic exercise/wk (no more than 2 consecutive days without physical activity)	ADA, AHA
Adverse nutrition	Diets low in fat (<30%) and saturated fat <7%; lower glycemic index (when necessary with caloric restriction); 1.2–2 g sodium/d; alcohol up to 2 drinks/d (1 drink/d for women; 1 drink = 354 mL (12 oz) beer or 120 mL (4 oz) wine, or 44 mL (1.5 oz) distilled spirit)	ADA, AHA, ATP III, OEI, JNC VII

Abbreviations: ATP III, Adult Treatment Panel III; JNC VII, the seventh report of the Joint National Committee on Detection, Evaluation and Treatment of High Blood Pressure; OEI, Obesity Education Initiative.

[a] Per advisory from National Cholesterol Education Program.[33]

[b] ADA and AHA,[70] JNC 7,[71] ATP III,[32] for OEI.[72]

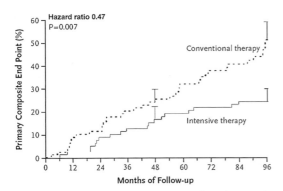

Fig. 16. Multifactorial intervention and cardiovascular disease in patients with type 2 diabetes: STENO-2. (*Adapted from* Gaede P, Vedel P, Larsen N, et al. Multifactorial intervention and cardiovascular disease in patients with type 2 diabetes. N Engl J Med 2003;348:383–93; with permission.)

important aim of the multifactorial intervention approach is to actively involve the patient with appropriate education and provide tools for self-care. In addition to dietary advice and weight loss, smoking cessation and regular exercise should be emphasized. Pharmacologic intervention should be targeted to specific goals with an appreciation for potential side effects of such goal-driven therapy, particularly with respect to glycemic therapy. The cost-effectiveness of a multifactorial approach to therapy also deserves attention. In the Steno-2 study, the discounted quality-adjusted life expectancy was 1.66 quality-adjusted life years (QALY) higher for intensive compared with conventional treatment, resulting in an incremental cost-effectiveness of 2538 euros per QALY gained.[76]

CURRENT STATE OF AFFAIRS AND FUTURE DIRECTIONS

This review clearly documents evidence from large randomized controlled trials, the benefits of comprehensive risk reductions in patients with to lower CV events. So the question arises as to how well this is being incorporated in clinical practice. A recent study reported on the improving trends seen in the management of diabetes mellitus and attendant CV disease based on NHANES data.[77] Changes in HbA$_{1c}$, blood pressure, and total cholesterol were estimated between 1988 and 1994 and between 2005 and 2006 using regression analysis and data from the NHANES. HbA$_{1c}$ fell by 0.68% among US adults with diagnosed diabetes. Among those with diabetes and hypertension, systolic and diastolic blood pressure fell by 5.66 and 8.15 mm Hg, respectively. Among those with diabetes and high cholesterol,

total cholesterol fell by 36.41 mg/dL. These improvements were projected to improve life expectancy for persons with newly diagnosed diabetes by a year. Similar estimates were recently published in a study conducted in the United Kingdom.[78]

Analysis of data with long-term follow-up of large cohorts with diabetes mellitus has raised certain interesting aspects relevant to long-term management. It would seem that early and aggressive goal-directed therapy may potentially have beneficial effects in terms of delaying macrovascular events either by deterring renal failure and or by the legacy effect. In the ADVANCE study, with a protocol involving a multifactorial goal-directed therapy, there is a late separation in the Kaplan-Meier curves for major macrovascular events and death from any cause. Although this was not significant for the duration of follow-up reported in the trial, this might represent the beginning of a long-term risk reduction that might become evident with a longer duration of follow-up. The lessons learned from the extended follow-up of the UKPDS and the Steno-2 study clearly emphasizes the importance of long-term sustained efficacy of comprehensive risk reduction in the patient with diabetes. It would seem that a paradigm of early identification and comprehensive risk reduction with therapy directed toward achieving well-defined targets may prove to be both beneficial and economical in reducing the risk of CV and other complications in patients with diabetes.

Prevention of Diabetes Mellitus as a Therapeutic Strategy

Prevention of type 2 diabetes might be an attainable goal and might have a much larger effect and be more economical given the scale of the problem at present. The prevention of diabetes, especially with therapeutic lifestyle interventions, may indeed be the most attractive strategy because the interventions needed are generally less expensive and would translate to large reductions in health care expenditure with the potential for reduction of macrovascular events. Supportive evidence in favor of diabetes prevention comes from observational studies such as the Nurses' Health Study, in which 84,941 women were followed up from 1980 to 1996. Almost 90% of the cases of incident diabetes were found in women with obesity, lack of exercise, poor diet, and tobacco abuse.[79] The Western Working Group, NCEP, ADA, and other major groups have emphasized the importance of the metabolic syndrome as a potential prediabetic state.[13,32,34] Simple measures such as weight reduction and regular activity can reduce the risk of developing diabetes mellitus and potentially reduce CV disease in this population at risk. During transition from euglycemia to overt diabetes, many patients go through a phase of impaired glucose tolerance or impaired fasting glucose level, defined by an oral glucose tolerance test finding of 140 to 190 mg/dL and a fasting plasma glucose level of 110 to 125 mg/dL, respectively. There is now substantial trial evidence showing that the onset of diabetes can be prevented or at least delayed in this cohort of individuals (Finnish Diabetes Prevention study,[80] Diabetes Prevention Program (DPP),[81] STOP-NIDDM[82]).

The DPP trial randomized 3234 obese subjects between the ages of 25 and 85 years at high risk of diabetes (BMI $\geq$24 kg/m,[2] fasting plasma glucose 96–125 mg/dL and 2-hour plasma glucose between 140 and 199 mg/dL) to intensive lifestyle changes versus metformin (850 mg twice a day) plus information on diet and exercise versus placebo. The study was terminated a year ahead of schedule by the Data and Safety Monitoring Board noting that fewer subjects in the intensive lifestyle group developed diabetes at an average follow-up of 3 years (14% vs 22% and 29% in the metformin and placebo groups, respectively). A 10-year follow-up to the DPP trial, the Diabetes Prevention Program Outcomes, was recently published by Knowler and colleagues.[83] In this study, 85% of subjects originally enrolled in DPP joined the long-term follow-up and were offered group-implemented lifestyle intervention. Subjects who were originally assigned to the metformin group continued to receive it. After a 10-year follow-up period, the incidence of diabetes in the lifestyle modification and metformin groups was significantly reduced (34% and 18%, respectively). Based on studies mentioned earlier and other supporting data, the ADA guidelines include the prevention of diabetes in individuals with impaired glucose tolerance or impaired fasting glucose as a goal. The assumption is that prevention of diabetes will also lead to prevention of atherosclerosis, which is yet to be shown from prospective trials.

SUMMARY

It is well established that patients with diabetes are at increased risk of CV disease morbidity and mortality. Although the CV risk of individuals with diabetes might be spread over a range depending on concurrent risk factors, the baseline risk attributable to the diabetic state alone is high. The treatment of diabetes has evolved over the years from being focused purely on glycemic control to a more sophisticated approach addressing multiple CV risk factors that tend to coaggregate in these individuals. There are now sufficient evidence-based data to support multifactorial risk intervention with specific targets for goal-directed therapy for both secondary and primary prevention. These interventions have shown survival benefit in addition to prevention of micro- and macrovascular complications. Although in general these studies have shown a 15% to 30% relative risk reduction in CV events, the absolute risk of CV events remains high in the intervention group. Moreover, the incidence of diabetes is reaching epidemic proportions in concert with the obesity epidemic, and morbidity and mortality related to diabetes will continue to have a major effect on the health care status of the world population and health care budget of nations. Interventions directed at prevention of diabetes or at the very least delaying onset of diabetes should be an important aspect in the health care strategy and research in confronting the oncoming epidemic.

REFERENCES

1. Wild S, Roglic G, Green A, et al. Global prevalence of diabetes: estimates for the year 2000 and projections for 2030. Diabetes Care 2004;27:1047–53.
2. CDC. National Health and Nutrition Examination Survey 1999–2000 data files. Available at: http://www.cdc.gov/nchs/nhanes/nhanes1999-2000/nhanes99_00.htm. Accessed December 9, 2010.
3. International Diabetes Federation. IGT/IFG consensus statement. Report of an expert consensus workshop, August 1–4, 2001. Stoke Poges, United Kingdom. Impaired glucose tolerance and impaired fasting glycemia: the current status on definition and intervention. Diabet Med 2002;19:708–23.
4. Haffner SM, Lehto S, Ronnemaa T, et al. Mortality from coronary heart disease in subjects with type 2 diabetes and in nondiabetic subjects with and without prior myocardial infarction. N Engl J Med 1998;339:229–34.
5. National Cholesterol Education Program (NCEP) Expert Panel on Detection, Evaluation, and Treatment of High Blood Cholesterol in Adults (Adult Treatment Panel III). Third Report of the National Cholesterol Education Program (NCEP) Expert Panel on Detection, Evaluation, and Treatment of High Blood Cholesterol in Adults (Adult Treatment Panel III) final report. Circulation 2002;106:3143–421.
6. Saydah SH, Eberhardt MS, Loria CM, et al. Age and the burden of death attributable to diabetes in the United States. Am J Epidemiol 2002;156:714–9.
7. Bhatt DL, Eagle KA, Ohman EM, et al. Comparative determinants of 4-year cardiovascular event rates in stable outpatients at risk of or with atherothrombosis. JAMA 2010;304(12):1350–7.

8. Schramm TK, Gislason GH, Kober L, et al. Diabetes patients requiring glucose-lowering therapy and nondiabetics with a prior myocardial infarction carry the same cardiovascular risk: a population study of 3.3 million people. Circulation 2008;117:1945–54.

9. Spencer EA, Pirie KL, Stevens RJ, et al. Diabetes and modifiable risk factors for cardiovascular disease: the prospective Million Women Study. Eur J Epidemiol 2008;23(12):793–9.

10. Sarwar N, Gao P, et al, Emerging risk factors collaboration. Diabetes mellitus, fasting blood glucose concentration, and risk of vascular disease: a collaborative meta-analysis of 102 prospective studies. Lancet 2010;375(9733):2215–22.

11. Gu K, Cowie CC, Harris MI. Diabetes and decline in heart disease mortality in US adults. JAMA 1999; 281:1291–7.

12. Ford ES, Giles WH, Dietz WH. Prevalence of the metabolic syndrome among US adults: findings from the Third National Health and Nutrition Examination Survey. JAMA 2002;287:356–9.

13. Fagan TC, Deedwania PC. The cardiovascular dysmetabolic syndrome. Am J Med 1998;105(1A):77S–82S.

14. Ford ES, Li C, Sattar N. Metabolic syndrome and incident diabetes: current state of the evidence. Diabetes Care 2008;31:1898.

15. Sattar N, McConnachie A, Shaper AG, et al. Can metabolic syndrome usefully predict cardiovascular disease and diabetes? Outcome data from two prospective studies. Lancet 2008;371:1927.

16. Abbasi F, McLaughlin I, Lamendola C, et al. The relationship between glucose disposal in response to physiological hyperinsulinemia and basal glucose and free fatty acid concentrations in healthy volunteers. J Clin Endocrinol Metab 2000; 85:1252–4.

17. Taskinen MR, Smith U. Lipid disorders in NIDDM: implications for treatment. J Intern Med 1998;244:361–70.

18. Garg A. Treatment of diabetic dyslipidemia. Am J Cardiol 1998;81:47B–51B.

19. Veniant MM, Sullivan MA, Kim SK, et al. Defining the atherogenicity of large and small lipoproteins containing apolipoprotein B100. J Clin Invest 2000; 106:1501–10.

20. Stamler J, Vaccaro I, Neaton JD, et al. Diabetes, other risk factors, and 12-yr cardiovascular mortality for men screened in the multiple risk factor intervention trial. Diabetes Care 1993;16:434–44.

21. Turner RC, Millns H, Neil HA, et al. Risk factors for coronary artery disease in non-insulin dependent diabetes mellitus: United Kingdom Prospective Diabetes Study (UKPDS: 23). BMJ 1998;316:823–8.

22. Garg A, Grundy SM. Management of dyslipidemia in NIDDM. Diabetes Care 1990;13:153–69.

23. Pyorola K, Pederson TR, Kjekshus J, et al. Cholesterol lowering with simvastatin improves prognosis of diabetic patients with coronary heart disease: a sub-group analysis of the Scandinavian Simvastatin Survival Study (4S). Diabetes Care 1997;20: 614–20.

24. Goldberg RB, Mellies MJ, Sacks FM, et al, for the CARE investigators. Cardiovascular events and their reduction with pravastatin in diabetic and glucose-intolerant myocardial infarction survivors with average cholesterol and recurrent events (CARE) trial. Circulation 1998;98:2513–9.

25. Shepherd J, Barter P, Carmena R, et al. Effect of lowering LDL cholesterol substantially below currently recommended levels in patients with coronary heart disease and diabetes: the Treating to New Targets (TNT) study. Diabetes Care 2006;29:1220–6.

26. Shepherd J, Kastelein JP, Bittner VA, et al, Treating to New Targets Steering Committee and Investigators. Intensive lipid lowering with atorvastatin in patients with coronary artery disease, diabetes, and chronic kidney disease. Mayo Clin Proc 2008; 83(8):870–9.

27. Collins R, Armitage J, Parish S, et al. MRC/BHF Heart Protection Study of cholesterol-lowering with simvastatin in 5963 people with diabetes: a randomised placebo-controlled trial. Lancet 2003; 361(9374):2005–16.

28. Colhoun HM, Betteridge DJ, Durrington PN, et al, CARDS investigators. Primary prevention of cardiovascular disease with atorvastatin in type 2 diabetes in the Collaborative Atorvastatin Diabetes Study (CARDS): multicenter randomized placebo-controlled trial. Lancet 2004;364(9435):685–96.

29. Koskinen P, Manninen V, Huttunen JK, et al. Coronary heart disease incidence in NIDDM patients in the Helsinki Heart Study. Diabetes Care 1992;15: 820–5.

30. Keech A, Simes RJ, Barter P, et al, FIELD Study Investigators. Effects of long-term fenofibrate therapy on cardiovascular events in 9795 people with type 2 diabetes mellitus (the FIELD study): randomized controlled trial. Lancet 2005;366:1849–61.

31. The ACCORD Study Group. Effects of combination lipid therapy in type 2 diabetes mellitus. N Engl J Med 2010;362:1563–74.

32. Expert Panel on Detection, Evaluation, and Treatment of High Blood Cholesterol in Adults. Executive Summary of the Third Report of the National Cholesterol Education Program (NCEP) Expert Panel on Detection, Evaluation, and Treatment of High Blood Cholesterol in Adults (Adult Treatment Panel III). JAMA 2001;285:2486–97.

33. Grundy SM, Cleeman JI, Bairey Merz CN, et al. Implications of recent clinical trials for the National Cholesterol Education Program Adult Treatment Panel III guidelines. Circulation 2004;110:227–39.

34. American Diabetes Association. Standards of medical care in diabetes–2010. Diabetes Care 2010;33(Suppl 1):S11–61.

35. Ferrannini E, Buzzigoli G, Bonadona R. Insulin resistance in essential hypertension. N Engl J Med 1987; 317:350–7.

36. Swislocki AL, Hoffman BB, Raven GM. Insulin resistance, glucose intolerance and hyperinsulinemia in patients with hypertension. Am J Hypertens 1989; 2:419–23.

37. UK Prospective Diabetes Study Group (1998) Tight blood pressure control and risk of macrovascular and microvascular complications of type 2 diabetes: UKPDS 38. Br Med J 1998;317:703–13.

38. Hansson L, Zanchetti A, Carruthers SG, et al. Effects of intensive blood pressure lowering and low-dose aspirin in patients with hypertension: principal results of the hypertension optimal treatment (HOT) randomised trial. Lancet 1998;351:1755–62.

39. The ACCORD study group. Effects of intensive blood-pressure control in type 2 diabetes mellitus. N Engl J Med 2010;362:1575–85.

40. Patel A, MacMahon S, et al, ADVANCE Collaborative Group. Effects of a fixed combination of perindopril and indapamide on macrovascular and microvascular outcomes in patients with type 2 diabetes mellitus (the ADVANCE trial): a randomised controlled trial. Lancet 2007;370(9590):829–40.

41. Wright JT Jr, Jones DW, Green LA, et al. The seventh report of the Joint National Committee on prevention, detection, evaluation and treatment of high blood pressure: the JNC 7 Report. JAMA 2003;289:2560–71.

42. Bakris GL, Williams M, Dworkin L, et al. Preserving renal function in adults with hypertension and diabetes: a consensus approach. Am J Kidney Dis 2000;36(3):646–61.

43. Heart Outcomes Prevention Evaluation (HOPE) Study Investigators. Effects of ramipril on cardiovascular and microvascular outcomes in people with diabetes mellitus: results of the HOPE Study and MICRO-HOPE substudy. [published correction appears in Lancet 2000;356:850]. Lancet 2000; 355:253–9.

44. K/DOQI clinical practice guidelines for chronic kidney disease: evaluation, classification, and stratification. Kidney disease outcome quality initiative. Am J Kidney Dis 2002;39(Suppl 1):S1–266.

45. Weber MA, Bakris GL, Jamerson K, et al. Cardiovascular events during differing hypertension therapies in patients with diabetes. J Am Coll Cardiol 2010;56: 77–85.

46. United Kingdom Prospective Diabetes Study Group. Intensive blood-glucose control with sulphonylureas or insulin compared with conventional treatment and risk of complications in patients with type 2 diabetes (UKPDS 33). Lancet 1998;352: 837–53.

47. United Kingdom Prospective Diabetes Study Group. Effect of intensive blood glucose control with metformin on complications in overweight patients with type 2 diabetes (UKPDS 34). Lancet 1998;352: 854–65.

48. Khaw KT, Wareham N, Luben R, et al. Glycated hemoglobin, diabetes, and mortality in men in Norfolk cohort of European prospective investigation of cancer and nutrition (EPIC-Norfolk). BMJ 2001; 322(7277):15–8.

49. DECODE Study Group, European Diabetes Epidemiology Group. Is the current definition for diabetes relevant to mortality risk from all causes and cardiovascular and noncardiovascular diseases? Diabetes Care 2003;26(3):688–96.

50. The Action to Control Cardiovascular Risk in Diabetes Study Group. Effects of intensive glucose lowering in type 2 diabetes. N Engl J Med 2008; 358:2545–59.

51. The ADVANCE Collaborative Group. Intensive blood glucose control and vascular outcomes in patients with type 2 diabetes. N Engl J Med 2008;358:2560–72.

52. Dormandy JA, Charbonnel B, Eckland DJ, et al. Secondary prevention of macrovascular events in patients with type 2 diabetes in the PROactive Study (PROspective pioglitAzone Clinical Trial In macroVascular Events): a randomised controlled trial. Lancet 2005;366:1279–89.

53. Nissen SE, Wolski K. Effect of rosiglitazone on the risk of myocardial infarction and death from cardiovascular causes. N Engl J Med 2007;356: 2457–71.

54. Home PD, Pocock SJ, Beck-Nielsen H, et al. Rosiglitazone evaluated for cardiovascular outcomes in oral agent combination therapy for type 2 diabetes (RECORD): a multicentre, randomised, open-label trial. Lancet 2009;373:2125–35.

55. Nissen SE, Wolski K. Rosiglitazone revisited: an updated meta-analysis of risk for myocardial infarction and cardiovascular mortality. Arch Intern Med 2010; 170(14):1191–201.

56. Nathan DM, Buse JB, Davidson MB, et al. Medical management of hyperglycemia in type 2 diabetes: a consensus algorithm for the initiation and adjustment of therapy: a consensus statement of the American Diabetes Association and the European Association for the Study of Diabetes. Diabetes Care 2009;32:193–203.

57. Holman RR, Paul SK, Bethel A, et al. 10-year follow-up of intensive glucose control in type 2 diabetes. N Engl J Med 2008;359:1577–89.

58. Collaborative Group of the Primary Prevention Project. Low-dose aspirin and vitamin E in people at cardiovascular risk: a randomized trial in general practice. Lancet 2002;357:89–95.

59. Baigent C, Blackwell L, et al, Antithrombotic Trialists' (ATT) Collaboration. Aspirin in the primary and secondary prevention of vascular disease: collaborative meta-analysis of individual participant data from randomised trials. Lancet 2009;373:1849–60.

60. ETDRS Investigators. Aspirin effects on mortality and morbidity in patients with diabetes mellitus. Early Treatment Diabetic Retinopathy Study report 14. JAMA 1992;268:1292–300.

61. Belch J, MacCuish A, Campbell I, et al. The prevention of progression of arterial disease and diabetes (POPADAD) trial: factorial randomized placebo controlled trial of aspirin and antioxidants in patients with diabetes and asymptomatic peripheral arterial disease. BMJ 2008;337:a1840.

62. Wolff T, Miller T, Ko S. Aspirin for the primary prevention of cardiovascular events: an update of the evidence for the U.S. Preventive Services Task Force. Ann Intern Med 2009;150:405–10.

63. US Preventive Services Task Force. Aspirin for the prevention of cardiovascular disease: U.S. Preventive Services Task Force recommendation statement. Ann Intern Med 2009;150:396–404.

64. De Berardis G, Sacco M, Evangelista V, et al. ACCEPT-D Study Group. Aspirin and simvastatin combination for cardiovascular events prevention trial in diabetes (ACCEPT-D): design of a randomized study of the efficacy of low-dose aspirin in the prevention of cardiovascular events in subjects with diabetes mellitus treated with statins. Trials 2007;8:21.

65. British Heart Foundation. ASCEND: a study of cardiovascular events in diabetes. Available at: http://clinicaltrials.gov/ct2/show/NCT00135226. Accessed September 19, 2010.

66. Pignone M, Alberts MJ, Colwell JA, et al. Aspirin for primary prevention of cardiovascular events in people with diabetes. J Am Coll Cardiol 2010; 55(25):2878–86.

67. Antithrombotic Trialists' Collaboration. Collaboration meta-analysis of randomized trials of antiplatelet therapy for prevention of death, myocardial infarction, and stroke in high risk patients. BMJ 2002; 324:71–86.

68. Pi-Sunyer X, Blackburn G, Brancati FL, et al. Reduction in weight and cardiovascular disease risk factors in individuals with type 2 diabetes: one-year results of the Look AHEAD trial. Diabetes Care 2007;30:1374–83.

69. Mozaffarian D, Rimm EB. Fish intake, contaminants and human health: evaluating the risks and the benefits. JAMA 2006;297:1885–99.

70. Buse JB, Ginsberg HN, Bakris GL, et al. Primary prevention of cardiovascular diseases in people with diabetes mellitus: a scientific statement from the American Heart Association and the American Diabetes Association. Circulation 2007;115(1):114–26.

71. Chobanian AV, Bakris GL, Black HR, et al. The Seventh Report of the Joint National Committee on Prevention, Detection, Evaluation, and Treatment of High Blood Pressure: the JNC 7 report. JAMA 2003;289(19):2560–72.

72. Pi-Sunyer FX, Dietz WH, Becker DM, et al. Clinical guidelines on the identification, evaluation, and treatment of overweight and obesity in adults: the evidence report. Bethesda (MD): National Heart, Lung, and Blood Institute; 1998.

73. Gaede P, Vedel P, Larsen N, et al. Mutlifactorial intervention and cardiovascular disease in patients with type 2 diabetes. N Engl J Med 2003;348:383–93.

74. Lauritzen T, Griffin S, Borch-Johnsen K, et al. The ADDITION study: proposed trial of the cost-effectiveness of an intensive multifactorial intervention on morbidity and mortality among people with type 2 diabetes detected by screening. Int J Obes Relat Metab Disord 2000; 24(Suppl 3):S6–11.

75. Janssen PG, Gorter KJ, Stolk RP, et al. Randomised controlled trial of intensive multifactorial treatment for cardiovascular risk in patients with screen-detected type 2 diabetes: 1-year data from the ADDITION Netherlands study. Br J Gen Pract 2009;59:43–8.

76. Gaede P, Valentine WJ, Palmer AJ, et al. Cost-effectiveness of intensified versus conventional multifactorial intervention in type 2 diabetes: results and projections from the Steno-2 study. Diabetes Care 2008;31:1510–5.

77. Hoerger TJ, Zhang P, Segel JE, et al. Improvements in risk factor control among persons with diabetes in the United States: evidence and implications for remaining life expectancy. Diabetes Res Clin Pract 2009;86:225–32.

78. Hu FB, Manson JE, Stampfer MJ, et al. Diet, lifestyle, and the risk of type 2 diabetes mellitus in women. N Engl J Med 2001;345(11):790–7.

79. Leal J, Gray AM, Clarke PM. Development of life-expectancy tables for people with type 2 diabetes. Eur Heart J 2009;30:834–9.

80. Lindstrom J, Eriksson JG, Valle TT, et al. Prevention of diabetes mellitus in subjects with impaired glucose tolerance in the Finnish Diabetes Prevention Study: results from a randomized clinical trial. J Am Soc Nephrol 2003;14:S108–13.

81. The DPP Research Group. Reduction in the incidence of type 2 diabetes with lifestyle intervention or metformin. N Engl J Med 2002;346:393–403.

82. Chiasson JL, Josse RG, Gomis R, et al. Acarbose for prevention of type 2 diabetes mellitus: the STOP-NIDDM randomised trial. Lancet 2002;359: 2072–7.

83. Knowler WC, Fowler SE, Hamman RF, et al. 10-year follow-up of diabetes incidence and weight loss in the Diabetes Prevention Program Outcomes Study. Lancet 2009;374(9702):1677–8.

84. Haffner SM, Alexander CM, Cook TJ, et al. Reduced coronary events in simvastatin-treated patients with coronary heart disease and diabetes or impaired

fasting glucose levels: subgroup analyses in the Scandinavian Simvastatin Survival Study. Arch Intern Med 1999;159:2661–7.

85. Keech A, Colquhoun D, Best J, et al. Secondary prevention of cardiovascular events with long-term pravastatin in patients with diabetes or impaired fasting glucose: results from the LIPID trial. Diabetes Care 2003;26:2713–21.

86. Tenenbaum A, Motro M, Fisman EZ, et al. Bezafibrate for the secondary prevention of myocardial infarction in patients with metabolic syndrome. Arch Intern Med 2005;165:1154–60.

Antiplatelet Therapy in Coronary Heart Disease Prevention

Kumaran Kolandaivelu, MD, PhD[a,b],
Deepak L. Bhatt, MD, MPH[c,d,e,f,g],*

KEYWORDS

• Antiplatelet • Prevention • Cardiovascular • Coronary

Platelets are central to the pathogenesis of coronary heart disease (CHD).[1] An ever-growing number of antiplatelet therapies used in different doses and combinations have helped manage atherothrombosis, both acutely and in primary and secondary prevention.[2-6] Despite modern therapy, nearly 800,000 individuals suffer annually from an initial coronary event in the United States alone; almost 500,000 experience a recurrent event.[7] This review provides a current appraisal of antiplatelet drug use in CHD prevention, and discusses key barriers to achieving their full potential in real-world practice.

ANTIPLATELET THERAPIES

Following vascular disruption, as occurs with acute plaque rupture or after percutaneous coronary intervention (PCI), platelets tether, activate, adhere, and aggregate to reactive subendothelial components (**Fig. 1**).[8] Generation and release of several autocrine and paracrine molecules are central in this process. Thromboxane A_2 (TXA_2), generated through prostaglandin H synthase 1

(also known as cyclooxygenase-1 or COX-1)-dependent pathways, potentiates activation via thromboxane receptors.[9,10] Adenosine 5'-diphosphate (ADP) released from platelet granules and erythrocytes bind specific ADP receptors ($P2Y_1$ and $P2Y_{12}$), activating platelets through distinct, parallel pathways.[10] Thrombin, generated by the coagulation cascade, potently activates platelets via protease activated receptors (PARs; predominantly PAR1).[2] These steps culminate in glycoprotein (GP) IIb/IIIa activation, fibrinogen-bridging, and platelet aggregation.[1]

Antiplatelet drugs inhibit various aspects of platelet response. Mechanistic and pharmacokinetic differences alter their usefulness in CHD prevention. Although some agents are less efficacious, others lead to excess bleeding, the most feared complication of antiplatelet therapies.[8] Balancing clot prevention with hemorrhagic risk is a crucial aspect of long-term antiplatelet management.[11,12] Although aspirin and clopidogrel (Plavix) remain the only antiplatelet therapies approved for CHD prevention, several others are discussed for which there is evidence to support initiation during

Conflicts of interest: D.L. Bhatt declares research grant support from Astra Zeneca, Bristol-Myers Squibb, Eisai, Sanofi Aventis, and The Medicines Company. K.K. declares no competing interests.

a Division of Cardiology, Brigham and Women's Hospital, 75 Francis Street, Boston, MA 02115, USA
b Division of Health Sciences and Technology, Massachusetts Institute of Technology, 77 Massachusetts Avenue, Cambridge, MA 02139, USA
c Division of Cardiology, VA Boston Healthcare System, 1400 VFW Parkway, Boston, MA 02132, USA
d Integrated Interventional Cardiovascular Program, Brigham and Women's Hospital, 75 Francis Street, Boston, MA 02115, USA
e Integrated Interventional Cardiovascular Program, VA Boston Healthcare System, 1400 VFW Parkway, Boston MA 02132, USA
f TIMI Study Group, Brigham and Women's Hospital, 75 Francis Street, Boston, MA 02115, USA
g Department of Medicine, Harvard Medical School, 25 Shattuck Street, Boston, MA 02115, USA
* Corresponding author. Division of Cardiology, VA Boston Healthcare System, 1400 VFW Parkway, Boston, MA 02132.
E-mail address: dlbhattmd@post.harvard.edu

Cardiol Clin 29 (2011) 71–85
doi:10.1016/j.ccl.2010.10.001
0733-8651/11/$ — see front matter. Published by Elsevier Inc.

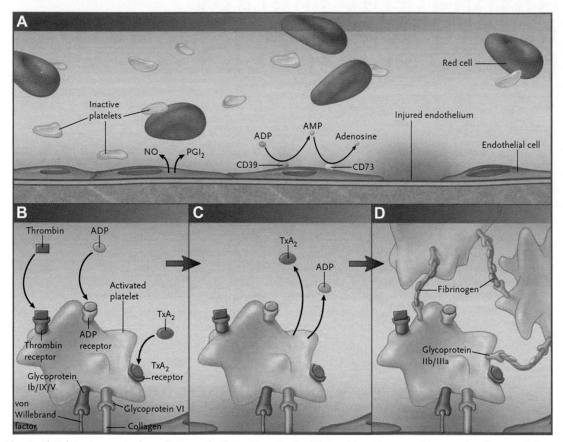

Fig. 1. Platelets are central mediators of atherothrombosis. (*A*) Inactive, they partition to the flow periphery, serving as efficient scouts of vascular integrity. On vascular disruption, as with acute plaque rupture or after PCI, they tether and activate to reactive subendothelial components such as collagen and bound von Willebrand Factor (vWF). (*B*) They are further activated through a variety of signaling molecules such as thromboxane A$_2$ (TxA$_2$), ADP, and thrombin through specialized receptors. (*C*) On activation, they release newly generated or pre-formed mediators into the thrombotic milieu that serve as autocrine and paracrine activators, amplifying the process. (*D*) In a final common step, glycoprotein (GP) IIb/IIIa receptors are activated, facilitating fibrinogen and vWF bridging and platelet aggregation. Antiplatelet agents act by inhibiting various steps in this complex process. (*From* Bhatt DL. Intensifying platelet inhibition — navigating between Scylla and Charybdis. N Engl J Med 2007;357:2079; with permission.)

acute episodes of care, but whose efficacy in preventing further ischemic events continues well after the precipitating event has quiesced, thus blurring formal definitions of prevention.

Aspirin

Aspirin is the most widely used antiplatelet agent. After ingestion, it reaches peak plasma levels in 30 minutes.[9] At low doses, it acetylates platelet COX-1, resulting in irreversible, near total inhibition of TXA$_2$ production.[10] Given platelets' inability to synthesize new COX-1, aspirin's antiplatelet effect long outlasts its plasma clearance, requiring regeneration of the platelet pool for return of platelet function (7–10 days for full repletion).[13,14]

Several trials have investigated aspirin use in CHD prevention and meta-analyses help shape our understanding of its benefits and risks.[15,16] In patients with prior myocardial infarction (MI), the Antithrombotic Trialists (ATT) Collaboration found a 25% relative risk reduction in recurrent vascular events (MI, stroke, vascular death) with aspirin use.[15] Overall mortality decreased one-sixth with antiplatelet therapy.[15] Similar relative risk reductions persist in broader populations, such as in those with a history of unstable angina (UA) or stroke.[15,16] Aspirin is clearly indicated in secondary prevention of CHD.

The effect of aspirin in primary prevention settings, where absolute cardiovascular event rates are an order of magnitude lower (~1 per

1000 patients versus ~10–60 per 1000), is less obvious.[12,16] A recent analysis of data from 95,000 participants from primary prevention trials found a 12% reduction in vascular events (absolute reduction from 0.57% to 0.51%), with an 18% reduction in coronary events attributable mostly to nonfatal MI.[16] There was no mortality benefit and absolute major bleeding increased from 0.07% to 0.10%.[16]

Balancing these competing risks of clotting and bleeding is essential for optimal antiplatelet use (**Fig. 2**A).[8,9] As vascular risk increases, so does the absolute benefit of aspirin (see **Fig. 2**B).[16] Moreover, benefit seems roughly proportional to risk.[16] In contrast, bleeding risk is often assumed constant or age dependent.[11,12,15] Risk models suggest aspirin use is indicated in patients with coronary event rates in excess of 0.6% and possibly as high as 1.5% to 2% per year, whereas in those with annual risk less than 0.5%, bleeding risk supersedes.[10,11] Reality is far more complex because bleeding risks are not constant. The same factors that increase cardiovascular risk increase propensity to bleed (**Fig. 3**A).[16] Moreover, some individuals are at exceptional bleeding risk (eg, those with gastrointestinal complications, particularly the elderly; see **Fig. 3**B).[9,12] Improved risk scores and paradigms are needed to help providers and patients make these difficult, everyday treatment decisions.

Choosing the right dose of antiplatelet therapy can help maximize benefit and minimize risk, yet optimal aspirin dose remains uncertain. At doses of 30 to 50 mg, platelet TXA_2 production is completely inhibited. However, there is a suggestion that doses less than 75 mg may be less effective than doses greater than 75 mg.[15] Because small reductions in TXA_2 inhibition yield large reductions in inhibitory effect, this lower limit may in part reflect individual variability in pharmacokinetics or drug effect.[10] Although true biochemical aspirin nonresponsiveness is now considered rare, broader aspirin resistance can be attributed to several factors including variable pharmacokinetics, increased platelet turnover, or drug-drug interactions.[17] For example, enteric coatings significantly reduce absorption rate and bioavailability, and nonsteroidal antiinflammatory drugs (NSAIDs) directly compete for COX-1 binding, decreasing aspirin's efficacy.[9] That much of aspirin's nonresponsiveness is lost in closely monitored settings indicates the important role of patient adherence (discussed later).[17]

Increasing dose can, in part, overcome antiplatelet nonresponsiveness, yet there is an upper bound to efficacy and safety. Higher aspirin doses result in pleiotropic systemic effects through broader COX-1 and less specific COX-2 inhibition.[9] Despite theoretic advantages in reducing vascular inflammation, higher dose aspirin (up to 1500 mg) have not been found efficacious in CHD prevention, perhaps because of concurrent reductions in endothelial prostacyclin.[4,9,15] Moreover, gastric prostaglandin suppression in combination with platelet inhibition can increase bleeding risk.[9,14] Given the aggregate findings, current recommendations are to use 162 to 325 mg in acute settings, reducing to 75 to 162 mg for longitudinal prevention in patients with sufficiently high risk of cardiovascular disease (>6%–10% over 10 years).[18]

Thienopyridine $P2Y_{12}$ Inhibitors

Thienopyridines irreversibly block platelet $P2Y_{12}$ receptors, inhibiting ADP-mediated activation for a platelet's lifespan.[2,5] Ticlopidine (a first-generation agent) reduced vascular events and mortality in broad categories of patients.[4] However, twice-daily dosing and its potential for severe side effects (severe neutropenia and thrombotic thrombocytopenic purpura [TTP]) have led to its near-universal replacement with clopidogrel.[2]

Clopidogrel

Clopidogrel is intestinally absorbed as a prodrug, most of which is quickly degraded by plasma esterases.[17] The remainder is hepatically converted via sequential cytochrome P-450 (CYP) steps to a short-lived active metabolite.[19] Depending on loading dose administered (600 mg vs 300 mg), platelet inhibition is achieved in 2 to 6 hours in most patients. Higher loading doses were not consistently more effective.[20]

CAPRIE investigated daily clopidogrel (75 mg) as an alternative to aspirin (325 mg) in high-risk patients with manifest CHD, stroke, or symptomatic peripheral artery disease (PAD) and found an 8.7% relative reduction in vascular events (**Fig. 4**A).[21] Bleeding risk was unchanged. Thus, clopidogrel can be used safely for CHD prevention in aspirin-intolerant patients at sufficiently high risk. Given the substantial cost differential between aspirin ($15 per year) and clopidogrel ($1200 per year), universal application is not justified, although as clopidogrel approaches generic availability, this issue may be revisited.[22]

CURE showed that adding clopidogrel to aspirin therapy (dual antiplatelet therapy [DAPT]) for up to 1 year reduced vascular events by 20% (11.4% to 9.3%) in patients presenting with acute coronary syndromes (ACS), with even greater benefits in those undergoing PCI (31% relative risk reduction; PCI-CURE).[23,24] Although major bleeding increased with DAPT

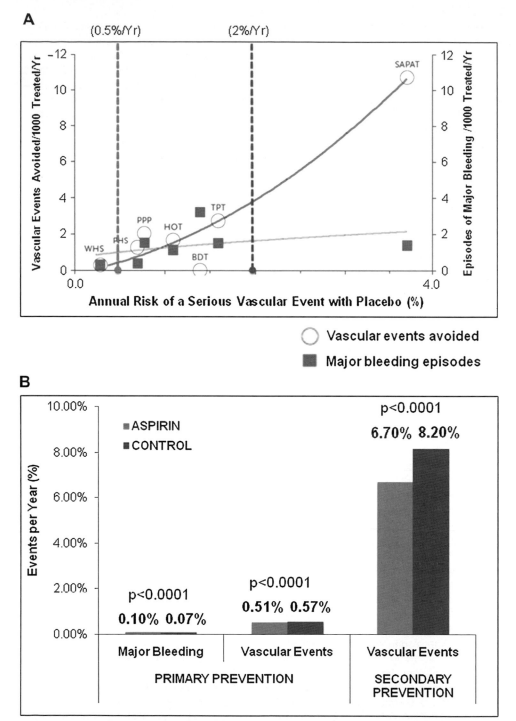

Fig. 2. Balancing the risks of vascular events and major bleeding episodes is a central theme to antiplatelet use. (*A*) A plot of vascular and bleeding event rates observed in major primary prevention aspirin trials as a function of untreated vascular risk. Aspirin use is clearly indicated when vascular risks are greater than 2% per year (and as low as 0.6% per year in some analyses). When vascular risk is less than 0.5% per year, bleeding risk supersedes. In between these percentages, clinical uncertainty remains. (*From* Patrono C, Garcia Rodriguez LA, Landolfi R, et al. Low-dose aspirin for the prevention of atherothrombosis. N Engl J Med 2005;353:2380; with permission.) (*B*) A recent analysis performed by the Antithrombotic Trialists' Collaboration found significant reductions in serious vascular events when aspirin was used in secondary as well as primary prevention. However, as shown, the absolute benefit in primary prevention was far smaller and must be balanced with major bleeding. (*Data from* Baigent C, Blackwell L, Collins R, et al. Aspirin in the primary and secondary prevention of vascular disease: collaborative meta-analysis of individual participant data from randomised trials. Lancet 2009; 373:1849–60.)

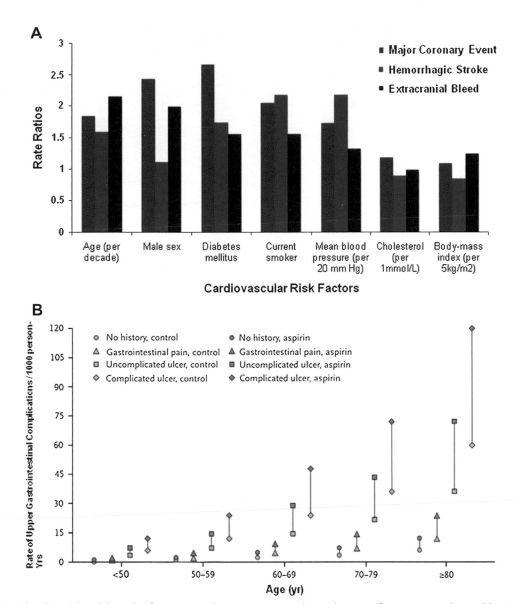

Fig. 3. Bleeding risks, although often assumed constant or age dependent, are far more complex and better risk scores are needed to help guide clinical decisions to use or not use antiplatelet therapy in patients at increased risk of bleeding. (*A*) Bleeding risk is highly dependent on cardiovascular risk factors. (*Data from* Baigent C, Blackwell L, Collins R, et al. Aspirin in the primary and secondary prevention of vascular disease: collaborative meta-analysis of individual participant data from randomised trials. Lancet 2009; 373:1849–60.) (*B*) Bleeding risk increases substantially as a function of age and gastrointestinal symptoms. (*From* Patrono C, Garcia Rodriguez LA, Landolfi R, et al. Low-dose aspirin for the prevention of atherothrombosis. N Engl J Med 2005;353:2381; with permission.)

(2.7% to 3.7%), life-threatening and intracranial bleeding were similar. Thus, clopidogrel use in conjunction with aspirin in ACS leads to long-term event reductions with or without PCI and its use is indicated.[23]

The benefits of DAPT do not apply to all high-risk patients. CHARISMA investigated clopidogrel plus low-dose aspirin versus low-dose aspirin alone in stable patients for secondary or primary prevention.[25] Patients with ACS or recent stenting were excluded. Although the primary end point was neutral in the overall population studied, there was a significant increase in moderate bleeding with dual therapy. Moreover, subgroup analysis suggested that patients on primary prevention had no evidence for benefit, although were still at risk for bleeding (see **Fig. 4**B). However, benefit was suggested in the patients on secondary

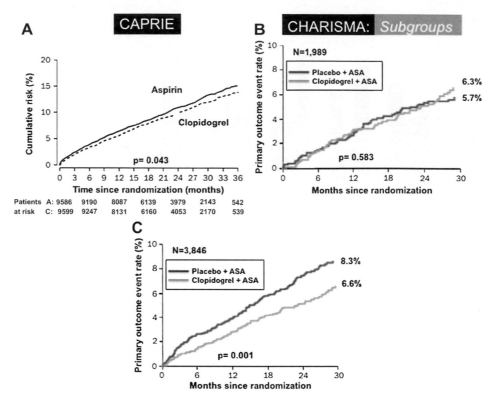

Fig. 4. As vascular risk increases, more intense therapies become justified. (*A*) CAPRIE found clopidogrel was more effective than aspirin in patients with established cardiovascular disease as shown in the 3-year Kaplan-Meier curves, although these modest benefits do not justify routine aspirin replacement given the current increased cost of clopidogrel. Dual therapy with aspirin and clopidogrel was not significantly better than aspirin alone in the main CHARISMA trial, which considered patients with established disease or multiple risk factors. Post-hoc subgroup analysis, found that although benefits were not seen in the primary prevention subgroup (*From* CAPRIE Steering Committee. A randomised, blinded, trial of clopidogrel versus aspirin in patients at risk of ischaemic events (CAPRIE). Lancet 1996;348:1333, with permission.), (*B*) the group of patients receiving dual therapy for secondary prevention for ischemic events did have a reduction in MI, stroke, or cardiovascular death; (*C*) shown are the Kaplan-Meier curves for patients with prior MI. These findings must be confirmed prospectively. (*From* Bhatt DL, Flather MD, Hacke W, et al. Patients with prior myocardial infarction, stroke, or symptomatic peripheral arterial disease in the CHARISMA trial. J Am Coll Cardiol 2007;49:1987; with permission.)

prevention, particularly those with prior ischemic events (see **Fig. 4**C).[26] Analysis of the CHARISMA data also showed that the incremental risk of bleeding with clopidogrel plus aspirin versus aspirin alone was largely during the first year of therapy.[26,27] In patients who tolerated therapy for the first year without bleeding problems, the subsequent risk of bleeding was similar to that seen with aspirin alone. It is important that these subgroup hypotheses be confirmed through well-powered prospective testing, particularly as MATCH found that combined clopidogrel and aspirin use following ischemic stroke compared with clopidogrel alone led to excessive life-threatening bleeding without significant benefit.[28]

The potential risk of DAPT, when applied too broadly, and uncertainty about its use in long-term secondary prevention, raises the current controversy in how long patients should remain on combination therapy once initiated.[29] Although at least 1 month of therapy is required after bare metal stent implantation (ideally a year in those at low bleeding risk), a period of at least a year is required after drug-eluting stenting (DES) given persistent risks of late stent thrombosis.[29] The latter issue requires further delineation and is actively being addressed by the DAPT trial. Further complicating the issue is the observation that second-generation DES may have a lower risk of stent thrombosis than first-generation devices.

Variability in clopidogrel responsiveness (**Fig. 5**A) and its association with worse clinical outcomes is a great concern, particularly after stent placement.[30,31] For example, gene-products derived from polymorphisms in *CYP2C19* and *ABCB1* lead to altered hepatic metabolism and intestinal absorption, respectively, decreased clopidogrel response, and are associated with higher rates of vascular events.[19,32] Conversely, the CYP2C19*17 allele accelerates metabolism and was shown to increase propensity to bleed.[33] In addition to genetic determinants, environmental factors including hypertension, diabetes, hyperlipidemia, smoking, and increasing age influence clopidogrel response.[32] Drug-drug interactions, for example, proton pump inhibitors (PPIs), statins, and calcium-channel blockers, can alter clopidogrel metabolism, generating controversy about the safety of combined use. Often, these interactions have been associated with decreased measures of clopidogrel response, the clinical significance of which is unclear.[17] Given the lack of evidence to suggest clinical harm when considered in large randomized fashion, the beneficial effects of these medications seem to overshadow the theoretic risks.[34]

The potential effect of clopidogrel nonresponsiveness has led to approaches to overcome it, most simply through using higher doses of clopidogrel. Recently, CURRENT OASIS-7 showed that higher clopidogrel doses (600 mg loading followed by 150 mg daily for 1 week, then 75 mg maintenance) were better than standard regimens in preventing stent thrombosis, although when applied indiscriminately to patients managed medically, bleeding rates increased.[35] Methods of personalizing therapy may help to target more intense therapies to those most likely to need them (discussed later). However, clopidogrel nonresponsiveness can be only partially overcome with higher doses.[35]

Prasugrel

Prasugrel (Effient) is rapidly converted to an active metabolite via plasma esterases and a single CYP activation step, thus shortening its time to onset (1 hour) and increasing its potency.[2] At maintenance and loading doses of 60 mg and 10 mg, respectively, it exhibits less interindividual variability compared with clopidogrel (either 300 or 600 mg loading and 75 or 150 mg maintenance).[36]

In TRITON-TIMI 38, prasugrel (60 mg/10 mg) reduced cardiovascular events 20% compared with clopidogrel (300 mg/75 mg) when added to aspirin in patients with ACS undergoing PCI.[37] However, bleeding increased (including fatal and intracranial bleeds). In patients more than 75 years old and those less than 60 kg, benefit of therapy was lost.[37] Patients with prior transient ischemic attack or stroke suffered net harm.[37] Prasugrel was recently approved by the US Food and Drug Administration for patients with ACS in planned

PCI, with a black-box warning in these subsets. TRILOGY-ACS should help define if lower doses of prasugrel are beneficial in these high-risk groups.[2] Its use in clopidogrel nonresponders remains to be studied (discussed later).

Nonthienopyridine P2Y$_{12}$ Inhibitors

Direct reversible inhibitors of P2Y$_{12}$ have recently been tested in large clinical trials. Given their short-lived effect on platelet inhibition when stopped, these agents may help dissociate intensity of therapy and risk of uncontrollable bleeding.

Ticagrelor

Ticagrelor (Brilinta) is an adenosine triphosphate analogue that reversibly blocks P2Y$_{12}$ receptors without requiring metabolic conversion, thus achieving consistent platelet inhibition within 2 hours.[13] When stopped, platelet function returns to baseline within 1 to 2 days. This attractive feature, however, requires ticagrelor be administered twice daily.[13]

PLATO compared ticagrelor (180 mg loading; 90 mg twice daily maintenance) with clopidogrel (300–600 mg/75 mg) in combination with aspirin in patients with ACS.[38] After 1 year, relative vascular events decreased 16% and there was no difference in rates of major bleeding. Overall mortality decreased significantly (5.9% to 4.5%; $P<.001$).[38] When coronary artery bypass graft (CABG)-related bleeding (a planned procedure) was excluded, ticagrelor use was associated with increased major bleeding (4.5% vs 3.8%; $P = .03$) as might be expected.[38] This, along with its more frequent dosing schedule, could influence its effect when applied in real-world settings and its application in CHD prevention awaits further study.[39]

Intravenous Formulations: Cangrelor and Elinogrel

Cangrelor reversibly inhibits the P2Y$_{12}$ receptor, but is parenterally administered.[2] It achieves predictable, steady platelet inhibition within minutes, and when stopped, is metabolized rapidly in the plasma. Platelet function normalizes within 60 minutes.[13]

Cangrelor (followed by transition to oral clopidogrel with a 600 mg load administered 1 hour after stopping the infusion) was recently compared with clopidogrel use alone in patients (primarily with ACS) undergoing PCI and was not found superior, although it was found to be noninferior (CHAMPION PCI and CHAMPION PLATFORM trials).[40,41] Moreover, its intravenous (IV) formulation precludes long-term use. However, and

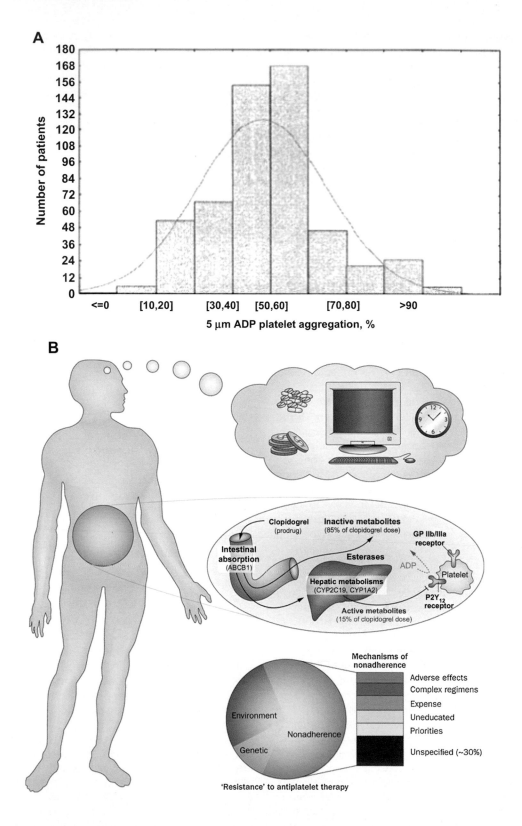

A

Number of patients

5 µm ADP platelet aggregation, %

B

Clopidogrel
(prodrug)

Inactive metabolites
(85% of clopidogrel dose)

GP IIb/IIIa
receptor

Intestinal
absorption
(ABCB1)

Esterases

ADP

Platelet

Hepatic metabolisms
(CYP2C19, CYP1A2)

P2Y₁₂
receptor

Active metabolites
(15% of clopidogrel dose)

Mechanisms of
nonadherence

Adverse effects
Complex regimens
Expense
Uneducated
Priorities

Unspecified (~30%)

Environment

Nonadherence

Genetic

'Resistance' to antiplatelet therapy

with relevance to longitudinal management, its equivalence with clopidogrel and dose-dependence makes it a potential bridging therapy in patients requiring invasive procedures (cardiac or otherwise), a prospect currently being tested in the BRIDGE study.[2] Methods of transitioning between IV and oral agents must be clarified; for example, cangrelor/$P2Y_{12}$ binding may affect clopidogrel loading.[42] Elinogrel, also a direct, reversible $P2Y_{12}$ inhibitor in phase II testing, is available in both IV and oral formulations offering the potential for seamless transitions between routes.[3,13]

GPIIB/IIIA Inhibitors

GPIIB/IIIA inhibitors block fibrinogen cross-linking with GPIIB/IIIA receptors. Three IV formulations have been approved for management of high-risk ACS and PCI.[2,3] These agents effectively reduced composite vascular end points in large, randomized clinical trials. However, most trials occurred before effective application of $P2Y_{12}$ inhibitors, which have now largely supplanted the need for GPIIb/IIIa inhibitors.[3] Currently, GPIIb/IIIa inhibitors are best reserved for provisional use. Early promise of GPIIb/IIIa antagonism led to development of various oral GPIIb/IIIa antagonists (of relevance to long-term prevention). Several have been tested, although as a class they resulted in excess bleeding without cardiovascular benefits.[43] Further development was abandoned.

Phosphodiesterase Inhibitors

Phosphodiesterase (PDE) inhibitors (dipyridamole [Persantine] and cilostazol [Pletal]) inhibit cyclic nucleotide PDE activity, thereby increasing intracellular cyclic nucleotides with pleiotropic effects on platelet inhibition and vasodilation.[4,10] Early formulations of dipyridamole resulted in inconsistent absorption and poor bioavailability, potentially accounting for variability in clinical effects.[15,44] Recent trials have focused on its use in cerebrovascular disease. Extended-release formulations, when combined with aspirin, significantly reduce

vascular event rates more than aspirin alone (ESPS 2 and ESPRIT trials), with efficacy similar to clopidogrel although with a greater risk of serious bleeding (PROFESS trial).[45,46] Use of these newer formulations in CHD has yet to be defined.

Cilostazol has been studied as an adjunct to standard DAPT regimens (so-called triple antiplatelet therapy [TAPT]).[47] In small studies (both ACS and PCI), TAPT with cilostazol reduced vascular events, stent thrombosis, even total mortality, without excess bleeding.[47] Moreover, cilostazol was found to reduce variability in clopidogrel response and decrease restenosis after stenting.[2,47] Although intriguing, these findings must be replicated in larger, more diverse randomized trials before being broadly applied, particularly given the high rate of side effects associated with cilostazol and mortality concerns associated with PDE inhibitor use in patients with heart failure.[48]

Protease Activated Receptor Inhibitors

PAR inhibitors have the theoretic advantage of localizing antiplatelet effects to the vicinity of active thrombin generation and clot, potentially reducing the risk of systemic bleeding.[10] Early testing demonstrated similar rates of bleeding when added as a third agent to standard DAPT. Currently, there are 2 oral formulations being testing in secondary prevention trials: SCH530348 with a half-life of 5 to 10 days resulting in platelet inhibition for around 1 month (through the TRA-2P-TIMI 50 trial) and E5555 with a significantly shorter half-life (through the LANCELOT CAD trial).[10]

SPECIAL POPULATIONS

Parallel to novel antiplatelet development, much remains to be done to realize the full benefit of therapies that are already proven. Randomized controlled trials serve as powerful proof of efficacy, yet strict inclusion and exclusion criteria can produce significant bias. Thus, the

Fig. 5. (*A*) Significant variability exists in individual responses to clopidogrel, as shown in the distribution of platelet aggregation to 5 μM adenosine. Antiplatelet nonresponsiveness and its proven effect on clinical outcomes has led to pharmacogenomic and pharmacodynamic approaches to personalize therapy, typically through the use of increased dosing, alternate antiplatelet agents, or added antiplatelet agents. (*From* Serebruany VL, Steinhubl SR, Berger PB, et al. Variability in platelet responsiveness to clopidogrel among 544 individuals. J Am Coll Cardiol 2005;45:247; with permission.) (*B*) Despite proven biochemical nonresponsiveness, significant real-world barriers exist to achieving the full potential of these important medications. For example, patient nonadherence to antiplatelet therapy is an enormous issue, confounding measures of platelet response and our understanding of evidence-based therapies. Treating nonadherent patients as if they were nonresponsive could result in increased health care costs and net harm. (*From* Kolandaivelu K, Bhatt DL. Overcoming 'resistance' to antiplatelet therapy: targeting the issue of nonadherence. Nat Rev Cardiol 2010;7;464; with permission.)

applicability of evidence-based antiplatelet use in underrepresented populations must be considered.

Elderly

The elderly are an expanding subset who are at exceptionally high risk both for cardiovascular events and bleeding.[49] In primary prevention settings, risk for coronary events increases 85% with each decade, and the risk of ischemic stroke increases 2.5-fold.[16] Intracranial and extracranial bleeding risks also increase by nearly 60% and 115%, respectively.[16] As combined risk increases, the importance of optimal antiplatelet use is stressed. Yet, the elderly continue to be underrepresented in clinical trials given excess comorbidities, concern for hemorrhage, and potential drug-drug interactions.[49] Although 40% of patients presenting with ACS are more than 75 years old, less than 20% of trial participants in pooled analyses are elderly. Fewer than one-third of recent trials shaping our clinical understanding of antiplatelet use have shown significant treatment benefit in elderly subgroups.[49]

In acute and secondary prevention settings, it is generally accepted that standard antiplatelet therapies should not be withheld in elderly patients. However, examples such as TRITON-TIMI 38 (where the subgroup of patients older than 75 years failed to derive net treatment benefit) show the need for closer evaluation. In primary prevention settings, benefits of antiplatelet agents are even less certain. For example, in a 2009 update, the US Preventative Services Task Force (USPSTF) concluded there was insufficient evidence to provide recommendations on aspirin use in individuals more than 80 years of age.[12] In the absence of evidence, individual bleeding risks and patient preferences must be considered. ASPREE, a study investigating primary prevention aspirin use in patients more than 70 years of age may help add clarity.[50]

Women

Currently in the United States, more women die from heart attacks annually than men, yet they too are underrepresented in trials.[51,52] Despite improved inclusion rates, women continue to account for only 25% of enrollment in CHD prevention trials, despite representing 46% of patients with CHD.[51] The effect of low enrollment on evidence-based recommendations is unclear, and makes further analysis (eg, ethnic and race differences) difficult. These biases are especially concerning given recognized gender-based differences in CHD. For example, CHD in women peaks

around 10 years after that in men and nearly 40% of women die within 1 year of a first MI compared with 25% of men (likely because of the confounding issue of age, rather than gender per se).[12] More fundamentally, cardiovascular risk prediction in women is less well characterized.[52]

Although treatment in individuals with secondary and high-risk CHD is gender indifferent, the USPSTF recommends (barring excess bleeding risk) that aspirin is used when 10-year stroke risk exceeds 3%, 8%, and 11% in lower-risk women aged 55–59 years, 60–69 years, and 70–79 years, respectively.[12] Moreover, doses of 81 mg or 100 mg every other day may be sufficient given gender differences in pharmacokinetics.[52] However, in the absence of definitive evidence and given the potential for interindividual variability, standard daily dosing (75 to 162 mg) remains reasonable.[53] With respect to clopidogrel, it seems to be similarly efficacious in both men and women in the cardiovascular clinical trials to date.[54]

Comorbidities

Comorbid diseases modify CHD and bleeding risks, increase potential drug-drug interactions, and can affect antiplatelet pharmacokinetics through altered metabolism and/or elimination (as in renal or hepatic failure). Although far from inclusive, diabetes, heart failure, and those conditions requiring anticoagulation are highly prevalent among patients with CHD and deserve special mention.

Diabetes
Diabetes increases CHD risk 4-fold.[55] Given augmented risk, the American Diabetes Association (ADA) recommended aspirin use in patients with diabetes more than 40 years of age as primary prevention.[55] Meta-analyses incorporating nearly 4000 individuals failed to show consistent reductions in vascular events or mortality with aspirin use, although bleeding increased 50% relative to patients without diabetes.[55] A recent expert consensus statement recommended that low-dose therapy is reasonable in men more than 50 years of age and in women more than 60 years of age with 1 or more risk factors, although should not be used in younger patients with diabetes without additional risk (10-year CHD <5%; American College of Cardiology Foundation ACCF)/ American Heart Association (AHA) class III, level of evidence C).[55] Furthermore, effective risk factor reduction may lower CHD risk sufficiently to no longer merit therapy, a point to consider in patients without diabetes as well. ASCEND and ACCEPT-D are ongoing primary prevention trials dedicated to

patients with diabetes, and may shed further light on this important subgroup.

Secondary prevention in patients with diabetes certainly merits treatment and increasingly potent therapies may be warranted. For example, dual therapy with aspirin and prasugrel (rather than clopidogrel) led to a 40% reduction in MI in patients with diabetes with ACS undergoing PCI, compared with only an 18% reduction in patients without diabetes.[56] Whether or not these benefits will persist when compared with higher doses of clopidogrel is currently being tested (OPTIMUS-3).[57]

Anticoagulation

Anticoagulation, and in particular warfarin, is widely used to manage procoaguable states. In atrial fibrillation stroke prevention, for example, warfarin was superior to DAPT, which was superior to aspirin alone (ACTIVE-W and ACTIVE-A trials, respectively).[58] Thus, anticoagulant and antiplatelet therapies may be indicated concurrently, despite augmented bleeding risks.[59] In the Get with the Guidelines (GWTG) registry, around 5% of patients presenting with ACS received triple therapy (DAPT + warfarin), mostly for atrial fibrillation in conjunction with stenting.[60] Despite the potential benefit of this strategy in reducing embolic stroke risk, only one-fifth of those with atrial fibrillation actually received triple therapy.[60] Lack of treatment uniformity is concerning, and driven by an inability to adequately balance risk in increasingly complex scenarios as well as a lack of clinical data effectively addressing these issues. However, when warfarin is used with DAPT, low-dose aspirin should be used and international normalized ratios (INRs) should be carefully targeted between 2.0 to 2.5 to limit excessive bleeding.[60] Consideration should also be given for prophylactic PPI use with triple therapy.[61] Newer oral anticoagulants, such as dabigatran, may offer alternative safer approaches than warfarin in the future.[62]

Heart failure

Antiplatelets are indicated for secondary CHD prevention in many patients with heart failure given the prevalence of ischemic cardiomyopathy (ICMP).[63] Moreover, heart failure itself is often considered a procoagulant state and even in the absence of atherothrombotic disease, antithrombotic therapies may be prescribed.[63] Although warfarin is commonly used (often without strong indication), its associated bleeding risk has led to consideration of antiplatelet therapies, even for non-ICMP (NICMP). The safety and efficacy of aspirin in these settings is controversial given a potential reduction in acetyl cholinesterase

inhibitor efficacy that has been inconsistently observed.[63] In the recent WATCH trial, warfarin use was associated with fewer heart failure admissions than aspirin.[63] Thus, it is reasonable to avoid chronic aspirin therapy in patients with nonischemic heart failure who are at low risk for cardiovascular events, particularly ones with recurrent heart failure exacerbations.

Low-income Countries

Applicability of evidence-based interventions to the broader global population is unclear. For example, 80% of global deaths attributable to CHD occur in low- and middle-income countries.[64] The low cost of aspirin makes it ideal in these settings, yet, in some regions, as few as 65% of individuals take aspirin after a heart attack and as few as 30% after a stroke.[65] Moreover, even basic additions such as statins begin to outstrip limited resources in impoverished regions.[64] Clearly, novel antiplatelet drugs would be infeasible, regardless of their evidence.

Combination pills (polypills), incorporating aspirin with other evidence-based therapies, may have promise in low-income settings, although their use is not straightforward given issues about potential drug-drug interactions and compliance.[66] Given the limited possibilities for follow-up, surveillance, and in-depth risk stratification, the population-wide safety of a polypill approach remains to be seen. Moreover, as additional therapies become generic (such as clopidogrel), whether they can be incorporated cost effectively into polypill strategies is unclear.

TOWARD PERSONALIZED THERAPY

Although much remains to be done to define antiplatelet use in special populations, personalized medicine is the logical extension of this ongoing effort and new pharmacogenomic and pharmacodynamic approaches are being considered as methods of tailoring antiplatelet therapies to fit individual needs. As discussed, specific polymorphisms can alter clopidogrel responsiveness and also correlate with poor outcomes. However, whether gene profiling for such polymorphisms will allow therapies to be prospectively modified to improve clinical outcomes remains unproved.[67] One concern is the effect of environmental factors on response variability.[17] Pharmacodynamic tools that can monitor platelet responsiveness may help integrate both genetic and environmental factors into a single measure.[17,31] However, current tools remain nonstandardized and have high interassay variability. Only recently have pharmacodynamic approaches been rigorously compared to determine their efficacy in predicting outcomes.[17,31] Although the POPular study found some assays were better predictors than others, all had modest receiver operating curves and none could predict risk of bleeding.[68] Intraindividual variability further confounds application of these tools, particularly as response levels measured during acute episodes of care need not reflect those in outpatient settings.[17]

Despite many issues, the potential for personalized antiplatelet therapy is foreseeable. In a small study, the vasodilator-stimulator phosphoprotein (VASP) index was used prospectively to alter clopidogrel dosing with PCI, resulting in improved cardiovascular outcomes without increased bleeding.[69] Several larger ongoing trials (such as ARCTIC, DANTE, GRAVITIAS, and TRIGGER-PCI) should help define the role of these approaches in prospective management.[3] If effective, these tools could usher a new era of personalized antiplatelet therapy, hopefully at acceptable costs.

BARRIERS TO ANTIPLATELETS IN PREVENTION

Regardless of the evidence supporting antiplatelet drugs or their optimal use, no therapy is effective if a patient does not receive it. Provider nonprescription and patient nonadherence pose significant barriers to real-world antiplatelet use in CHD prevention.

Antiplatelet Nonprescription

In a registry of high-risk patients, 15% to 20% were not receiving antiplatelet therapy for secondary prevention, and nearly 50% with multiple risk factors were not on primary prevention therapy.[70] Practice variability has led to several quality initiatives to facilitate guideline adoption, already with measurable clinical improvements. In 1 initiative, for example, medication use in patients presenting with ACS was tracked. Basic provider education and feedback resulted in a significant, but only partial, increase in clopidogrel use from 50% to 72% in 2 years.[71]

Antiplatelet Nonadherence

The dangers of patient nonadherence to antiplatelet therapy are becoming increasingly recognized and the implications for CHD prevention are enormous (see **Fig. 5**B).[17] In one analysis, 7% of patients presenting with ACS reported aspirin nonadherence within 3 months of discharge; 12% were nonadherent to clopidogrel.[72] Another database found nearly 28% of patients failed to fill clopidogrel prescriptions after discharge.[73]

Thienopyridine nonadherence after stenting has been shown to increase mortality 9-fold in the first year; even a 1-day lapse in filling discharge clopidogrel prescription was associated with excess stent thrombosis.[74,75] In primary prevention, rates of noncompliance are even higher. For example, in patients with diabetes with asymptomatic PAD, 5-year drug use dropped by 50%.[76]

Reasons for nonadherence are complex and multifactorial, and aspects of therapy other than efficacy can influence patient decisions. For example, although severe bleeding is a major concern in trials, nuisance bleeding is far more common and, although often unreported, may increase nonadherence.[77] Alternatively, complex regimens (such as TAPT or agents requiring frequent dosing) may perform very differently when applied in real-world settings.[17,39] Costs and insurance coverage must also be considered.[17] As ability to personalize antiplatelet therapy approaches, the confounding role that nonadherence has on measured responsiveness must be addressed, because more potent, expensive therapies to overcome misdiagnosed nonresponsiveness may increase potential for net harm.[17]

SUMMARY

Antiplatelet therapy is an essential part of CHD prevention. As atherothrombotic risks increase, so do the beneficial effects of therapy and increasingly potent regimens seem justified. Novel advances in drug mechanisms, along with the foreseeable potential of personalized therapy, offer a way to dissociate clotting and bleeding risks and may revolutionize treatment paradigms. However, addressing basic issues such as dosage, duration, and proof of efficacy in real-world populations must not lag. Barriers such as slow adoption of guidelines and patient nonadherence pose fundamental threats to antiplatelet efficacy and must also be a focus of longitudinal care.

REFERENCES

1. Davi G, Patrono C. Platelet activation and atherothrombosis. N Engl J Med 2007;357(24):2482–94.
2. Michelson AD. Antiplatelet therapies for the treatment of cardiovascular disease. Nat Rev Drug Discov 2010;9(2):154–69.
3. Desai NR, Bhatt DL. The state of periprocedural antiplatelet therapy after recent trials. JACC Cardiovasc Interv 2010;3(6):571–83.
4. Patrono C, Baigent C, Hirsh J, et al. Antiplatelet drugs: American College of Chest Physicians

evidence-based clinical practice guidelines (8th edition). Chest 2008;133(Suppl 6):199S–233S.

5. Bhatt DL, Topol EJ. Scientific and therapeutic advances in antiplatelet therapy. Nat Rev Drug Discov 2003;2(1):15–28.

6. Nagarakanti R, Sodhi S, Lee R, et al. Chronic antithrombotic therapy in post-myocardial infarction patients. Cardiol Clin 2008;26(2):277–88, vii.

7. Lloyd-Jones D, Adams RJ, Brown TM, et al. Heart disease and stroke statistics–2010 update: a report from the American Heart Association. Circulation 2010;121(7):e46–215.

8. Bhatt DL. Intensifying platelet inhibition–navigating between Scylla and Charybdis. N Engl J Med 2007;357(20):2078–81.

9. Patrono C, Garcia Rodriguez LA, Landolfi R, et al. Low-dose aspirin for the prevention of atherothrombosis. N Engl J Med 2005;353(22):2373–83.

10. Patrono C, Rocca B. The future of antiplatelet therapy in cardiovascular disease. Annu Rev Med 2010;61:49–61.

11. Sanmuganathan PS, Ghahramani P, Jackson PR, et al. Aspirin for primary prevention of coronary heart disease: safety and absolute benefit related to coronary risk derived from meta-analysis of randomised trials. Heart 2001;85(3):265–71.

12. Calonge N, Petitti DB, DeWitt TG, et al. Aspirin for the prevention of cardiovascular disease: US Preventive Services Task Force recommendation statement. Ann Intern Med 2009;150(6):396–404.

13. Sakhuja R, Yeh RW, Bhatt DL. Antiplatelet agents in acute coronary syndromes. Curr Probl Cardiol 2010; 35(3):123–70.

14. Campbell CL, Smyth S, Montalescot G, et al. Aspirin dose for the prevention of cardiovascular disease: a systematic review. JAMA 2007;297(18): 2018–24.

15. Baigent C, Sudlow C, Collins R, et al. Antithrombotic Trialists' Collaboration. Collaborative meta-analysis of randomised trials of antiplatelet therapy for prevention of death, myocardial infarction, and stroke in high risk patients. BMJ 2002;324(7329): 71–86.

16. Baigent C, Blackwell L, Collins R, et al. Aspirin in the primary and secondary prevention of vascular disease: collaborative meta-analysis of individual participant data from randomised trials. Lancet 2009;373(9678):1849–60.

17. Kolandaivelu K, Bhatt DL. Overcoming 'resistance' to antiplatelet therapy: targeting the issue of nonadherence. Nat Rev Cardiol 2010;7(8):461–7.

18. Smith SC Jr, Allen J, Blair SN, et al. AHA/ACC guidelines for secondary prevention for patients with coronary and other atherosclerotic vascular disease: 2006 update: endorsed by the National Heart, Lung, and Blood Institute. Circulation 2006; 113(19):2363–72.

19. Mega JL, Close SL, Wiviott SD, et al. Cytochrome p-450 polymorphisms and response to clopidogrel. N Engl J Med 2009;360(4):354–62.

20. von Beckerath N, Taubert D, Pogatsa-Murray G, et al. Absorption, metabolization, and antiplatelet effects of 300-, 600-, and 900-mg loading doses of clopidogrel: results of the ISAR-CHOICE (Intracoronary Stenting and Antithrombotic Regimen: Choose Between 3 High Oral Doses for Immediate Clopidogrel Effect) trial. Circulation 2005;112(19):2946–50.

21. CAPRIESteeringCommittee. A randomised, blinded, trial of clopidogrel versus aspirin in patients at risk of ischaemic events (CAPRIE). Lancet 1996; 348(9038):1329–39.

22. Gaspoz JM, Coxson PG, Goldman PA, et al. Cost effectiveness of aspirin, clopidogrel, or both for secondary prevention of coronary heart disease. N Engl J Med 2002;346(23):1800–6.

23. Yusuf S, Zhao F, Mehta SR, et al. Effects of clopidogrel in addition to aspirin in patients with acute coronary syndromes without ST-segment elevation. N Engl J Med 2001;345(7):494–502.

24. Mehta SR, Yusuf S, Peters RJ, et al. Effects of pretreatment with clopidogrel and aspirin followed by long-term therapy in patients undergoing percutaneous coronary intervention: the PCI-CURE study. Lancet 2001;358(9281):527–33.

25. Bhatt DL, Fox KA, Hacke W, et al. Clopidogrel and aspirin versus aspirin alone for the prevention of atherothrombotic events. N Engl J Med 2006; 354(16):1706–17.

26. Bhatt DL, Flather MD, Hacke W, et al. Patients with prior myocardial infarction, stroke, or symptomatic peripheral arterial disease in the CHARISMA trial. J Am Coll Cardiol 2007;49(19):1982–8.

27. Berger PB, Bhatt DL, Fuster V, et al. Bleeding complications with dual antiplatelet therapy among patients with stable vascular disease or risk factors for vascular disease: results from the Clopidogrel for High Atherothrombotic Risk and Ischemic Stabilization, Management, and Avoidance (CHARISMA) trial. Circulation 2010;121(23):2575–83.

28. Menon BK, Frankel MR, Liang L, et al. Rapid change in prescribing behavior in hospitals participating in Get with the guidelines-stroke after release of the management of atherothrombosis with clopidogrel in high-risk patients (MATCH) clinical trial results. Stroke 2010;41(9):2094–7.

29. Windecker S, Meier B. Late coronary stent thrombosis. Circulation 2007;116(17):1952–65.

30. Serebruany VL, Steinhubl SR, Berger PB, et al. Variability in platelet responsiveness to clopidogrel among 544 individuals. J Am Coll Cardiol 2005; 45(2):246–51.

31. Sweeny JM, Gorog DA, Fuster V. Antiplatelet drug 'resistance'. Part 1: mechanisms and clinical measurements. Nat Rev Cardiol 2009;6(4):273–82.

32. Shuldiner AR, O'Connell JR, Bliden KP, et al. Association of cytochrome P450 2C19 genotype with the antiplatelet effect and clinical efficacy of clopidogrel therapy. JAMA 2009;302(8):849–57.

33. Sibbing D, Koch W, Gebhard D, et al. Cytochrome 2C19*17 allelic variant, platelet aggregation, bleeding events, and stent thrombosis in clopidogrel-treated patients with coronary stent placement. Circulation 2010;121(4):512–8.

34. Juurlink DN. Proton pump inhibitors and clopidogrel: putting the interaction in perspective. Circulation 2009;120(23):2310–2.

35. Mehta SR, Bassand JP, Chrolavicius S, et al. Dose comparisons of clopidogrel and aspirin in acute coronary syndromes. N Engl J Med 2010;363(10): 930–42.

36. Wiviott SD, Trenk D, Frelinger AL, et al. Prasugrel compared with high loading- and maintenance-dose clopidogrel in patients with planned percutaneous coronary intervention: The Prasugrel in Comparison to Clopidogrel for Inhibition of Platelet Activation and Aggregation-Thrombolysis in Myocardial Infarction 44 trial. Circulation 2007;116(25): 2923–32.

37. Wiviott SD, Braunwald E, McCabe CH, et al. Prasugrel versus clopidogrel in patients with acute coronary syndromes. N Engl J Med 2007;357(20):2001–15.

38. Wallentin L, Becker RC, Budaj A, et al. Ticagrelor versus clopidogrel in patients with acute coronary syndromes. N Engl J Med 2009;361(11):1045–57.

39. Bhatt DL. Antiplatelet therapy: Ticagrelor in ACS—what does PLATO teach us? Nat Rev Cardiol 2009; 6(12):737–8.

40. Bhatt DL, Lincoff AM, Gibson CM, et al. Intravenous platelet blockade with cangrelor during PCI. N Engl J Med 2009;361(24):2330–41.

41. Harrington RA, Stone GW, McNulty S, et al. Platelet inhibition with cangrelor in patients undergoing PCI. N Engl J Med 2009;361(24):2318–29.

42. Steinhubl SR, Oh JJ, Oestreich JH, et al. Transitioning patients from cangrelor to clopidogrel: pharmacodynamic evidence of a competitive effect. Thromb Res 2008;121(4):527–34.

43. Chew DP, Bhatt DL, Sapp S, et al. Increased mortality with oral platelet glycoprotein IIb/IIIa antagonists: a meta-analysis of phase III multicenter randomized trials. Circulation 2001;103(2):201–6.

44. De Schryver EL, Algra A, van Gijn J. Dipyridamole for preventing stroke and other vascular events in patients with vascular disease. Cochrane Database Syst Rev 2006;(2):CD001820.

45. Halkes PH, van Gijn J, Kappelle LJ, et al. Aspirin plus dipyridamole versus aspirin alone after cerebral ischaemia of arterial origin (ESPRIT): randomised controlled trial. Lancet 2006;367(9523):1665–73.

46. Sacco RL, Diener HC, Yusuf S, et al. Aspirin and extended-release dipyridamole versus clopidogrel for recurrent stroke. N Engl J Med 2008;359(12): 1238–51.

47. Croce K. Antiplatelet therapy after percutaneous coronary intervention: should another regimen be "TAPT?". Circ Cardiovasc Interv 2010;3(1):3–5.

48. Cheng JW. Cilostazol. Heart Dis 1999;1(3):182–6.

49. Dauerman HL, Bhatt DL, Gretler DD, et al. Bridging the gap between clinical trials of antiplatelet therapies and applications among elderly patients. Am Heart J 2010;159(4):508–17. e501.

50. Nelson MR, Reid CM, Ames DA, et al. Feasibility of conducting a primary prevention trial of low-dose aspirin for major adverse cardiovascular events in older people in Australia: results from the ASPirin in Reducing Events in the Elderly (ASPREE) pilot study. Med J Aust 2008;189(2):105–9.

51. Melloni C, Berger JS, Wang TY, et al. Representation of women in randomized clinical trials of cardiovascular disease prevention. Circ Cardiovasc Qual Outcomes 2010;3(2):135–42.

52. Mosca L, Banka CL, Benjamin EJ, et al. Evidence-based guidelines for cardiovascular disease prevention in women: 2007 update. Circulation 2007;115(11):1481–501.

53. Pearson TA, Blair SN, Daniels SR, et al. AHA guidelines for primary prevention of cardiovascular disease and stroke: 2002 update: consensus panel guide to comprehensive risk reduction for adult patients without coronary or other atherosclerotic vascular diseases. American Heart Association Science Advisory and Coordinating Committee. Circulation 2002;106(3):388–91.

54. Berger JS, Bhatt DL, Cannon CP, et al. The relative efficacy and safety of clopidogrel in women and men a sex-specific collaborative meta-analysis. J Am Coll Cardiol 2009;54(21):1935–45.

55. Pignone M, Alberts MJ, Colwell JA, et al. Aspirin for primary prevention of cardiovascular events in people with diabetes. J Am Coll Cardiol 2010; 55(25):2878–86.

56. Wiviott SD, Braunwald E, Angiolillo DJ, et al. Greater clinical benefit of more intensive oral antiplatelet therapy with prasugrel in patients with diabetes mellitus in the trial to assess improvement in therapeutic outcomes by optimizing platelet inhibition with prasugrel - Thrombolysis in Myocardial Infarction 38. Circulation 2008;118(16): 1626–36.

57. Angiolillo DJ. Antiplatelet therapy: new data on prasugrel from AHA 2009 - OPTIMUS-3 and SWAP trials. Paper presented at: AHA 2009. Orlando (FL), November 16, 2009.

58. Connolly SJ, Pogue J, Hart RG, et al. Effect of clopidogrel added to aspirin in patients with atrial fibrillation. N Engl J Med 2009;360(20):2066–78.

59. Khurram Z, Chou E, Minutello R, et al. Combination therapy with aspirin, clopidogrel and warfarin

following coronary stenting is associated with a significant risk of bleeding. J Invasive Cardiol 2006;18(4):162–4.

60. Depta JP, Cannon CP, Fonarow GC, et al. Patient characteristics associated with the choice of triple antithrombotic therapy in acute coronary syndromes. Am J Cardiol 2009;104(9):1171–8.

61. Bhatt DL, Scheiman J, Abraham NS, et al. ACCF/ACG/AHA 2008 expert consensus document on reducing the gastrointestinal risks of antiplatelet therapy and NSAID use: a report of the American College of Cardiology Foundation Task Force on Clinical Expert Consensus Documents. J Am Coll Cardiol 2008;52(18):1502–17.

62. Connolly SJ, Ezekowitz MD, Yusuf S, et al. Dabigatran versus warfarin in patients with atrial fibrillation. N Engl J Med 2009;361(12):1139–51.

63. Konstam MA. Antithrombotic therapy in heart failure: WATCHful wondering. Circulation 2009;119(12):1559–61.

64. Gaziano TA. Cardiovascular disease in the developing world and its cost-effective management. Circulation 2005;112(23):3547–53.

65. Mendis S, Abegunde D, Yusuf S, et al. WHO study on Prevention of REcurrences of Myocardial Infarction and StrokE (WHO-PREMISE). Bull World Health Organ 2005;83(11):820–9.

66. Yusuf S, Pais P, Afzal R, et al. Effects of a polypill (Polycap) on risk factors in middle-aged individuals without cardiovascular disease (TIPS): a phase II, double blind, randomised trial. Lancet 2009;373(9672):1341–51.

67. Bhatt DL. Tailoring antiplatelet therapy based on pharmacogenomics: how well do the data fit? JAMA 2009;302(8):896–7.

68. Breet NJ, van Werkum JW, Bouman HJ, et al. Comparison of platelet function tests in predicting clinical outcome in patients undergoing coronary stent implantation. JAMA 2010;303(8):754–62.

69. Bonello L, Camoin-Jau L, Arques S, et al. Adjusted clopidogrel loading doses according to vasodilator-stimulated phosphoprotein phosphorylation index decrease rate of major adverse cardiovascular events in patients with clopidogrel resistance: a multicenter randomized prospective study. J Am Coll Cardiol 2008;51(14):1404–11.

70. Bhatt DL, Steg PG, Ohman EM, et al. International prevalence, recognition, and treatment of cardiovascular risk factors in outpatients with atherothrombosis. JAMA 2006;295(2):180–9.

71. Mehta RH, Roe MT, Chen AY, et al. Recent trends in the care of patients with non-ST-segment elevation acute coronary syndromes: insights from the CRUSADE initiative. Arch Intern Med 2006;166(18):2027–34.

72. Ho PM, Spertus JA, Masoudi FA, et al. Impact of medication therapy discontinuation on mortality after myocardial infarction. Arch Intern Med 2006;166(17):1842–7.

73. Ho PM, Peterson ED, Wang L, et al. Incidence of death and acute myocardial infarction associated with stopping clopidogrel after acute coronary syndrome. JAMA 2008;299(5):532–9.

74. Spertus JA, Kettelkamp R, Vance C, et al. Prevalence, predictors, and outcomes of premature discontinuation of thienopyridine therapy after drug-eluting stent placement: results from the PREMIER registry. Circulation 2006;113(24):2803–9.

75. Ho PM, Tsai TT, Maddox TM, et al. Delays in filling clopidogrel prescription after hospital discharge and adverse outcomes after drug-eluting stent implantation: implications for transitions of care. Circ Cardiovasc Qual Outcomes 2010;3(3):261–6.

76. Belch J, MacCuish A, Campbell I, et al. The prevention of progression of arterial disease and diabetes (POPADAD) trial: factorial randomised placebo controlled trial of aspirin and antioxidants in patients with diabetes and asymptomatic peripheral arterial disease. BMJ 2008;337:a1840.

77. Serebruany VL, Atar D. Assessment of bleeding events in clinical trials—proposal of a new classification. Am J Cardiol 2007;99(2):288–90.

Lipid-Lowering Therapy with Statins for the Primary and Secondary Prevention of Cardiovascular Disease

Joel A. Lardizabal, MD[a], Prakash Deedwania, MD[b],*

KEYWORDS

- Lipid-lowering • Statin • Cardiovascular disease
- Coronary heart disease • Stroke • Primary prevention
- Secondary prevention

Nearly one-third of the annual global mortality is attributed to cardiovascular disease (CVD), making it the leading cause of death worldwide. Overall, coronary heart disease (CHD) is the predominant cause of death from CVD followed by stroke, accounting for approximately 7.2 million and 5.7 million annual deaths, respectively.[1] Approximately 18 million individuals are afflicted with CHD in the United States, and over a million Americans suffer from acute coronary events every year. On the other hand, stroke has a prevalence of nearly 6.5 million, with an incidence of 600,000 new cases diagnosed each year in the United States.[2]

As one of the established risk factors for CVD, dyslipidemia plays a significant role in the pathogenesis of both CHD and stroke. Lipid-lowering therapy, primarily with HMG-CoA reductase inhibitors (statins), has well-established benefits in the management of these conditions. Mortality from CVD has been on a declining trend, and this is principally ascribed to evidence-based therapies and risk-reduction strategies, including the use of statins. The burden of CVD, however, remains high, and clarifying the role of statin therapy in the primary and secondary prevention of high-risk cardiovascular conditions can improve the use of these agents in appropriate patients, which can potentially lessen the adverse public health and economic impact of the CVD epidemic.

LIPIDS AND ATHEROSCLEROSIS

Atherosclerosis is the central pathophysiologic mechanism primarily responsible for the development of most CVD conditions, including CHD and stroke. Atherosclerosis is believed to result from chronic inflammation and injury to the vessel wall. The prevailing theory on atherosclerosis points to the critical role of inflammation in atherogenesis. The pivotal step in initiation of inflammatory response is the oxidation of low-density lipoprotein (LDL) cholesterol, which subsequently initiates the

The authors have nothing to disclose.

[a] Division of Cardiology, Department of Medicine, University of California-San Francisco (Fresno Medical Education Program), 155 North Fresno Street, Fresno, CA 93701, USA

[b] Division of Cardiology, Department of Medicine, Veterans Affairs Central California Health Care System/ University of California, San Francisco, Fresno Program, 2615 East Clinton Avenue, Fresno, CA 93703, USA

* Corresponding author. Division of Cardiology, Department of Medicine, Veterans Affairs Central California Health Care System/ University of California, San Francisco, Fresno Program, 2615 East Clinton Avenue, Fresno, CA 93703.

E-mail address: deed@fresno.ucsf.edu

Cardiol Clin 29 (2011) 87–103

doi:10.1016/j.ccl.2010.10.002

0733-8651/11/$ — see front matter. Published by Elsevier Inc.

cascade of events leading to atherosclerosis. Lipid oxidation is largely mediated by reactive oxygen species derived from the lipoxygenase and myeloperoxidase pathways. These oxidized LDL particles contain arachidonic acid and are readily recognized by the innate immune system.[3,4] These particles are then taken up by monocytes, forming the classic foam cell, which eventually gets deposited into the vessel wall. This process further stimulates lipid deposition and formation of the atherosclerotic plaque. Progressive plaque deposition leads to chronic vessel stenosis, whereas rupture of this atherosclerotic lesion results in acute vascular syndromes.

On the other hand, progression of the atherosclerotic process is inhibited by high-density lipoprotein (HDL) cholesterol, primarily through the reverse transport of cholesterol from lipid-laden macrophages in the vascular wall, as well as through its antiinflammatory effects.[5] The inhibition of LDL oxidation and the scavenging of these proinflammatory oxidized lipids may in part explain the antiinflammatory effects of HDL. In addition, HDL has also been shown to prevent the release of tumor necrosis factor, inhibit the activation of complement, and reduce macrophage infiltration.[4]

A HISTORICAL PERSPECTIVE ON LIPID-MODULATING THERAPY

The relationship between hypercholesterolemia and atherosclerosis has been well known since the 1940s,[6] but it was not until 1951 that the link between CVD and abnormalities in lipoprotein fractions (eg, low HDL and high LDL levels) was first described.[7] Following reports of the antiatherosclerotic benefits of lipid-modifying therapy, drugs specifically designed for lowering cholesterol levels were developed, the fibrates being the first therapeutic class of agents used for such purposes.

In 1965, the World Health Organization (WHO) initiated a large, randomized controlled trial of nearly 16,000 hypercholesterolemic men without overt CHD who were treated with either clofibrate or placebo. After more than 5 years of follow-up, this primary prevention study found that the 9% reduction in cholesterol levels associated with clofibrate therapy resulted in a 25% decrease in myocardial infarction (MI) and a 20% lowering of CHD incidence. There was, however, an unexpected 25% increase in non-CHD mortality with clofibrate, predominantly from hepatobiliary causes.[8]

In 1966, the Coronary Drug Project (CDP) started the enrollment of more than 8300 patients with CHD who were randomized to receive either clofibrate, niacin, estrogen, or dextrothyroxine or placebo. The estrogen and dextrothyroxine arms were discontinued early because of increased mortality and thrombotic events. After 5 years of follow-up, this secondary prevention trial found no evidence of mortality benefit for clofibrate. It instead showed that this fibric acid derivative increased the incidence of CVD events and gallstones. As such, the investigators recommended against the use of clofibrate in patients with CHD.[9]

The CDP did, however, demonstrate a significant (albeit modest) reduction in recurrent MI with niacin treatment. The 5-year mortality outcome was unchanged by niacin therapy, and this was partly ascribed to the compliance issues encountered during the study period. Remarkably, 15-year follow-up showed a significant 11% lower death rate with niacin when compared with placebo, a late benefit that was found 9 years after discontinuation of the drug.[10] Despite the beneficial effects seen with niacin, the CDP investigators recommended that caution be exercised in prescribing this agent because of the side effects possibly linked to it.

The higher adverse event rates in the treatment arms of the CDP prompted subsequent research on the modes of action of the different cholesterol-modulating agents and stimulated the development of safer, more effective drugs. In the late 1970s, the Pooling Project[11] made the assertion that LDL, among the different lipoprotein fractions, had the strongest association with CHD. Meanwhile, the Framingham Study demonstrated the cardioprotective role of HDL, noting that it was inversely related to CHD risk independent of LDL levels.[12]

The Lipid Research Clinics Coronary Primary Prevention Trial (LRC-CPPT),[13] in 1973, started the recruitment of more than 3800 asymptomatic, hypercholesterolemic men who were randomized to receive either placebo or cholestyramine, a bile acid sequestrant (the newest class of lipid-lowering agents at the time). The study found that 5 years of cholestyramine therapy resulted in a 12% reduction in LDL levels, which was in turn associated with a significant 19% decrease in CHD events. Furthermore, the LRC-CPPT study showed that cholestyramine use yielded a small increase in HDL level, which accounted for an additional (albeit less profound) 2% reduction of CHD risk, independent of LDL or total cholesterol levels.

In 1981, the Helsinki Heart Study[14] conducted a randomized primary prevention trial on more than 4000 hypercholesterolemic men using gemfibrozil, a fibric acid derivative that had a more favorable safety and tolerability profile compared with clofibrate. Early data revealed that gemfibrozil therapy induced a rapid increase in HDL levels by nearly 16%, as well as significant reductions in levels of LDL by 10%, triglycerides by 43%, and non-HDL cholesterol by 14%. After 5 years of follow-up, the study revealed a significant 34% lowering in CHD incidence with gemfibrozil, although mortality rate was unaffected.

Although concerns regarding the safety and efficacy of drug treatment hounded the earlier WHO Cooperative Trial and the CDP Study, the LRC-CPPT and the Helsinki Heart Study cemented the beneficial role of lipid-modulating therapy in the primary prevention of CHD. It was also during this period that LDL and non-HDL cholesterol fractions emerged as the primary targets of pharmacologic treatment. The focus shifted toward development of new LDL-lowering agents that were more effective than those currently available at the time (fibrates, niacin, and bile acid sequestrants). In the 1980s, the statins were introduced as the latest class of cholesterol-modulating therapeutic agents.

Lovastatin, the first commercially developed statin, was approved for clinical use in 1987. Initial studies on both healthy volunteers[15] and those with hypercholesterolemia[16] showed a 28% to 45% reduction in LDL levels from baseline. Head-to-head trials were conducted in the late 1980s comparing statins with the other classes of lipid-lowering agents. The Lovastatin Study Group III, for instance, randomized 260 patients with severe primary hyperlipidemia to either lovastatin (20 mg or 40 mg twice daily) or cholestyramine (12 g twice daily) and found a 50% greater reduction in LDL levels and significantly lower incidence of adverse events with high-dose lovastatin compared with cholestyramine after 12 weeks of treatment.[17] Lower-dose lovastatin was also more efficacious than cholestyramine but to a lesser degree compared with the higher-dose regimen. The Lovastatin Study Group IV,[18] on the other hand, compared lovastatin with probucol (another bile acid resin) in 290 hypercholesterolemic patients and demonstrated that statin therapy was associated with an 80% greater reduction in LDL levels and a 25% greater lowering in triglyceride levels. The Finnish Multicenter Study compared lovastatin therapy with gemfibrozil treatment in 334 patients with hypercholesterolemia and showed that lovastatin was 2 to 4 times more effective than gemfibrozil in reducing LDL concentrations.[19]

The Familial Atherosclerosis Treatment Study (FATS)[20] was performed to assess whether or not intensive lipid-lowering strategies would translate to improvement in arteriographic and clinical outcomes. The trial randomized 146 patients at high risk for CHD events into treatments with lovastatin and colestipol, niacin and colestipol, or conventional therapy. Coronary arteriography, performed at baseline and at 30 months, showed that both lovastatin- and niacin-based regimens were associated with significantly better atherosclerotic indices compared with conventional therapy. Notably, lovastatin-based therapy was associated with a 14% less incidence in progression and an 18% increase in the frequency of regression of atherosclerotic lesions compared with the niacin-based treatment. After 2.5 years of follow-up, the study demonstrated that intensive lipid-lowering therapy with either lovastatin- or niacin-based regimens was associated with a 73% reduction in major CHD events compared with conventional therapy.

These findings confirmed the superior efficacy and safety profile of statins, which facilitated the evolution of lipid-lowering therapy from the earlier classes of LDL-lowering drugs to the modern era where statin class has become the preferred, standard agents (**Fig. 1**) and has since revolutionized the medical treatment of CVD.

MECHANISMS OF STATIN EFFECTS

The HMG-CoA reductase enzyme catalyzes the first committed step of cholesterol synthesis in the mevalonate pathway. Statins lower LDL levels primarily through the inhibition of this specific enzyme. The more potent agents have been shown to reduce LDL levels by up to 55%. In addition, statins also decrease triglyceride levels to a lesser degree (up to 20%), presumably through the inhibition of its synthesis in the liver and enhancement of lipoprotein lipase enzyme activity in the adipocytes.[21,22] Furthermore, statins are known to modestly increase levels of HDL (up to 10%). The precise mechanism by which statins increase HDL levels is not known; however, it is thought to result from apolipoprotein A1 gene induction through the activation of peroxisome proliferator–activated receptors.[23] It is also postulated that certain lipid-independent effects of statins (commonly referred to as pleiotropic effects) contribute to some degree to their antiatherothrombotic properties. Among the purported mechanisms are modulation of inflammatory response, improvement of endothelial function, and inhibition of coagulation.[24]

The reduction in LDL levels and the overall improvement in lipid profile associated with drug therapy have been shown to halt the progression and facilitate the regression of atherosclerotic lesions. This concept was established by the early coronary arteriographic studies on lipid-lowering therapy that used different classes of agents, including statins (**Table 1**). Regression of plaque

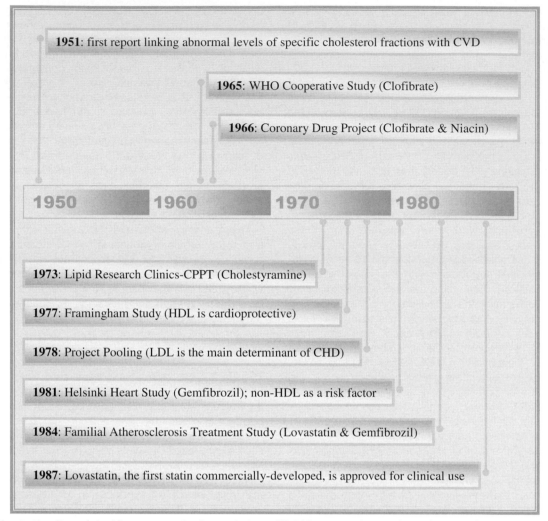

Fig. 1. Timeline of significant events in the evolution of lipid-lowering therapy from the age of fibrates to the current era of statins.

was observed in mild, moderate, or severe lesions. However, these changes (when expressed in absolute terms) seem remarkably small, and a large majority of stenoses do not improve even with intensive lipid-modulating regimens. Nevertheless, the use of lipid-lowering agents was associated with substantial reductions in clinical event rates, which seemed out of proportion to the observed arteriographic changes.[25]

It was later found that most of the acute coronary events were attributed to mild and moderate lesions, which may abruptly progress to severe occlusions as a result of plaque rupture or disruption, resulting in unstable angina or MI.[26] The vulnerable plaque is characterized by a large lipid core, predominance of lipid-laden macrophages, and a thin fibrous cap. In early experimental studies, lipid-lowering therapy has been shown to deplete cholesterol levels from the core lipid pool and significantly reduce the number of lipid-laden macrophages. The stabilization of vulnerable plaque was believed to be responsible for the sizeable reduction in clinical event rates seen in the lipid-lowering trials.[25]

Recent clinical trials corroborate the efficacy of statins in halting the progression and inducing the regression of atherosclerosis within relatively short periods of time. In the Reversal of Atherosclerosis with Aggressive Lipid Lowering (REVERSAL) trial[27] of more than 500 patients with CHD, 18 months of high-intensity statin treatment using atorvastatin was found to be associated with significant reduction in the rate of progression of coronary atherosclerotic burden. In this study, significantly slower rates of atherosclerotic progression, as measured by intravascular ultrasonography (IVUS), were

Table 1
Summary of arteriographic outcomes and frequencies of reported clinical events in the early lipid-lowering trials

Study	Control Subjects			Treatment Subjects			Clinical Event Reduction
	Progression (%)	Regression (%)	Mean Change in Percent Stenosis	Progression (%)	Regression (%)	Mean Change in Percent Stenosis	
NHLBI	49	7	—	32	7	—	33%
CLAS	61	2	—	39	16	—	25%
PORCH	65	6	—	37	14	—	35% (SS)
Lifestyle	32	32	+3.4	14	41	−2.2 (SS)	0 vs 1
FATS (N+C)	46	11	+2.1	25	39	−0.9 (SS)	80% (SS)
FATS (L+C)				22	32	−0.7 (SS)	70%
CLAS II	83	6	—	30	18	—	43%
UC-SCOR	41	13	+0.8	20	33	−1.5 (SS)	1 vs 0
STARS (D)	46	4	+5.8	10	38	−1.1 (NS)	69% (SS)
STARS (D+R)				12	33	−1.9 (SS)	89%
SCRIP	—	10	—	—	21	—	50%
Heidelberg	42	4	+3.0	20	30	−1.0 (SS)	

A positive (+) value represents "progression;" a negative (−) value represents "regression."
Abbreviations: C, colestipol; D, diet; L, lovastatin; N, niacin; NS, not significant; R, resin (colestipol or cholestyramine); SS, statistically significant.
Data from Brown BG, Zhao XQ, Sacco DE, et al. Lipid lowering and plaque regression. New insights into prevention of plaque disruption and clinical events in coronary disease. Circulation 1993;87:1781–91.

especially noted in patients with greater reductions in LDL and C-reactive protein (CRP) levels. Also, in nearly 1000 asymptomatic individuals with subclinical atherosclerosis, the Measuring Effects on Intima-Media Thickness: an Evaluation of Rosuvastatin (METEOR)[28] trial showed that statin treatment significantly slowed the rate of increase of carotid intima-media thickness (a measure of atherosclerosis) on ultrasonography, a change that was evident as early as 12 months within initiation of therapy.[29] Furthermore, in more than 500 patients with CHD, A Study to Evaluate the Effect of Rosuvastatin on Intravascular Ultrasound-Derived Coronary Atheroma Burden trial (ASTEROID) found that 2 years of high-intensity statin therapy resulted in a significant reduction in coronary atheroma volume and overall plaque burden as measured by IVUS.[30]

More recent experimental data also substantiate the plaque-stabilizing effects of statins, which is the presumed mechanism for the prevention of most adverse CVD events. Animal and human studies have demonstrated that statin therapy results in significant reductions in lipid content, LDL oxidation, inflammation, and apoptosis in atherosclerotic plaques. The lipid depletion and reduction of inflammatory activity within the plaque are accompanied by increased collagen content and expression of antiinflammatory mediators. These processes represent the statin-induced molecular changes in plaque composition that favor stability.[31]

STATINS AND PRIMARY PREVENTION OF CVD EVENTS

In epidemiologic terms, primary prevention refers to the avoidance of development of a particular disease or event through treatment or interventions directed toward the risk factors of said condition. Because the lipoproteins (specifically LDLs) are pivotal in the atherosclerotic process, it was thought that lipid-lowering therapy using statins could reduce the risk of coronary events in individuals who are at risk but have not had a previous CVD event.

The role of statin therapy in primary prevention in patients with abnormally elevated cholesterol levels is well documented. The West of Scotland Coronary Prevention Study (WOSCOPS)[32] assessed the effects of statin therapy on major CHD events in more than 6500 hyperlipidemic patients with no previous history of MI. After a 5-year follow-up, the trial revealed that pravastatin treatment was associated with significant reductions in nonfatal MI by 31% and cardiovascular mortality by 32%. This finding was further validated by the more recent Management of Elevated Cholesterol

in the Primary Prevention Group of Adult Japanese (MEGA)[33] trial. The study demonstrated a 48% reduction in MI and a 28% reduction in total mortality with pravastatin therapy in nearly 8000 hyperlipidemic patients without prior history of MI or stroke. Both WOSCOPS and MEGA trials also found a nonsignificant 11% to 17% decrease in stroke incidence with pravastatin.

Statins were also shown to have a primary preventive role in those who have moderate cholesterol levels. The Air Force/Texas Coronary Atherosclerosis Prevention Study (AFCAPS/TexCAPS)[34] enrolled more than 6600 patients with average cholesterol levels and free of overt CVD, who were followed for occurrence of first CHD event. After 5 years of follow-up, the trial found that lovastatin therapy was associated with a 40% reduction in MI and a 37% decrease in combined CHD event rates. This finding was congruent with that of the earlier and smaller Asymptomatic Carotid Artery Progression Study (ACAPS) of more than 900 asymptomatic patients with moderate cholesterol levels, which showed that lovastatin therapy was associated with a 64% reduction in CHD event rates.[35]

The lipid-lowering arm of the Anglo-Scandinavian Cardiac Outcomes Trial (ASCOT-LLA) randomized more than 10,300 hypertensive patients with average or lower than average cholesterol profile and have at least 3 other risk factors to treatment with either low-dose atorvastatin or placebo. The study was prematurely terminated after 3.3 years when it found a significant 36% reduction in fatal CHD and nonfatal MI, as well as a 27% decrease in fatal and nonfatal stroke in the atorvastatin group.[36] Further analysis of trial also demonstrated that atorvastatin was associated with less wave reflection and less augmentation of carotid blood pressure in well-controlled hypertensive individuals, suggesting a possible favorable interaction between statin treatment and antihypertensive therapy, which may be a contributing factor to the observed beneficial cardiovascular effects.[37]

A meta-analysis of 10 randomized primary prevention trials involving nearly 64,000 patients found that statin therapy, on average, reduces the risks of MI by 27%, stroke by 12%, and overall mortality by 7% (**Fig. 2**). Of note, the study found no increase in major adverse effects such as cancer or rhabdomyolysis with statins, confirming the overall safety of these agents.[38]

Recently, the potential beneficial effect of statin therapy in asymptomatic patients was evaluated by the Justification for the Use of Statins in Prevention: an Intervention Trial Evaluating Rosuvastatin (JUPITER),[39] which enrolled nearly 18,000

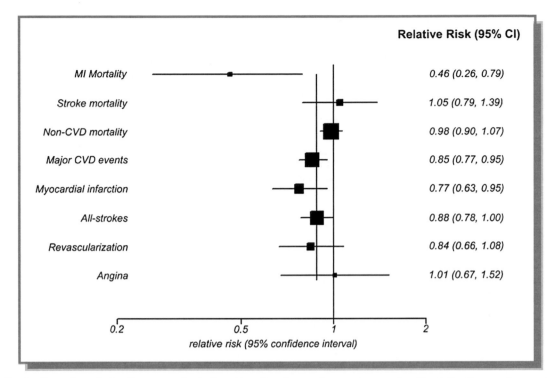

Relative Risk (95% CI)

MI Mortality	0.46 (0.26, 0.79)
Stroke mortality	1.05 (0.79, 1.39)
Non-CVD mortality	0.98 (0.90, 1.07)
Major CVD events	0.85 (0.77, 0.95)
Myocardial infarction	0.77 (0.63, 0.95)
All-strokes	0.88 (0.78, 1.00)
Revascularization	0.84 (0.66, 1.08)
Angina	1.01 (0.67, 1.52)

relative risk (95% confidence interval)

Fig. 2. Plotted pooled estimates and relative risks of major cardiovascular events with statin therapy in a meta-analysis of 10 primary prevention trials. (*From* Mills EJ, Rachlis B, Wu P, et al. Primary prevention of cardiovascular mortality and events with statin treatments: a network meta-analysis involving more than 65,000 patients. J Am Coll Cardiol 2008;52:1769–81; with permission.)

apparently healthy subjects with normal cholesterol levels and elevated CRP levels. The study was terminated early after only 1.9 years of follow-up when preliminary results showed that treatment with rosuvastatin led to significant reductions of 54% in MI, 51% in stroke, and 20% in total mortality in this group of seemingly low-risk individuals.

A later analysis of JUPITER data clarified that only a quarter of the patients enrolled in the trial are considered low risk, and most of them are at least in the intermediate risk category based on Framingham and Reynolds risk scores (34% were in the 5%–10% and 41% were in the 10%–20% range of 10-year CHD risk). When stratified according to underlying risk, no benefit was observed in the low-risk patients. Only those in the intermediate risk category derived a significant 45%–49% reduction in CVD events from statin therapy.[40]

There have been significant concerns raised regarding the clinical applicability or utility of the JUPITER trial. Some of the concerns raised include methodological design flaws, including the ill-defined basis for the early termination of the study, potential clinical and epidemiologic inconsistencies in the data, and similar rates of cardiovascular mortality in the treatment and control groups.[41] Clearly, more data are required

from other studies duplicating the results of the JUPITER trial before widespread application in the clinical setting is considered.

STATINS AND SECONDARY PREVENTION OF CVD EVENTS

Secondary prevention refers to the measures and therapies intended to avert the recurrence of disease or event in an individual who already had such condition. Although the clinical significance and economic consequences of treating healthy patients with lipid-lowering agents remains uncertain, the benefit of statin therapy in the secondary prevention of CHD events is well established. Although data establishing the link between hyperlipidemia and cerebrovascular disease are not as robust as that establishing the link between hyperlipidemia and CHD, the stroke outcomes in most secondary studies have been favorably affected with statin therapy.

The Scandinavian Simvastatin Survival Study (4S)[42] was the first large randomized clinical trial to demonstrate such advantageous effect. The study enrolled 4444 patients with established CHD, who were observed for more than 5 years. The trial showed that long-term treatment with simvastatin was associated with significant reductions in the rates of overall mortality by 30%, coronary mortality by 42%, major coronary events by 34%, and cerebrovascular events by 37%. Furthermore, this study was one of the first to point out that the benefit of statins also extended to women and older individuals.

The 4S was followed by the Cholesterol and Recurrent Events (CARE)[43] study involving more than 4000 MI patients with average cholesterol levels. This trial found that after 5 years of treatment, pravastatin therapy lowered major CHD events by 24%, the need for coronary revascularization by 23%, and stroke incidence by 31%. Of note, the benefit conferred by statin treatment on CVD events was greater in women than in men and larger in those with higher baseline LDL levels.

The CARE trial, however, was unable to definitively show that statin therapy reduces the risk of death. The mortality benefit of statins was subsequently established by the Long-Term Intervention with Pravastatin in Ischemic Disease (LIPID)[44] study. In more than 9000 CHD patients with a broad range of cholesterol levels, the LIPID trial was able to demonstrate that treatment with pravastatin for more than 6 years was associated with significant decreases in the rates of overall mortality by 22%, coronary death by 24%, MI by 29%, coronary revascularization by 20%, and stroke by 19%.

Similar results were seen in the Heart Protection Study, a large randomized trial involving over 20,500 patients with CVD who were treated with simvastatin for 5 years. Substantial survival advantages and morbidity reductions were seen with statin therapy after the follow-up period, including significant decreases in the rates of all-cause mortality by 13%, coronary death by 18%, nonfatal MI by 38%, coronary revascularization by 24%, major CHD events by 27%, and stroke by 25%. Furthermore, the study also found that the magnitude of benefit from statin therapy was dependent on the individual's overall CVD risk rather than lipid profile alone.

In a meta-analysis of 25 clinical trials involving nearly 70,000 CHD patients with a wide range of pretreatment LDL levels, it was estimated that statin therapy reduces total mortality by 16%, CHD mortality by 23%, and major CHD events by 25% (**Fig. 3**). These beneficial effects extended to women and the elderly and even at baseline LDL levels below 100 mg/dL.[45]

High-Intensity Versus Low-Intensity Statin Therapy

A key issue when discussing statin therapy in the secondary prevention of CVD events is the intensity of treatment, and still needing to be resolved is the important clinical question asking "how low should you go?" The results of several clinical trials have shown that higher-dose statin therapy is generally correlated with a greater reduction in atherosclerosis progression, and this was best demonstrated in the REVERSAL trial.[27] In this study of more than 500 patients with CHD, high-intensity statin treatment (atorvastatin, 80 mg daily) was associated with significant reduction in the rate of progression of coronary atherosclerotic burden (measured using IVUS) compared with moderate-intensity (pravastatin, 40 mg daily) therapy.

Patients at the highest risk for CHD events were shown to derive substantial benefit from high-intensity statin treatment, even with only short-term therapy. In the Myocardial Ischemia Reduction with Aggressive Cholesterol Lowering (MIRACL)[46] trial, more than 3000 patients hospitalized for acute coronary syndrome (ACS) were given either placebo or high-dose atorvastatin (80 mg daily), regardless of baseline LDL levels. The study found that after only 4 months of treatment, the addition of high-dose statin to the usual ACS therapies resulted in a 24% lowering of recurrent ischemic events.

Similarly, in more than 4000 patients with ACS, the Pravastatin or Atorvastatin Evaluation and Infection Therapy—Thrombolysis In Myocardial Infarction 22 (PROVE IT-TIMI 22) trial showed that intensive statin therapy (using atorvastatin, 80 mg daily) was superior to moderate-intensity treatment (using pravastatin, 40 mg daily) in preventing subsequent CHD events. The study found that intensive therapy lowered the first occurrence of major CVD events or death by 17% after 30 days, 18% after 90 days, and 16% after 2 years of follow-up.[47] Moreover, recurrent CVD events were also reduced by 19% with high-dose statin treatment during the same follow-up period.[48]

In high-risk individuals, a more intensive statin regimen also translates to better clinical outcomes, even if the LDL levels are within "normal" ranges. The Treat to New Targets (TNT) trial enrolled more than 10,000 patients with CHD and LDL levels less than 130 mg/dL, who were given either 10 mg or 80 mg of atorvastatin daily. After 5 years of follow-up, the study found that high-dose statin therapy was associated with significant decreases of 22% in total CVD events and 21% in coronary events[49] (**Table 2**). Nearly half of the TNT population had previous coronary bypass surgery,[50] and in this subgroup of patients, intensive statin therapy resulted in further reductions of 27% in major CVD events and repeat revascularization by 30%.

Study	Statin Therapy, No./Total No.	Placebo Use, No./Total No.	RR (95% CI Fixed)	Weight, %	RR (95% CI Fixed)
Pravastatin					
CARE[3]	212/2081	274/2078		9.5	0.77 (0.65-0.91)
LIPID[4]	557/4512	715/4502		24.8	0.78 (0.70-0.86)
PLAC-I[16,17]	14/281	29/278		1.0	0.48 (0.26-0.88)
PMSG[19]	0/530	7/532		0.3	0.07 (0.00-1.17)
PROSPER/CHD[13]	166/1306	211/1259		7.4	0.76 (0.63-0.92)
Subtotal	**949/8710**	**1236/8649**		**43.0**	**0.76 (0.70-0.82)**
Test for heterogeneity: $\chi^2_4=5.16$; $P=.27$					
Test for overall effect: $z=-6.77$; $P<.001$					
Pravastatin (after PTCA)					
PREDICT[15]	7/347	5/348		0.2	1.40 (0.45-4.38)
Subtotal	**7/347**	**5/348**		**0.2**	**1.40 (0.45-4.38)**
Test for heterogeneity: $\chi^2_0=0.0$					
Test for overall effect: $z=0.58$; $P=.6$					
Simvastatin					
4S[2]	431/2221	623/2223		21.6	0.69 (0.62-0.77)
CIS[21]	2/129	7/125		0.2	0.28 (0.06-1.31)
HPS/CHD[12]	717/6694	927/6692		32.1	0.77 (0.71-0.85)
Subtotal	**1150/9044**	**1557/9040**		**54.0**	**0.74 (0.69-0.79)**
Test for heterogeneity: $\chi^2_2=3.88$; $P=.14$					
Test for overall effect: $z=-8.51$; $P<.001$					
Fluvastatin					
Riegger et al[26]	2/187	5/178		0.2	0.38 (0.07-1.94)
Subtotal	**2/187**	**5/178**		**0.2**	**0.38 (0.07-1.94)**
Test for heterogeneity: $\chi^2_0=0.0$					
Test for overall effect: $z=-1.16$; $P=.2$					
Fluvastatin (after PTCA/PCI)					
FLARE[27]	6/409	17/425		0.6	0.37 (0.15-0.92)
LIPS[14]	42/844	60/833		2.1	0.69 (0.47-1.01)
Subtotal	**48/1253**	**77/1258**		**2.7**	**0.62 (0.44-0.88)**
Test for heterogeneity: $\chi^2_1=1.56$; $P=.21$					
Test for overall effect: $z=-2.66$; $P=.008$					
Total	**2156/19541**	**2880/19473**		**100**	**0.75 (0.71-0.79)**
Test for heterogeneity: $\chi^2_1=13.83$; $P=.24$					
Test for overall effect: $z=-11.14$; $P<.001$					

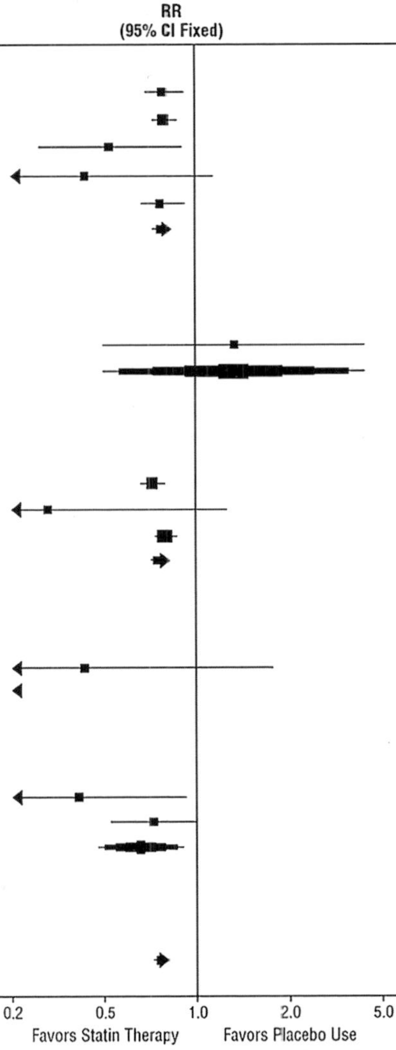

0.2   0.5   1.0   2.0   5.0

Favors Statin Therapy   Favors Placebo Use

Fig. 3. Comparison of relative risks for CHD mortality and nonfatal MI between statin therapy and placebo from the different secondary prevention trials. (*From* Wilt TJ, Bloomfield HE, MacDonald R, et al. Effectiveness of statin therapy in adults with coronary heart disease. Arch Intern Med 2004;164:1430; with permission. Copyright 2004 American Medical Association. All rights reserved.)

Table 2
Estimated hazard ratios for the individual cardiovascular outcomes with high-intensity statin therapy compared with low-intensity statin therapy in the TNT trial

Outcome	10 mg of Atorvastatin (N = 5006)	80 mg of Atorvastatin (N = 4995)	Hazard Ratio (95% CI)	P Value
		no with first event (%)		
Primary outcome				
Total major cardiovascular events	548 (10.9)	434 (8.7)	0.78 (0.69–0.89)	<0.001
Death from CHD	127 (2.5)	101 (2.0)	0.80 (0.61–1.03)	0.09
Nonfatal, nonprocedure–related MI	308 (6.2)	243 (4.9)	0.78 (0.66–0.93)	0.004
Resuscitation after cardiac arrest	26 (0.5)	25 (0.5)	0.96 (0.56–1.67)	0.89
Fatal or nonfatal stroke	155 (3.1)	117 (2.3)	0.75 (0.59–0.96)	0.02
Secondary outcomes				
Major coronary event	418 (8.3)	334 (6.7)	0.80 (0.69–0.92)	0.002
Cerebrovascular event	250 (5.0)	196 (3.9)	0.77 (0.64–0.93)	0.007
Hospitalization for congestive heart failure	164 (3.3)	122 (2.4)	0.74 (0.59–0.94)	0.01
Peripheral artery disease	282 (5.6)	275 (5.5)	0.97 (0.83–1.15)	0.76
Death from any cause	282 (5.6)	284 (5.7)	1.01 (0.85–1.19)	0.92
Any cardiovascular event	1677 (33.5)	1405 (28.1)	0.81 (0.75–0.87)	<0.001
Any coronary event	1326 (26.5)	1078 (21.6)	0.79 (0.73–0.86)	<0.001

Data from LaRosa, Grundy, Waters, et al. Intensive lipid lowering with atorvastatin in patients with stable coronary dis. New Engl J Med 2005;352:1432.

Correspondingly, the Incremental Decrease in End Points through Aggressive Lipid Lowering (IDEAL)[51] trial compared the treatment strategies of high-dose atorvastatin (80 mg daily) versus usual-dose simvastatin (20 mg daily) in 8888 patients with CHD. After nearly 5 years of follow-up, the study demonstrated significant reductions of 13% in major CVD events and 16% in coronary events with high-dose atorvastatin therapy.

Statins in Other High-Risk CVD Conditions

There is accumulating evidence that indicate possible morbidity and mortality benefits of adding lipid-modifying therapy in patients with other high-risk CVD conditions such as diabetes mellitus, peripheral vascular disease (PVD), and chronic kidney disease (CKD).

Analysis of data on diabetic patients enrolled in the LIPID, CARE, and 4S secondary prevention trials showed that statin therapy was associated with significant reductions in CHD events by 28% and stroke by 32% across a wide range of pretreatment LDL levels.[52] The Heart Protection Study also found a 22% lowering in coronary events and stroke in patients with diabetes who were treated with simvastatin, irrespective of comorbidities and baseline cholesterol levels.[53] The prospective, randomized, multicenter Collaborative Atorvastatin Diabetes Study (CARDS)[54] subsequently corroborated these findings in more than 2800 diabetic patients with average cholesterol levels without preexisting CVD, demonstrating curtailment in CHD events by 36%, stroke by 48%, and mortality by 27% with atorvastatin treatment. Data from the CARDS study provided the convincing evidence that supports the role of statin therapy for the primary prevention of CVD events in all diabetic patients.

Patients with CHD and metabolic syndrome, in particular, derive incremental benefit from higher-dose statin therapy, whether or not diabetes is present (**Fig. 4**). More than 5500 patients with CHD in the TNT trial had metabolic syndrome, and this group of patients had a 44% higher incidence of CVD events compared with those without metabolic syndrome. In the patients with metabolic syndrome, 5 years of treatment with high-dose atorvastatin (80 mg daily) resulted in a 29% reduction in CVD events compared with a low-dose regimen (10 mg daily).[55]

A post-hoc analysis of the Heart Protection Study also revealed a similar degree of improvement in CVD outcomes in those with PVD. In

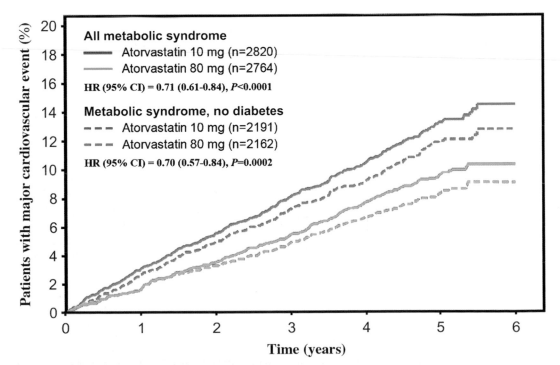

Fig. 4. Time to first major cardiovascular event in nondiabetic patients with metabolic syndrome in the TNT trial. (*Adapted from* Deedwania P, Barter P, Carmena R, et al. Reduction of low-density lipoprotein cholesterol in patients with coronary heart disease and metabolic syndrome: analysis of the Treating to New Targets Study. Lancet 2006;368:919–28; with permission.)

more than 6700 patients enrolled in the study, statin therapy decreased CVD events by 22% and noncoronary revascularization by 20%, effects that appeared independent of lipid lowering.[56] Results of smaller trials further suggest that statin use may be linked with improvements in walk performance, leg function, and symptoms in individuals with PVD.[57-59]

The TNT study showed that CHD patients with CKD had a 35% higher incidence of CVD events compared with those with normal glomerular filtration rate (GFR). A subanalysis of data from TNT[60] on more than 3000 patients with CHD and concomitant CKD revealed a 32% reduction in the risk of major CVD events with high-dose compared with low-dose atorvastatin therapy. Furthermore, both statin regimens resulted in increases in GFR over time, but a significantly greater improvement in renal function was observed with intensive atorvastatin therapy, suggesting a dose-related effect.[61]

A systematic review of 26 trials involving over 25,000 patients with CKD not requiring dialysis[62] revealed that the reduction of LDL levels achieved with statin therapy was associated with significant decreases in nonfatal CVD events by 25%, CVD deaths by 20%, and total mortality by 19%. These findings, however, were not observed in those with end-stage CKD. The German Diabetes and Dialysis Study (GDDS)[63] and A Study to Evaluate the Use of Rosuvastatin in Subjects on Regular Hemodialysis: An Assessment of Survival and Cardiovascular Events (AURORA)[64] trial both found no significant beneficial effect of statin therapy on CVD outcomes in patients requiring maintenance dialysis. One possible explanation for the negative results was that initiating lipid-lowering therapy in patients who already have end-stage renal disease may be too late to translate into consistent improvement of outcomes.

MANAGEMENT GUIDELINES ON STATIN THERAPY IN CVD PREVENTION

For primary prevention of CHD and stroke in low-risk patients, the National Cholesterol Education Program: Adult Treatment Panel III (NCEP-ATP III) guidelines recommend initiation of lipid-lowering drug therapy if LDL level is more than 190 mg/dL (optional if LDL>160 mg/dL). Pharmacologic treatment, to date, is not advocated for healthy individuals with LDL level less than 160 mg/dL, unless 2 or more CVD risk factors are present (**Table 3**).[65]

For patients with established CHD, the prevailing secondary prevention guidelines recommend prompt initiation of statin therapy to achieve a goal of LDL level less than 100 mg/dL, using intensity sufficient enough to achieve a 30% to 40% reduction in LDL levels in high-risk individuals. A target LDL goal of less than 70 mg/dL using high-dose statin treatment is also considered desirable.[66] In addition, in patients with ACS, including those who underwent revascularization, it is strongly advocated that statin therapy be started regardless of baseline LDL levels.[67] Similarly, the current guidelines on the secondary prevention of cerebrovascular disease recommend

Table 3
The NCEP-ATP III goals for LDL cholesterol and cutpoints for therapeutic lifestyle changes and drug therapy in different risk categories

Risk Category	LDL Goal	LDL Level at Which to Initiate Therapeutic Lifestyle Changes (TLCs)	LDL Level at Which to Consider Drug Therapy
CHD or CHD Risk equivalents (10-year risk >20%)	<100 mg/dL	>100 mg/dL	≥130 mg/dL (100-129 mg/dL: drug optional)
2+ Risk factors (10-year risk ≤20%)	<130 mg/dL	>130 mg/dL	10-year risk 10%-20%: ≥130 mg/dL 10-year risk <10%: ≥ 60 mg/dL
0-1 Risk factor[a]	<160 mg/dL	>160 mg/dL	190 mg/dL (160-189 mg/dL: LDL-lowering drug optional)

[a] Risk factors include cigarette smoking, hypertension, family history of premature CHD, age (men>45 years; women>55 years), and low HDL cholesterol (high HDL cholesterol>60 mg/dL counts as a "negative" risk factor, which removes 1 risk factor from the total count).
Data from ATP III Guidelines at-a-Glance Quick Desk Reference. Bethesda, MD: National Institutes of Health; May 2001. NIH publication no. 01-3305.

statin therapy with a target LDL goal of less than 100 mg/dL for those with CHD or symptomatic atherosclerotic disease and LDL cholesterol level less than 70 mg/dL for higher-risk persons with multiple risk factors.[68]

Because diabetes mellitus, PVD, and CKD are considered CHD equivalents, the management guidelines set forth by the American Heart Association/American College of Cardiology, American Diabetes Assocation,[69] and National Kidney Foundation[70] all advocate an aggressive secondary prevention approach to lipid-lowering therapy in these patients, recommending the use of statins to achieve a target LDL level of at least less than 100 mg/dL, similar to that of patients with established CHD.

There have always been propositions for an expanded use of statin agents in a greater proportion of the general population since the publication of the earliest evidence of the beneficial effects of lipid-lowering therapy in the primary prevention setting. Recently, this has been fueled even further by the results of the JUPITER trial. It remains to be seen whether or not future updates to the current clinical preventive management guidelines will extend the use of statins to healthy, normocholesterolemic, intermediate-to high-risk individuals (eg, those similar to the JUPITER trial population). Although statins are proved to be safe and serious adverse effects are rare, they are not completely benign. One still has to consider the risk-benefit ratio of this approach in asymptomatic persons. Also, in an economic climate emphasizing the need for significant curtailment in healthcare expenditure, the substantial fiscal drain associated with treating large numbers of normal people without CVD risk factors requires further evaluation and consideration.

There have also been proposals for a more aggressive approach to lipid-lowering therapy for secondary prevention. Some have criticized the NCEP-ATP III recommendations for not setting lower LDL target levels. However, this may be forthcoming in the new guidelines as most of the data supporting intensive lipid-lowering therapy to achieve lower LDL target levels have only become available after the publication of the NCEP-ATP III guidelines. Although there is no arguing against the fact that greater lipid-lowering is associated with a higher magnitude of improvement in outcomes, the reality is a large number of patients are not able to achieve LDL levels less than 70 mg/dL, even with the newer, more potent lipid-lowering drugs. The issue of targeting a specific numeric value for LDL versus simply using high-dose statin treatment as the initial approach to therapy in high-risk patients with CVD is a subject of major debate.

ROLE OF LIPID-LOWERING AGENTS OTHER THAN STATINS

There are several additional options available for LDL reduction in patients who are either intolerant to statins or are unable to reach target goals with the maximal doses of the available statins. In such patients, combination therapy with bile acid resin, niacin, and cholesterol intestinal absorption inhibitor (eg, ezetimibe) can be considered. It is important to note that there are several limitations to the use of any of these medications. For example, the bile acid resins are not well tolerated and have significant side effects. Although treatment with niacin can be beneficial, its combination with statins increases the risk of myopathy and hepatotoxicity. Such combinations, therefore, are restricted only to high-risk patients when dual therapy is essential.

In contrast to the bile acid resins and niacin derivatives, the cholesterol absorption inhibitor ezetimibe has gained popularity because of the virtual lack of side effects. Furthermore, this agent does not seem to increase the adverse effects of statins when used in combination. The addition of ezetimibe to statin therapy generally produces a 15% to 18% additional reduction in LDL levels[71] and as such appeared reasonable in those who are in need of combination therapy. However, recent data from a number of studies have raised questions about the clinical benefit of reducing LDL with ezetimibe. The controversy started with the results of the Ezetimibe and Simvastatin in Hypercholesterolemia Enhances Atherosclerosis Regression (ENHANCE) trial[72] involving more than 700 patients with familial hypercholesterolemia, which showed no improvement in atherosclerosis parameters with the addition of ezetimibe compared with statin therapy alone, despite the achievement of target cholesterol goals. There have been similar studies showing similar disappointing results.[73,74]

Medical communities are eagerly awaiting the results of the definitive Improved Reduction of Outcomes: Vytorin Efficacy International Trial (IMPROVE-IT)[75] to finally close this article regarding the clinical utility of LDL reduction with ezetimibe. Until such data become available, most clinicians are routinely not using ezetimibe for their patients, unless no other effective therapy is feasible.

SUMMARY

Although the overall burden of CVD remains high, the adverse outcomes from it have been on a declining trend. The use of statins and other guideline-based therapies has contributed significantly to this development. The benefit of statin therapy in the primary prevention of CVD events is well documented. Recently, evidence of mortality and morbidity reduction from CVD with statin use has been observed in healthy, low-risk individuals. Although lipid-lowering therapy for primary prevention purposes in those with abnormal cholesterol profile is clearly justified, the value of treating normal individuals with these drugs remains uncertain. The role of statin therapy in the secondary prevention of CVD events is well established in patients with CHD and stroke. There is also data of desirable results in individuals with other CVD conditions such as diabetes mellitus, PVD, and CKD. The proposal to further lower the current target LDL treatment goals certainly has its merits. However, this may not be achievable in a number of patients. The strategy of simply using high-intensity statin therapy, rather than focusing on specific LDL levels alone, still requires further clarification. Combination of statin and ezetimibe therapy is well tolerated and efficacious, but no clinical benefit has been seen so far with this treatment approach.

REFERENCES

1. The global burden of disease: 2004 update. World Health Organization; 2008.
2. Lloyd-Jones D, Adams RJ, Brown TM, et al. American Heart Association Statistics Committee and Stroke Statistics Subcommittee. Executive summary: heart disease and stroke statistics—2010 update: a report from the american heart association. Circulation 2010;121(7):948—54.
3. Navab M, Ananthramaiah GM, Reddy ST, et al. The oxidation hypothesis of atherogenesis: the role of oxidized phospholipids and HDL. J Lipid Res 2004;45(6):993—1007.
4. Shah PK, Kaul S, Nilsson J, et al. Exploiting the vascular protective effects of high-density lipoprotein and its apolipoproteins: an idea whose time for testing is coming, part I. Circulation 2001;104: 2376—83.
5. Fuster V, Moreno PR, Fayad ZA, et al. Atherothrombosis and high-risk plaque: part I: evolving concepts. J Am Coll Cardiol 2005;46(6):937—54.
6. Gofman JW, Jones HB, Lindgren FT, et al. Blood lipids and human atherosclerosis. Circulation 1950; 2(2):161—78.
7. Barr DP, Russ EM, Eder HA. Protein-lipid relationships in human plasma. II. In atherosclerosis and related conditions. Am J Med 1951;11(4):480—93.
8. A co-operative trial in the primary prevention of ischaemic heart disease using clofibrate. Report

9. Clofibrate and niacin in coronary heart disease. JAMA 1975;231(4):360—81.
10. Canner PL, Berge KG, Wenger NK, et al. Fifteen year mortality in coronary drug project patients: long-term benefit with niacin. J Am Coll Cardiol 1986;8:1245—55.
11. Pooling project research group: relationship of blood pressure, serum cholesterol, smoking habit, relative weight, and ECG abnormalities to incidence of major coronary events: final report of the pooling project. J Chronic Dis 1978;31:201—306.
12. Gordon T, Castelli WP, Hjortland MC, et al. High density lipoprotein as a protective factor against coronary heart disease: the Framingham Study. Am J Med 1977;62:707—14.
13. The lipid research clinics coronary primary prevention trial results. II. The relationship of reduction in incidence of coronary heart disease to cholesterol lowering. JAMA 1984;251(3):365—74.
14. Frick MH, Elo O, Haapa K, et al. Helsinki Heart Study: primary-prevention trial with gemfibrozil in middle-aged men with dyslipidemia. Safety of treatment, changes in risk factors, and incidence of coronary heart disease. N Engl J Med 1987;317(20): 1237—45.
15. Tobert JA, Bell GD, Birtwell J, et al. Cholesterol-lowering effect of mevinolin, an inhibitor of 3-hydroxy-3-methylglutaryl-coenzyme a reductase, in healthy volunteers. J Clin Invest 1982;69(4):913—9.
16. Hoeg JM, Maher MB, Zech LA, et al. Effectiveness of mevinolin on plasma lipoprotein concentrations in type II hyperlipoproteinemia. Am J Cardiol 1986; 57(11):933—9.
17. The lovastatin study group III. A multicenter comparison of lovastatin and cholestyramine therapy for severe primary hypercholesterolemia. JAMA 1988; 260(3):359—66.
18. The lovastatin study group IV. A multicenter comparison of lovastatin and probucol for treatment of severe primary hypercholesterolemia. Am J Cardiol 1990;66(8):22B—30B.
19. Tikkanen MJ, Helve E, Jäättelä A, et al. Comparison between lovastatin and gemfibrozil in the treatment of primary hypercholesterolemia: the Finnish Multicenter Study. Am J Cardiol 1988;62(15):35J—43J.
20. Brown G, Albers JJ, Fisher LD, et al. Regression of coronary artery disease as a result of intensive lipid-lowering therapy in men with high levels of apolipoprotein B. N Engl J Med 1990;323(19):1289—98.
21. Saiki A, Murano T, Watanabe F, et al. Pitavastatin enhanced lipoprotein lipase expression in 3T3-L1 preadipocytes. J Atheroscler Thromb 2005;12(3): 163—8.
22. Jones PH, Davidson MH, Stein EA, et al. Comparison of the efficacy and safety of rosuvastatin versus

atorvastatin, simvastatin, and pravastatin across doses (STELLAR* Trial). Am J Cardiol 2003;92(2): 152–60.

23. Yano M, Matsumura T, Senokuchi T, et al. Statins activate peroxisome proliferator-activated receptor gamma through extracellular signal-regulated kinase 1/2 and p38 mitogen-activated protein kinase-dependent cyclooxygenase-2 expression in macrophages. Circ Res 2007;100(10):1442–51.

24. Ray KK, Cannon CP. The potential relevance of the multiple lipid-independent (pleiotropic) effects of statins in the management of acute coronary syndromes. J Am Coll Cardiol 2005;46(8):1425–33.

25. Brown BG, Zhao XQ, Sacco DE, et al. Lipid lowering and plaque regression. New insights into prevention of plaque disruption and clinical events in coronary disease. Circulation 1993;87(6):1781–91.

26. Ambrose JA, Winters SL, Arora RR, et al. Angiographic evolution of coronary artery morphology in unstable angina. J Am Coll Cardiol 1986;7(3): 472–8.

27. Nissen SE, Tuzcu EM, Schoenhagen P, et al. Reversal of atherosclerosis with aggressive lipid lowering (REVERSAL) investigators. Statin therapy, LDL cholesterol, C-reactive protein, and coronary artery disease. N Engl J Med 2005;352(1):29–38.

28. Crouse JR 3rd, Raichlen JS, Riley WA, et al. Effect of rosuvastatin on progression of carotid intima-media thickness in low-risk individuals with subclinical atherosclerosis: the METEOR Trial. JAMA 2007; 297(12):1344–53.

29. Bots ML, Palmer MK, Dogan S, et al. Intensive lipid lowering may reduce progression of carotid atherosclerosis within 12 months of treatment: the METEOR study. J Intern Med 2009;265(6):698–707.

30. Nissen SE, Nicholls SJ, Sipahi I, et al. Effect of very high-intensity statin therapy on regression of coronary atherosclerosis: the ASTEROID trial. JAMA 2006;295(13):1556–65.

31. Crisby M, Nordin-Fredriksson G, Shah PK, et al. Pravastatin treatment increases collagen content and decreases lipid content, inflammation, metalloproteinases, and cell death in human carotid plaques: implications for plaque stabilization. Circulation 2001;103(7):926–33.

32. Shepherd J, Cobbe SM, Ford I, et al. Prevention of coronary heart disease with pravastatin in men with hypercholesterolemia. N Engl J Med 1995; 333:1301–7.

33. Nakamura H, Arakawa K, Itakura H, et al. Primary prevention of cardiovascular disease with pravastatin in Japan (MEGA Study): a prospective randomised controlled trial. Lancet 2006;368(9542): 1155–63.

34. Downs JR, Clearfield M, Weis S, et al. Primary prevention of acute coronary events with lovastatin in men and women with average cholesterol levels: results of AFCAPS/TexCAPS. Air Force/ Texas Coronary Atherosclerosis Prevention Study. JAMA 1998;279(20):1615–22.

35. Furberg CD, Adams HP Jr, Applegate WB, et al. Effect of lovastatin on early carotid atherosclerosis and cardiovascular events. Asymptomatic Carotid Artery Progression Study (ACAPS) Research Group. Circulation 1994;90(4):1679–87.

36. Sever PS, Dahlöf B, Poulter NR, et al. Prevention of coronary and stroke events with atorvastatin in hypertensive patients who have average or lower-than-average cholesterol concentrations, in the Anglo-Scandinavian Cardiac Outcomes Trial–Lipid Lowering Arm (ASCOT-LLA): a multicentre randomised controlled trial. Lancet 2003;361(9364): 1149–58.

37. Manisty C, Mayet J, Tapp RJ, et al. Atorvastatin treatment is associated with less augmentation of the carotid pressure waveform in hypertension: a substudy of the Anglo-Scandinavian Cardiac Outcome Trial (ASCOT). Hypertension 2009;54(5):1009–13.

38. Mills EJ, Rachlis B, Wu P, et al. Primary prevention of cardiovascular mortality and events with statin treatments: a network meta-analysis involving more than 65,000 patients. J Am Coll Cardiol 2008;52(22): 1769–81.

39. Ridker PM, Danielson E, Fonseca FA, et al. JUPITER study group. Rosuvastatin to prevent vascular events in men and women with elevated C-reactive protein. N Engl J Med 2008;359(21):2195–207.

40. Ridker PM, MacFayden JG, Nordestgaard BG, et al. Rosuvastatin for primary prevention among individuals with elevated high-sensitivity C-reactive protein and 5% to 10% and 10% to 20% 10-year risk. Circ Cardiovasc Qual Outcomes 2010;3(5):447–52. [Epub ahead of print].

41. de Lorgeril M, Salen P, Abramson J, et al. Cholesterol lowering, cardiovascular diseases, and the rosuvastatin-JUPITER controversy: a critical reappraisal. Arch Intern Med 2010;170(12):1032–6.

42. The 4S Investigators. Randomised trial of cholesterol lowering in 4444 patients with coronary heart disease: the Scandinavian Simvastatin Survival Study (4S). Lancet 1994;344(8934):1383–9.

43. Sacks FM, Pfeffer MA, Moye LA, et al. The effect of pravastatin on coronary events after myocardial infarction in patients with average cholesterol levels. Cholesterol and Recurrent Events Trial investigators. N Engl J Med 1996;335(14):1001–9.

44. The Long-Term Intervention with Pravastatin in Ischaemic Disease (LIPID) Study Group. Prevention of cardiovascular events and death with pravastatin in patients with coronary heart disease and a broad range of initial cholesterol levels. N Engl J Med 1998;339(19):1349–57.

45. Wilt TJ, Bloomfield HE, MacDonald R, et al. Effectiveness of statin therapy in adults with coronary

heart disease. Arch Intern Med 2004;164(13): 1427–36.

46. Schwartz GG, Olsson AG, Ezekowitz MD, et al. Myocardial Ischemia Reduction with Aggressive Cholesterol Lowering (MIRACL) Study Investigators. Effects of atorvastatin on early recurrent ischemic events in acute coronary syndromes: the MIRACL study: a randomized controlled trial. JAMA 2001; 285(13):1711–8.

47. Cannon CP, Braunwald E, McCabe CH, et al. Intensive versus moderate lipid lowering with statins after acute coronary syndromes. N Engl J Med 2004;350: 1495–504.

48. Murphy SA, Cannon CP, Wiviott SD, et al. Reduction in recurrent cardiovascular events with intensive lipid-lowering statin therapy compared with moderate lipid-lowering statin therapy after acute coronary syndromes from the PROVE IT-TIMI 22 (Pravastatin or Atorvastatin Evaluation and Infection Therapy-Thrombolysis In Myocardial Infarction 22) trial. J Am Coll Cardiol 2009;54(25):2358–62.

49. LaRosa JC, Deedwania PC, Shepherd J, et al. TNT Investigators. Comparison of 80 versus 10 mg of atorvastatin on occurrence of cardiovascular events after the first event (from the Treating to New Targets [TNT] trial). Am J Cardiol 2010;105(3):283–7.

50. Shah SJ, Waters DD, Barter P, et al. Intensive lipid-lowering with atorvastatin for secondary prevention in patients after coronary artery bypass surgery. J Am Coll Cardiol 2008;51(20):1938–43.

51. Pedersen TR, Faergeman O, Kastelein JJ, et al. High-dose atorvastatin vs usual-dose simvastatin for secondary prevention after myocardial infarction: the IDEAL study: a randomized controlled trial. JAMA 2005;294(19):2437–45.

52. Keech A, Colquhoun D, Best J, et al. The LIPID Study Group. Secondary prevention of cardiovascular events with long-term pravastatin in patients with diabetes or impaired fasting glucose: results from the LIPID trial. Diabetes Care 2003;26: 2713–21.

53. Collins R, Armitage J, Parish S, et al. Heart Protection Study Collaborative Group. MRC/BHF heart protection study of cholesterol-lowering with simvastatin in 5963 people with diabetes: a randomised placebo controlled trial. Lancet 2003;361:2005–16.

54. Colhoun HM, Betteridge DJ, Durrington PN, et al. CARDS Investigators. Primary prevention of cardiovascular disease with atorvastatin in type 2 diabetes in the Collaborative Atorvastatin Diabetes Study (CARDS): multicentre randomised placebo-controlled trial. Lancet 2004;364:685–96.

55. Deedwania P, Barter P, Carmena R, et al. Reduction of low-density lipoprotein cholesterol in patients with coronary heart disease and metabolic syndrome: analysis of the Treating to New Targets study. Lancet 2006;368(9539):919–28.

56. Heart Protection Study Collaborative Group. Randomized trial of the effects of cholesterol-lowering with simvastatin on peripheral vascular and other major vascular outcomes in 20,536 people with peripheral arterial disease and other high-risk conditions. J Vasc Surg 2007;45(4):645–54.

57. McDermott MM, Guralnik JM, Greenland P, et al. Statin use and leg functioning in patients with and without lower-extremity peripheral arterial disease. Circulation 2003;107(5):757–61.

58. Giri J, McDermott MM, Greenland P, et al. Statin use and functional decline in patients with and without peripheral arterial disease. J Am Coll Cardiol 2006; 47(5):998–1004.

59. Mohler ER, Hiatt WR, Creager MA. Cholesterol reduction with atorvastatin improves walking distance in patients with peripheral arterial disease. Circulation 2003;108(12):1481–6.

60. Shepherd J, Kastelein JJ, Bittner V, et al. Intensive lipid lowering with atorvastatin in patients with coronary heart disease and chronic kidney disease: the TNT (Treating to New Targets) study. J Am Coll Cardiol 2008;51(15):1448–54.

61. Shepherd J, Kastelein JJ, Bittner V, et al. Effect of intensive lipid lowering with atorvastatin on renal function in patients with coronary heart disease: the Treating to New Targets (TNT) study. Clin J Am Soc Nephrol 2007;2(6):1131–9.

62. Navaneethan SD, Pansini F, Perkovic V, et al. HMG CoA reductase inhibitors (statins) for people with chronic kidney disease not requiring dialysis. Cochrane Database Syst Rev 2009;(2):CD007784.

63. Wanner C, Krane V, März W, et al. German Diabetes and Dialysis Study Investigators. Atorvastatin in patients with type 2 diabetes mellitus undergoing hemodialysis. N Engl J Med 2005;353(3):238–48.

64. Fellström BC, Jardine AG, Schmieder RE, et al. AURORA Study Group. Rosuvastatin and cardiovascular events in patients undergoing hemodialysis. N Engl J Med 2009;360(14):1395–407.

65. Grundy SM, Cleeman JI, Merz CN, et al. The Coordinating Committee of the National Cholesterol Education Program. Implications of recent clinical trials for the national cholesterol education program adult treatment panel III guidelines. Circulation 2004; 110:227–39.

66. Smith SC, Allen J, Blair SN, et al. AHA/ACC guidelines for secondary prevention for patients with coronary and other atherosclerotic vascular disease: 2006 update. Circulation 2006;113:2363–72.

67. Anderson JL, Adams CD, Antman EM, et al. ACC/AHA 2007 guidelines for the management of patients with unstable angina/non–ST-elevation myocardial infarction: a report of the American College of Cardiology/American Heart Association Task Force on Practice Guidelines (Writing Committee to Revise the 2002 Guidelines for the Management of Patients

With Unstable Angina/Non–ST-Elevation Myocardial Infarction): developed in collaboration with the American College of Emergency Physicians, American College of Physicians, Society for Academic Emergency Medicine, Society for Cardiovascular Angiography and Interventions, and Society of Thoracic Surgeons. J Am Coll Cardiol 2007;50:e1–157.

68. Sacco RL, Adams R, Albers G, et al. Guidelines for prevention of stroke in patients with ischemic stroke or transient ischemic attack: a statement for healthcare professionals from the American heart association/American stroke association council on stroke: co-sponsored by the council on cardiovascular radiology and intervention: the American academy of neurology affirms the value of this guideline. Circulation 2006;113(10):e409–49.

69. American Diabetes Association. Standards of medical care in diabetes–2008. Diabetes Care 2008;31(Suppl 1):S12–54.

70. National Kidney Foundation. K/DOQI clinical practice guidelines for managing dyslipidemias in chronic kidney disease. Am J Kidney Dis 2003; 41(4 Suppl 3):S1–2.

71. Armitage J. Commentary on NICE technology appraisal guidance on ezetimibe for the treatment of primary (heterozygous-familial and non-familial) hypercholesterolaemia. Heart 2008;94(5):643–5.

72. Kastelein JJ, Akdim F, Stroes ES, et al. ENHANCE investigators. Simvastatin with or without ezetimibe in familial hypercholesterolemia. N Engl J Med 2008;358(14):1431–43.

73. Taylor AJ, Villines TC, Stanek EJ, et al. Extended-release niacin or ezetimibe and carotid intima-media thickness. N Engl J Med 2009;361(22): 2113–22.

74. Rossebø AB, Pedersen TR, Boman K, et al. Intensive lipid lowering with simvastatin and ezetimibe in aortic stenosis. N Engl J Med 2008;359(13): 1343–56.

75. Cannon CP, Giugliano RP, Blazing MA, et al. Rationale and design of IMPROVE-IT (IMProved Reduction of Outcomes: Vytorin Efficacy International Trial): comparison of ezetimibe/simvastatin versus simvastatin monotherapy on cardiovascular outcomes in patients with acute coronary syndromes. Am Heart J 2008;156(5):826–32.

Focusing on High-Density Lipoprotein for Coronary Heart Disease Risk Reduction

Michael H. Davidson, MD[a,b,*]

KEYWORDS

- High-density lipoprotein cholesterol
- Coronary heart disease • High-density lipoprotein particles
- Reverse cholesterol transport • Risk reduction

An estimated 16.8 million persons, or 7.6% of the United States population, have coronary heart disease (CHD), and cardiovascular disease is responsible for 864,480 or 35.3% of all deaths on an annual basis.[1] Focused risk reduction therapies are indicated for patients with CHD to reduce recurrent events and improve survival rates for these patients. The association between low-density lipoprotein cholesterol (LDL-C) and high-density lipoprotein cholesterol (HDL-C) and the development of CHD is widely acknowledged. In addition, the cardiovascular benefit for lipid lowering below current cholesterol goal levels (LDL-C ≤70 mg/dL) for those with chronic CHD is now well established.[2] Current treatment strategies for reducing risk in CHD require a focus on increasing low HDL-C level because reducing LDL-C alone is insufficient in preventing CHD events.[3–5]

Low levels of HDL-C commonly occur in patients at high risk of CHD, including patients who are obese and those with the metabolic syndrome. It is estimated that low HDL-C levels (<40 mg/dL) are found in 39% of men and 15% of women 20 years of age and older, many of whom also have elevated LDL-C levels.[2] The National Cholesterol Education Program Adult Treatment Panel III identifies an LDL-C goal of less than 100 mg/dL and a non-HDL-C goal (for patients with triglycerides greater than 200 mg/dL) of 130 mg/dL for patients at high risk for CHD events.[6]

A low serum HDL-C level has been demonstrated to be a risk factor for CHD. Considerable data from over 35 years of the Framingham Heart Study have shown that subjects with the highest HDL-C levels exhibited the lowest risk of developing CHD.[7] The first report from the Framingham Study, which was based on 4 years of surveillance, demonstrated an inverse relationship between HDL-C and CHD incidence.[8] Follow-up studies demonstrated that study participants at the 80th percentile of HDL-C were found to have half the risk of CHD developing when compared with subjects at the 20th percentile of HDL-C. In addition, each 1% increase in HDL-C was linked to a 2% reduction in the development of CHD. Similarly, other studies have supported the role of low HDL-C as an independent risk factor for CHD including the Physicians' Health Study,[9] in which subjects with low HDL-C had increased risk for CHD, and the Israeli Ischemic Heart Disease Study, in which subjects with low total cholesterol and high HDL-C had the lowest rates of CHD-associated morbidity and mortality.[10]

a Department of Medicine, Section of Cardiology, Pritzker School of Medicine, University of Chicago, 5758 South Maryland Avenue, Chicago, IL 60637, USA
b Radiant Research, 515 North State Street, Suite 2700, Chicago, IL 60654, USA
* Department of Medicine, Section of Cardiology, Pritzker School of Medicine, University of Chicago, 5758 South Maryland Avenue, Chicago, IL 60637.
E-mail address: michaeldavidson@radiantresearch.com

Cardiol Clin 29 (2011) 105–122
doi:10.1016/j.ccl.2010.11.005
0733-8651/11/$ — see front matter © 2011 Elsevier Inc. All rights reserved.

However, while several animal studies and clinical trials support an atheroprotective role for HDL, most of the findings were obtained in the context of changes in other plasma lipids, limiting identification of the individual role of HDL in atherosclerosis prevention.[11]

Treatment of coronary artery disease (CAD) has traditionally focused on reducing LDL-C, and statin therapy is an acknowledged component of the treatment regimen in improving CAD outcomes.[12] However, a significant issue is that approximately 70% of CAD events have not been prevented in statin trials.[13,14] As a result, increasing HDL-C is recognized as a strategy for reducing CAD risk. Yet modification of HDL by pharmacologic therapy remains complex because the HDL-C concentration may not be an adequate biomarker for total HDL particles or indicate the antiatherothrombotic properties of HDL or effective reverse cholesterol transport (RCT). In addition, a combination of mass and functional aspects may be responsible for the cardioprotective mechanisms by which HDL reduces atherosclerosis.

Several large epidemiologic studies have demonstrated that the level of HDL-C is an independent risk factor for CAD, including substantial data from the Framingham Heart Study, which demonstrated that subjects with the highest HDL-C levels had the lowest risk of developing CAD.[7] Raising low levels of HDL-C, defined as less than 40 mg/dL (1 mg/dL = 0.02586 mmol/L) by the National Cholesterol Education Program Adult Treatment Panel III (NCEP ATP III),[6] is an important goal in targeting CAD risk reduction. Review of several large clinical trials, including the Framingham Heart Study, the Lipid Research Clinics (LRC) Prevalence Mortality Follow-Up Study, the LRC Primary Prevention Trial, and the Multiple Risk Factor Intervention Trial, identified that a 1-mg/dL increase in HDL-C results in a 2% to 3% reduction in risk.[15]

The relationship of low HDL-C levels and increased CAD risk is well substantiated in the literature. In a study of more than 3000 patients in the Myocardial Ischemia Reduction with Aggressive Cholesterol Lowering (MIRACL) trial, patients with the metabolic syndrome, characterized as the presence of 3 characteristics including a history of diabetes mellitus, a history of hypertension and/or blood pressure 130/85 mm Hg or more, a body mass index of 30 kg/m^2 or more, HDL-C levels less than 40 mg/dL (men) or less than 50 mg/dL (women), and triglycerides 150 mg/dL or more (38%; n = 1161), had a 19% incidence of a primary end-point event (death, nonfatal myocardial infarction, cardiac arrest, or recurrent unstable myocardial ischemia) (**Fig. 1**).[16]

In addition, low HDL-C levels have been found to be predictive of CAD events after acute coronary syndrome (ACS). In a study of more than 1000 patients with non−ST-segment elevation myocardial infarction ACS treated with drug-eluting stent implantation, the incidence of mortality and major adverse cardiac events at 30 days was higher in patients with low levels of HDL-C (<40 mg/dL in men and <45 mg/dL in

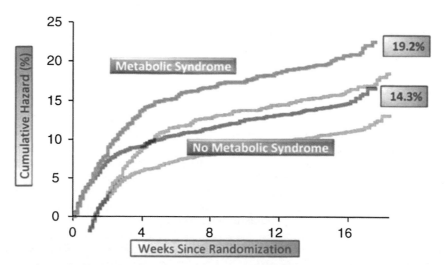

Fig. 1. Presence of metabolic syndrome, which is usually associated with low high-density lipoprotein (HDL) cholesterol, increases the risk of early recurrent events after acute coronary syndrome (hazard ratio, 1.40; 95% confidence interval, 1.16−1.67; P<.001). (*Data from* Schwartz GG, Olsson AG, Szarek M, et al. Relation of characteristics of metabolic syndrome to short-term prognosis and effects of intensive statin therapy after acute coronary syndrome: an analysis of the Myocardial Ischemia Reduction with Aggressive Cholesterol Lowering (MIRACL) trial. Diabetes Care 2005;28:2508−13.)

women) (P>.001 and P = .002, respectively; χ^2 analysis). A low baseline level of HDL-C was found to be a significant predictor of major adverse cardiac events and death (hazard ratio, 3.33; 95% confidence interval, 1.15–10.0) at 1 year.[17]

Several biologic properties and mechanisms of actions attributed to HDL-C suggest that it can serve as a potential basis for antiatherosclerotic activity (**Fig. 2**).[18] HDL has an antiatherogenic effect by affecting RCT and noncholesterol-dependent mechanisms (**Fig. 3**).[19] RCT involves the transfer of excess cholesterol from lipid-laden macrophages present in peripheral tissues, to the liver via HDL, with subsequent catabolism of cholesterol, or secretion into bile. Other noncholesterol-dependent mechanisms include altering endothelial dysfunction and LDL oxidation.

HDL METABOLISM

The metabolism of HDL is accomplished through several pathways involved in the generation and conversion of HDL. Mature HDL3 and HDL2 are generated from lipid-free apolipoprotein AI (Apo AI) or lipid-poor pre-β1 HDL as the precursors. These precursors are produced as nascent HDL by the liver or intestine, or are released from lipolyzed very-low-density lipoprotein (VLDL) and chylomicrons or by interconversion of HDL3 and HDL2 (**Fig. 4**).[20]

An important step for initial lipidation is adenosine triphosphate binding cassette A1 (ABC A1)-mediated lipid efflux from cells. Lecithin-cholesterol acyltransferase (LCAT)-mediated esterification of cholesterol generates spherical particles that continue to grow on ongoing cholesterol esterification and phospholipid transfer protein (PLTP)-mediated particle fusion and surface remnant transfer. Larger HDL2 particles are converted into smaller HDL3 particles on cholesteryl ester transfer protein (CETP)-mediated export of cholesteryl esters (CEs) from HDL onto Apo B-containing lipoproteins, on scavenger receptor class B type I (SR-BI)-mediated selective uptake of CEs into liver and steroidogenic organs, and on hepatic lipase–mediated and endothelial lipase (EL)-mediated hydrolysis of phospholipids (**Fig. 5**).[21] HDL lipids are catabolized either separately from HDL proteins (ie, by selective uptake or via CETP transfer) or together with HDL proteins (ie, via uptake through as-yet-unknown HDL receptors or Apo B receptors). The conversion of HDL2 into HDL3 and the PLTP-mediated conversion of HDL3 into HDL2 liberate lipid-free or poorly lipidated Apo AI. A part of lipid-free Apo AI undergoes glomerular filtration in the kidney and tubular reabsorption through cubilin.

NONPHARMACOLOGIC APPROACHES FOR RAISING HDL

As outlined in the NCEP ATP III guidelines, therapeutic lifestyle changes, including dietary measures to reduce saturated fatty acids and cholesterol, regular aerobic exercise, weight loss, and smoking cessation are often initial interventions to lower LDL-C and raise HDL-C.[6] Dietary modification, including of omega-3 fatty acids via fish consumption or supplementation with fish oils, have also demonstrated an effect in raising HDL-C. When therapeutic lifestyle changes are not adequate to increase serum HDL-C, pharmacologic therapy is often indicated.

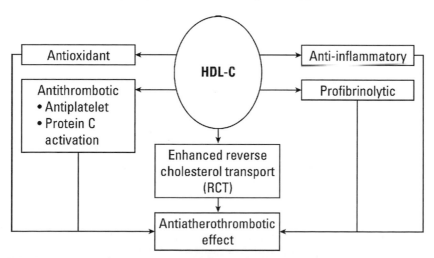

Fig. 2. Multiple biologic actions of HDL-C as a potential basis for antiatherosclerotic activity. (*Data from* Shah PK, Kaul S, Nilsson J, et al. Exploiting the vascular protective effects of high-density lipoprotein and its apolipoproteins: an idea whose time for testing is coming, part I. Circulation 2001;104:2376–83.)

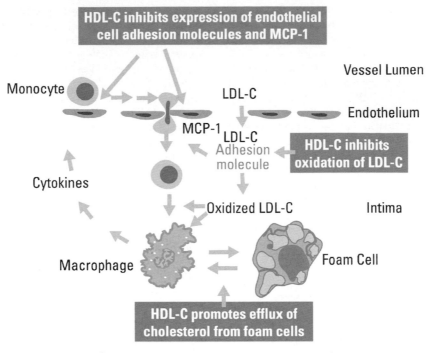

MCP-1 = monocyte chemoattractant protein-1.

Fig. 3. Potential antiatherogenic actions of HDL-C. LDL-C, low-density lipoprotein cholesterol. (*Data from* Barter PJ, Nicholls S, Rye KA, et al. Antiinflammatory properties of HDL. Circ Res 2004;95:764–72.)

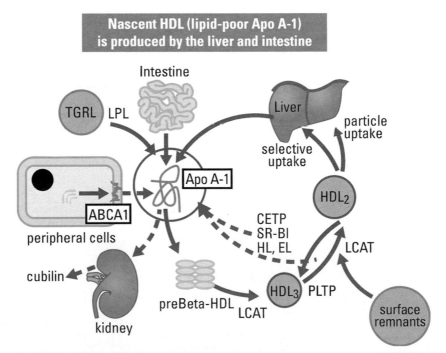

Fig. 4. HDL metabolism. ABCA1, adenosine triphosphate binding cassette A1; Apo A-1, apolipoprotein AI; CE, cholesteryl ester; CETP, cholesteryl ester transfer protein; EL, endothelial lipase; HL, hepatic lipase; LCAT, lecithin-cholesterol acyltransferase; LPL, lipoprotein lipase; PLTP, phospholipid transfer protein; SR-BI, scavenger receptor class B type I; TGRL, triglyceride-rich lipoprotein. (*Data from* Singh IM, Shishehbor MH, Ansell BJ, et al. High density lipoprotein as a therapeutic target: a systematic review. JAMA 2007;298:786–98.)

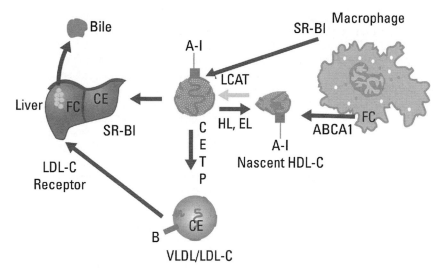

Fig. 5. HDL-C, RCT, and atherosclerosis. CE, cholesteryl ester; CETP, cholesteryl ester transfer protein; EL, endothelial lipase; FC, free cholesterol; HL, hepatic lipase; LCAT, lecithin-cholesterol acyltransferase; RCT, reverse cholesterol transport; SR-BI, scavenger receptor class B type I; VLDL, very-low-density lipoprotein. (*Data from* Cuchel M, Rader DJ. Genetics of increased HDL cholesterol levels: insights into the relationship between HDL metabolism and atherosclerosis. Arterioscler Thromb Vasc Biol 2003;23:1710–2.)

PHARMACOLOGIC THERAPY

When therapeutic lifestyle changes are not adequate to achieve target goals, several pharmacologic therapy options exist for the management of low HDL-C. **Table 1** outlines the principal drug classes that are used to increase HDL-C.[22] It is well established that 3-hydroxy-3-methylglutaryl coenzyme A (HMG-CoA) reductase inhibitors (statins) result in LDL-C lowering, which significantly affects cardiovascular morbidity and mortality. Statins are used in CHD to target the reduction of elevated LDL and to improve the lipid level profile. Other non-LDL lipid effects of statins, including decreasing triglycerides and raising HDL-C, may also contribute to the risk reduction. Additional therapies with significant non–LDL-lowering effects, such as fibrates and niacin, which

Table 1
Drugs that increase high-density lipoprotein cholesterol

Drug Class	HDL-C Increase	Side Effects	Contraindications	Clinical Trial Results
Statins	5%–15%	Myopathy, increased liver enzymes	Absolute: active or chronic liver disease, pregnancy Relative: certain drugs[a]	Reduced major coronary events, CHD deaths, need for coronary procedures, stroke, and total mortality
Fibrates	10%–20%	Dyspepsia, gallstones, myopathy, unexplained non-CHD deaths	Absolute: severe renal disease, severe hepatic disease	Reduced major coronary events
Niacin	15%–35%	Flushing, hepatotoxicity, hyperuricemia, upper gastrointestinal distress, hyperglycermia	Absolute: chronic liver disease, severe gout Relative: diabetes, hyperuricemia, peptic ulcer disease	Reduced major coronary events and possibly total mortality

[a] Including cytochrome P-450 inhibitors, cyclosporine, macrolide antibiotics, and various antifungal agents.
   Data from Toth PP. High density lipoprotein as a therapeutic target: clinical evidence and treatment strategies. Am J Cardiol 2005;96(9A):50K–58K.

lower triglycerides and raise HDL, also have been shown to reduce CHD events despite less potent effects on reducing LDL.[23] As highlighted in the NCEP ATP III guidelines, consideration should be given to combination therapy with a fibrate or nicotinic acid in addition to an LDL-lowering drug for high-risk patients with a low HDL-C level.

Statin Therapy

First-line management of patients with cardiovascular disease is achieved with statin therapy. In patients with low HDL-C, statins are very effective in reducing the absolute cardiovascular event rate; however, the residual risk often remains elevated. Statins typically increase HDL-C levels by approximately 5% to 10%. Although the mechanism(s) by which statins raise HDL-C remains unclear, statins appear to reduce the supranormal rates of endogenous CETP-mediated CE transfer from HDL by decreasing the number of Apo B lipoprotein available to accept CE from HDL. Statins also appear to enhance hepatic Apo AI production, which may not occur with high-dose atorvastatin (80 mg) in which there is less HDL-C increase compared with similar LDL-C lowering by simvastatin or rosuvastatin. The clinical relevance of the difference in the HDL-C increase between atorvastatin 80 mg and rosuvastatin 40 mg is being tested in the Study of Coronary Atheroma by Intravascular Ultrasound: Effect of Rosuvastatin Versus Atorvastatin (SATURN) trial, an intravascular ultrasound (IVUS) trial measuring plaque volume in CHD patients.[24]

Despite the established efficacy of statin therapy, a substantial number of CHD patients continue to have high residual risk for cardiovascular events. Statin trials have demonstrated reductions in the 5-year absolute risk of future CHD events with decreases in absolute risk reduction for patients with greater baseline risk, but often lower percent absolute risk reduction results, due to higher residual risk (**Fig. 6**).[25–27] However, despite substantial reductions in CHD morbidity and mortality that have been achieved with statins, data indicate that approximately two-thirds of all CHD events are not prevented with statin therapy.

Niacin Therapy

Niacin, or nicotinic acid, is a soluble B vitamin that has favorable effects on all major lipid subfractions but has limited use due to its side-effect profile. Although the exact mechanism of action of niacin is not well understood, it appears to reduce Apo B secretion, thereby lowering both VLDL and LDL, increasing Apo AI, and lowering lipoprotein a [Lp(a)]. Yet recent data suggest that niacin also increases the secretion of HDL Apo A1 by up-regulating both ABC A1 and Apo AI gene expression in the liver. This process results in the expression of very large HDL particles that, due to increased size, are more slowly catabolized. Niacin was one of the first lipid-altering drugs to demonstrate a reduction in CHD events in the Coronary Drug Project.[28] At present, niacin is identified as the most effective HDL-raising therapy. Although the mechanism by which niacin raises HDL is not well understood, the predominant

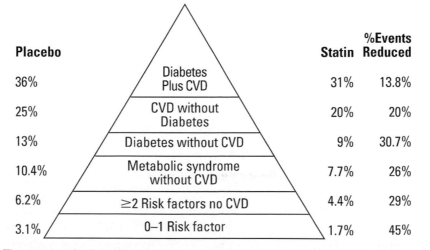

Placebo		Statin	%Events Reduced
36%	Diabetes Plus CVD	31%	13.8%
25%	CVD without Diabetes	20%	20%
13%	Diabetes without CVD	9%	30.7%
10.4%	Metabolic syndrome without CVD	7.7%	26%
6.2%	≥2 Risk factors no CVD	4.4%	29%
3.1%	0–1 Risk factor	1.7%	45%

The greater the baseline risk, the greater the absolute risk reduction but the lower the percent (%) absolute risk reduction due to higher residual risk

Fig. 6. Five-year absolute risk of future cardiovascular disease events. (*Data from* Refs.[25–27])

hypothesis is that niacin inhibits the holoparticle uptake of HDL, resulting in delayed catabolism. The uptake of SR-BI from HDL does not appear to be inhibited by niacin, and this seems to be the major route by which cholesterol ester is returned to the liver for biliary production (**Fig. 7**).[29] In clinical studies, niacin has been demonstrated to lower LDL by 10% to 20%, triglyceride (TG) by 20% to 40%, and Lp(a) by 10% to 30%, and to raise HDL by 15% to 30%. Niacin appears to increase HDL by decreasing the hepatic uptake of Apo AI, thereby delaying catabolism.

Despite niacin being widely used in the management of dyslipidemia, the side effect of flushing of the face and upper body can affect compliance to therapy. Flushing has been attributed as the major reason for discontinuation of therapy, estimated at rates as high as 25% to 40%. The cutaneous vasodilation skin flush typically starts in the face with a deep red coloration, usually accompanied by an intense feeling of warmth and itching, with occasional extension to the arms and chest. Although the duration of the flushing is generally less than 1 hour, the unpleasant sensation for patients can often affect compliance and lead to therapy discontinuation.

The flushing that is induced by niacin appears to be caused by the subcutaneous release of prostaglandin D_2 (PGD$_2$), which is mediated by niacin's action as a pharmacologic ligand for the adipocyte and macrophage G protein–coupled nicotinic acid receptor GPR109A (HM74A in humans, PUMA-G in mice), and to involve the formation of vasodilatory prostanoids (**Fig. 8**).[30] The exact cellular mechanisms responsible for flushing are not known, but epidermal Langerhans cells have been demonstrated to be essential mediators of the flushing response. Langerhans cells respond to niacin with an increase in calcium and the expression of prostanoid synthases, which are required for the formation of the prostaglandins (**Fig. 9**).[31–34]

The cutaneous release of PGD$_2$, with elevation of the PDG$_2$ metabolite 9α,11β-prostaglandin F$_2$, has been demonstrated to result in niacin-induced flushing. PGD$_2$ interacts in a paracrine manner with local capillary smooth muscle cells via the PGD$_2$ receptor 1 (DP1), resulting in cutaneous capillary vasodilation.[35]

Moderate doses of prostaglandin inhibitors have been demonstrated to reduce the cutaneous flushing response from niacin administration. Several additional strategies for reducing niacin-induced flushing include regular consistent dosing, use of extended-release formulations, patient education, dosing with meals or at bedtime, and avoidance of alcohol, hot beverages, spicy foods, and hot baths or showers close to or after dosing. In comparison with immediate-release niacin, extended-release niacin results in reduced flushing as it is taken once a day at bedtime, when most flushing symptoms will occur

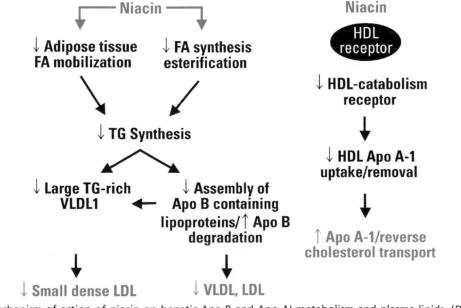

Fig. 7. Mechanism of action of niacin on hepatic Apo B and Apo AI metabolism and plasma lipids. (*Data from* Kamanna VS, Kashyap ML. Mechanism of action of niacin on lipoprotein metabolism. Curr Atheroscler Rep 2000;2:36–46.)

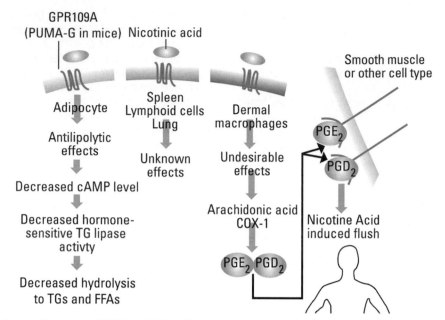

Fig. 8. Nicotinic acid receptor HM74A. cAMP, cyclic adenosine monophosphate; FFAs, free fatty acids; PG, prosta-glandin; TG, triglyceride. (*Data from* Pike NB. Flushing out the role of GPR109A (HM74A) in the clinical efficacy of nicotinic acid. J Clin Invest 2005;115:3400−3.)

when the patient is sleeping. However, the side-effect profile includes the potential for liver toxicity. Niacin should be discontinued if liver enzymes (aspartate aminotransferase and alanine amino-transferase) exceed 3 times the upper limit of normal. Other side effects include rash, flushing, gastrointestinal problems, worsening of esopha-geal reflux and gout, and headache. Promoting patient awareness of factors that can minimize niacin-induced flushing can help to enhance toler-ability to this valuable dyslipidemic agent with established cardiovascular benefits.

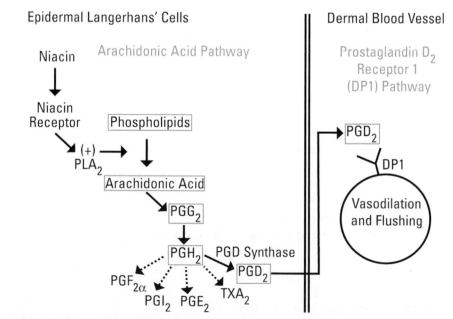

Fig. 9. An overview of the niacin-induced flushing pathway. PG, prostaglandin; PLA$_2$, phospholipase A$_2$; TXA$_2$, thromboxane A$_2$. Dashed arrows are normal parts of the arachidonic acid pathway that may or may not occur in Langerhans' cells. (*Data from* Refs.[31−34])

Statin Combination Therapy

The use of statin niacin therapy, statin-fibrate therapy, and novel therapies aimed at increasing low levels of HDL-C are often used to complement statin therapy. These additional statin combination therapies target other components of the dyslipidemic state to reduce the residual cardiovascular risk.

Statin-niacin combination therapy

Combination therapy with a statin and niacin has been used to reduce residual cardiovascular risk by targeting the lowering of LDL and increasing low HDL. Adding niacin to a statin is a likely combination, as niacin has the most significant effects on raising HDL. Several clinical trials using either immediate-release or extended-release niacin have demonstrated the efficacy and safety of this combination therapy in inhibiting the development of atherosclerosis. There has been increased interest in the use of combination therapy to maximize risk reduction in patients with dyslipidemia, due to the safety data of extended-release niacin in combination with a statin.

The Arterial Biology for the Investigation of the Treatment Effects of Reducing Cholesterol (ARBITER) 2 trial demonstrated that the addition of extended-release niacin to statin therapy resulted in an increase in HDL-C by 21% and slowed the progression of atherosclerosis via measurement of change in carotid intima-media thickness (CIMT) as compared with statin therapy alone in patients with known CHD and low HDL-C levels.[36]

Statin-fibrate combination therapy

Statin-fibrate combination therapy is effective in reducing LDL-C and TG, and in increasing HDL-C. Fibrates are peroxisome proliferator-activated receptor-alpha (PPAR-α) ligands that lead to increased lipoprotein lipase expression and decreased Apo CIII expression, which results in enhanced catabolism of TG-rich particles. The expression of Apo AI and A-II are also increased by fibrates, with a net result of decreasing hypertriglyceridemia and increasing HDL-C. Due to these effects, fibrate combination therapy is used for patients with hypertriglyceridemia and low HDL. The drug treatment options are similar in patients with high LDL-C and low HDL-C to those patients with isolated high LDL-C, with a somewhat greater emphasis on combination therapy that may beneficially modify HDL levels. In patients who are unable to achieve lipid goals with statin monotherapy, statin-fibrate combination therapy is considered a good therapeutic option.

However, statin-fibrate combination therapy has been a source of safety concerns due to the potential adverse effects on skeletal muscle, including myopathy. As a result, monitoring of liver function and creatine kinase (CK) is indicated with statin-fibrate combination therapy. The NCEP guidelines recommend discontinuing combination therapy (both statin and fibrate) if the CK is greater than 10 times the upper limit of normal associated with muscle symptoms such as tenderness, pain, or weakness.[6] Statin fibrate therapy is restricted, due to reports of rhabdomyolysis that mainly involved gemfibrozil and cerivastatin, which was voluntarily withdrawn from the market worldwide in 2001 after reports of fatal rhabdomyolysis. Fenofibrate or fenofibric acid is the fibrate of choice when used in combination with a statin because each is generally associated with a lower risk of myopathy than gemfibrozil. Several recent studies have demonstrated the efficacy and safety of fenofibric acid and statin therapy in patients with mixed dyslipidemia in reducing triglycerides and raising HDL-C compared with statin monotherapy.[37,38]

NOVEL HDL THERAPIES

This complex process involved in RCT provides multiple targets to modulate HDL metabolism with novel therapies. RCT involves the efflux of free cholesterol (FC) in the macrophage to discoidal pre-β1 HDL. Discoidal pre-β1 HDL is formed by Apo AI synthesized in the liver and intestine with the addition of phospholipid. These delipidated HDL particles pick up FC from cell membranes via the ABC A1 transporter to become discoidal α4 HDL. As this particle matures, it accumulates more FC from the cells (including macrophages) via the ABC G1 transporter. The FC is converted to CE by LCAT (LCAT adds a fatty acid from PC to FC) to form spherical α3 HDL, which contains both Apo AI and Apo AII. Via the action of lipoprotein lipase on triglyceride-rich lipoprotein, surface apolipoproteins (A1, AIV, and C apolipoproteins) are transferred to HDL via CETP and triglyceride is transferred to HDL in exchange for CE to form α2 HDL, which is further enlarged to α1 HDL. α1 HDL can be recycled back to pre-β1 HDL facilitated by EL and secretory phospholipase A2 (sPLA2). The α1 and α2 HDL can also donate CE to the liver via SR-BI. Once in the liver, CE is used for bile formation and is secreted into the intestine.

One simplified approach to modulating HDL metabolism is to consider potential therapies regarding the sequence of RCT; the efflux of FC from the macrophage to (1) increase cholesterol level in the acceptor, (2) increase circulatory levels of the acceptor for the FC, (3) decrease the catabolism of the lipid enriched acceptor, (4) increase the uptake of the acceptor in the liver, (5) enhance RCT as mediated by the intestine, and (6) modify the functionality of HDL to improve efflux capacity or other atheroprotective properties.[39]

Improving the Macrophage Free Cholesterol Efflux

The earliest step manifestations of the atherosclerotic process involve the cholesterol-loaded macrophage or foam cell. A challenging focus of antiatherosclerotic drug development has been selectively modifying the macrophage to more readily efflux FC to the HDL acceptor. Only FC is effluxed into the nascent HDL particle. However, increasing FC levels can be toxic to cells, leading to apoptosis and potentially enhanced atheroma development; this appears to be the case with some of the acyl-CoA cholesterol O-acyltransferase (ACAT) inhibitors. ACAT facilitate the conversion of FC to cholesterol ester while cholesterol ester hydrolase (CEH) converts cholesterol ester back from cholesterol. ACAT inhibitors were thought to be antiatherogenic by inhibiting FC conversion to lipid ester, resulting in more FC being available for efflux in HDL. However, 2 ACAT inhibitors, avasimibe and pactimibe, appear to increase plaque progression in human trials. The failure of these ACAT inhibitors has been disappointing, but there is one more ACAT inhibitor, NK-104, that continues in human trials evaluating plaque progression and inflammation by carotid magnetic resonance imaging. Another alternative strategy is to enhance CEH and animal studies in which CEH is overexpressed, supporting an antiatherosclerotic effect. Serum amyloid A (SAA) targets HDL to macrophages and up-regulates CEH. As a result, SAA may have antiatherogenic properties and, although a biomarker to increased risk, may become elevated in response to inflammatory stimuli in atherosclerotic plaques. CEH-enhancing peptides on SAA are yet to enter human trials.

Liver X receptor (LXR) is the nuclear receptor that up-regulates the ABC sterol transporters such as ABC A1 and ABC G1, which effluxes FC to either nascent (ABC A1) or mature HDL (ABC G1), protecting cells from cholesterol toxicity. LXR in the macrophage up-regulates the gene involved in FC efflux from the cells. Two receptor isoforms have been identified, LXRα and LXRβ. LXRα is ubiquitous, but LXRβ is more selectively found in the macrophage. Although LXR activation produces significant enhancement of RCT in animal models, this approach is hindered by the marked increase in hepatic steatosis associated with LXR agonism in the liver by up-regulation of SREBP1C, which stimulates lipogenesis. The steatosis appears to be related to LXRα but not LXRβ and, therefore, a selective LXRβ agonist may augment RCT without enduring hepatic lipogenesis, leading to steatosis.

Increasing Availability of FC Acceptor by Augmenting Apo AI

Increasing Apo A transgenically or infusing recombinant HDL (RHDL) in animal models promotes prominent regression of atherosclerosis and enhanced macrophage-specific RCT. Based on these animal models, this approach seems to offer the greatest clinical potential for HDL-based therapies. There are also several intriguing small human trials demonstrating that different approaches to increasing lipid-poor Apo AI acceptors induce regression of atherosclerosis in only 6 weeks in humans.

ETC-216 or Recombinant Apo AI Milano Complexed with Phospholipid

Apo AI Milano is a mutant Apo AI protein that was discovered in Italian families with low HDL-C but apparently decreased cardiovascular risk. ETC-216 infused in rabbits mobilized rabbit aortic cholesterol within hours. A small human IVUS trial showed that 5 weekly doses of ETC-216 significantly reduced atheroma by 4.2% compared with baseline, but hypersensitivity reactors and difficulty manufacturing ETC-216 has significantly delayed clinical development. In addition, transgenic animal experiments do not support the original concept that Apo AI Milano has greater FC efflux potential than wild-type Apo AI. IVUS was also used to assess the effect of infusion of reconstituted HDL on coronary atherosclerosis. The Atherosclerosis Safety and Efficacy (ERASE) Study[40] randomized 183 patients to placebo, 40 mg/kg, or 80 mg/kg of CSL-III, a reconstituted HDL consisting of Apo AI from human plasma combined with soybean phosphatidylcholine, which chemically and biologically resembles native HDL. Although liver function abnormalities resulted in early discontinuation of the higher dosage of CSL-III treatment, the short-term (4 weeks) infusion of CSL-III, 40 mg/kg resulted in statistically significant improvements in plaque characterization index on IVUS and coronary score on quantitative coronary angiography. However, no significant differences were found in change in atheroma volume or nominal change in plaque volume compared with placebo.

Although additional research is indicated, early results on the effect of manipulation of drug targets to infuse Apo AI are promising and may further contribute to a reduction in CHD events.[41] A reformulated version of CSC-111 (CSC-112) has been reported in preclinical studies to provide greater efflux capacity and likely less hepatotoxicity. At present, CSC-112 infusion therapy is in early human trials.

Another novel technique involves the collection of 1 L of plasma by apheresis. The technique includes over 2 hours of apheresis followed by selective lipid removed from HDL using organic solvents to produce lipid-poor pre-β HDL. The lipid-poor pre-β HDL, which is a more efficient acceptor of cholesterol, is then reinfused back into the patient. In another small human trial involving 28 patients with ACS, 7 weekly treatments resulted in a 5.2% decrease in atheroma volume compared with baseline. These small IVUS trials showed a similar 3.5% to 5% decrease in atheroma volume compared with baseline, but due to the small sample sizes was not statistically significantly different from placebo.

An oral drug trial with RVX-208 selectively induces nuclear transporter factors that induce hepatic and intestinal production of Apo AI. This compound significantly increases HDL-C by more than 40% in monkeys, and the serum of treated animals was shown to enhance cholesterol efflux from foam cells. Significant increases in total plasma Apo AI were demonstrated in a small and short-term human trial, but most of the increase was in pre-β HDL. RVX-208 was the first oral small molecule that stimulates Apo AII production to enter phase 2 trials. There are several Apo AI peptides that would potentially overcome some of the limitations with use of the entire Apo AI protein, such as cost of production and hypersensitivity. These 18- to 22-amino-acid peptides that mimic the region of Apo AI involved in lipid binding appear to inhibit LDL-induced monocyte activation and activation of LCAT. D4F is the most studied Apo AI mimetic. D4F does have some oral bioavailability and did affect HDL anti-inflammatory properties in humans at the highest dose, but appears to be poorly catabolized, and is unlikely to move forward until an alternative formulation is in development. Another Apo AI mimetic that is infused (Cerenis) is soon to enter a 500-patient IVUS trial.

Decrease the Catabolism of Lipid-Enriched Acceptor (Mature HDL) by CETP Inhibition

CETP inhibition represents a newer approach for elevating HDL-C. CETP plays an important role in cholesterol metabolism, as it is responsible for the transfer of CEs from HDL to VLDLs and LDLs (**Fig. 10**).[42] CETP is a very large protein and has a hydrophobic tunnel across the molecule that can accommodate neutral lipid. CETP is a shuttle-type structure that promotes an equal mass gradient transfer of triglyceride for cholesterol ester between HDL and Apo-B lipoprotein.[43] CETP appears to make things more uniformly distributed throughout the bloodstream and moves triglycerides where they are high (ie, VLDL) to where they are low (HDL and LDL) in exchange for an equal mass gradient of cholesterol ester. Animals that lack CETP have very high HDL and very low LDL. As a result, the role

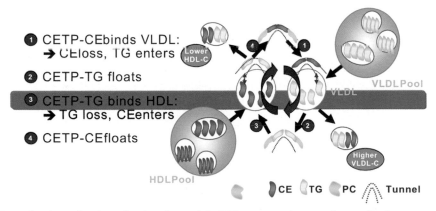

Fig. 10. CETP mechanism of action: the shuttle model. CETP operates by a carrier mechanism, accepting neutral lipids (triglyceride and cholesteryl ester) from a donor particle, shuttling them through the aqueous phase, and delivering them to an acceptor lipoprotein. (*Data from* Qiu X, Mistry A, Ammirati MJ, et al. Crystal structure of cholesteryl ester transfer protein reveals a long tunnel and four bound lipid molecules. Nat Struct Mol Biol 2007;14:106–13.)

of CETP is important in modulating HDL size by redistributing cholesterol ester from triglyceride-rich particles into HDL. The triglyceride-enriched HDL is further acted on by hepatic lipase to form a smaller dense HDL that is more rapidly catabolized. Therefore, inhibiting CETP by maintaining HDL particle size will reduce HDL catabolism. CETP is also involved in transporting triglycerides in exchange for cholesterol ester from triglyceride-rich particles to LDL, and therefore LDL becomes triglyceride enriched and further hydrolyzed by the lipases to form a small dense LDL. The atherogenicity of the lipoprotein particle is affected by many aspects of CETP as it attaches to the VLDL, takes in triglyceride, and exchanges cholesterol ester, shuttling that over to the HDL, and goes back and forth between these two particles. As a result, there is binding of the CETP to HDL to transport these different constituents from one lipoprotein to the other (see **Fig. 10**).[42]

Clinical trials with Japanese populations with CETP deficiency identified concurrent high levels of HDL-C, which led to the development of drugs targeting CETP activity to elevate HDL-C levels and potentially decrease cardiovascular risk (**Figs. 11** and **12**). However, results from recent clinical trials question the therapeutic use of at least one CETP inhibitor, torcetrapib, which was demonstrated to increase blood pressure and have no effect in decreasing the progression of coronary atherosclerosis.

Although initial studies with torcetrapib demonstrated significant increases in HDL-C levels of more than 50%, the risks of dose-dependent increases in blood pressure raised concern about the risk-benefit profile. Nevertheless, the concept of CETP inhibition may still represent a promising new focus to modulate CETP activity to alter atherogenesis.[39]

The potency of CETP inhibition in modulating HDL-C has been demonstrated in animal studies with mice and rabbits. Rabbits treated with the CETP inhibitor, torcetrapib, demonstrated increases in HDL from about 57 to 207 mg/dL. The effect of torcetrapib on the kinetics of CETP binding to HDL was analyzed, and the inhibitor effects attributed to the formation of a nonproductive complex between CETP and HDL. Studies in humans demonstrated that CETP inhibition was effective in increasing HDL-C and decreasing LDL-C beyond reductions seen with atorvastatin alone. Concurrent atorvastatin treatment with torcetrapib was shown to reduce Apo B-100 levels by enhancing VLDL Apo B-100 clearance and reducing production of intermediate-density lipoprotein and LDL Apo B-100.

Yet despite the impressive effects of CETP inhibition by torcetrapib in raising HDL-C levels, results from recent clinical trials raise skepticism over its therapeutic use. The Investigation of Lipid Level Management Using Coronary Ultrasound to Assess Reduction of Atherosclerosis by CETP Inhibition and HDL Elevation (ILLUSTRATE) trial assessed the effect of torcetrapib, 60 mg, plus atorvastatin compared with atorvastatin monotherapy on the progression of atherosclerosis in 1188 patients with CHD. Atorvastatin at an initial dose of 10 mg was titrated at 2-week intervals to 20 mg, 40 mg, or 80 mg to achieve target LDL-C levels.[44] After 24 months, there was an approximately 61% relative increase in HDL-C and a 20% relative decrease in LDL-C.

In another study, disease progression in 910 patients, as measured by repeated IVUS of the percent change of atheroma volume, was not significant in the treatment groups (0.19% in the atorvastatin-only group and 0.12% in the torcetrapib-atorvastatin group, $P = .72$). There was also no statistical difference in the change in 10 mm of the most diseased segment (reduction of 3.3 mm^3 in the atorvastatin-only group and of 4.2 mm^3 in the torcetrapib-atorvastatin group, $P = .12$). In addition, torcetrapib was also associated with an increase in systolic blood pressure of 4.6 mm Hg and an increase in all-cause mortality, resulting in the discontinuance of the trial.

In a phase 3 trial with approximately 15,000 patients at high risk for CHD, The Investigation of Lipid Level management to Understand its iMpact IN ATherosclerotic Events (ILLUMINATE) trial

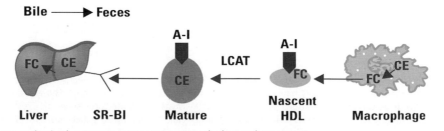

Fig. 11. Pharmacologic therapy to promote reverse cholesterol transport.

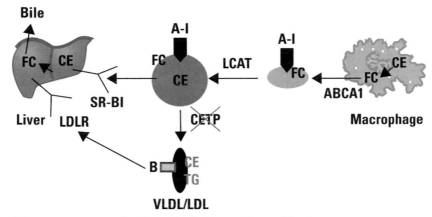

Fig. 12. CETP deficiency is associated with markedly increased HDL-C levels.

randomized subjects to treatment with torcetrapib (60 mg) plus atorvastatin versus atorvastatin alone (10–80 mg). However, the study was stopped because of significant increases in all-cause mortality in the torcetrapib/atorvastatin versus atorvastatin groups.[45]

The Rating Atherosclerotic Disease Change by Imaging with a New CETP Inhibitor (RADIANCE I) trial examined the effects of torcetrapib on carotid atherosclerosis in 850 patients with heterozygous familial hypercholesterolemia. The study used B-mode ultrasonography at baseline and at follow-up in patients randomized to atorvastatin monotherapy or atorvastatin at 20, 40, or 80 mg dose titrated at 4-week intervals to target LDL-C goals or to reach maximum tolerated dose, combined with torcetrapib 60 mg. After 24 months, the mean (±SD) HDL-C level was 52.4 ± 13.5 mg/dL and the mean LDL-C was 143.2 ± 42.2 mg/dL in the atorvastatin-only group, as compared with 81.5 ± 22.6 mg/dL and 115.1 ± 48.5 mg/dL in the torcetrapib-atorvastatin group. However, no significant differences were found in maximum CIMT increase (0.0053 ± 0.0028 mm per year in the atorvastatin-only group and 0.0047 ± 0.0028 mm per year in the torcetrapib-atorvastatin group, $P = .87$).[45] The results of the trial revealed that use of torcetrapib with atorvastatin, as compared with atorvastatin alone, did not cause further reduction of progression of atherosclerosis, as assessed by a combined measure of carotid arterial wall thickness. In addition, treatment was associated with the progression of disease in the common carotid segment, despite a large increase in HDL-C and substantial decreases in LDL-C and triglyceride.

Although torcetrapib increased the mortality rate in the ILLUMINATE trial, there remains cautious optimism that CETP inhibition is a viable option to raise HDL-C and lower LDL-C to reduce cardiovascular risk. The ILLUSTRATE trial (but not supported by RADIANCE-1 and -2 trials) demonstrated that greater reduction in percent atheroma volume occurred with higher levels of HDL-C on treatment. This finding suggests a positive benefit of torcetrapib on atherosclerosis, which was offset by the adverse effect on blood pressure and vascular toxicity. The off-target effects of torcetrapib are not shared, however, by at least 2 other CETP inhibitors, dalcetrapib and anacetrapib. In early human trials, torcetrapib was shown to increase blood pressure by 2 to 3 mm Hg, and in later trials such as ILLUMINATE, in high-risk patients the increase in blood pressure was approximately 4 to 5 mm Hg.[46] Torcetrapib, but not dalcetrapib, has been found to stimulate aldosterone production in a human adrenal cell line and stimulate 11β-hydroxylase, an enzyme involved in steroid genesis. The steroidogenic effect of torcetrapib in humans may explain the increased rate of sepsis and cancer in the ILLUMINATE trial. Torcetrapib and angiontensin-2 share several common properties centered on the CYP11B2 gene expression, which may explain the aldosterone and steroidogenic effect that led to the off-target toxicity (**Fig 13**).[47]

The mechanisms of action of dalcetrapib are different to torcetrapib with regard to CETP inhibition. Dalcetrapib binds to CETP and induces a conformational change in the CETP molecule that hinders its ability then to bind to HDL in the plasma (**Fig. 14**).[48] In comparison, torcetrapib binds to CETP, resulting in a triple complex of torcetrapib and HDL. In addition, dalcetrapib does not increase blood pressure in humans.

Furthermore, anacetrapib does not share the increase in aldosterone production in the adrenal

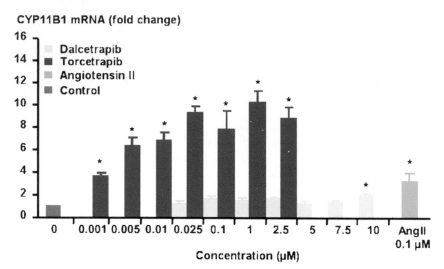

Fig. 13. Torcetrapib, but not dalcetrapib, induced 11 β-hydrolase (CYP11B1) mRNA in H295R cells after 24 hours. Mean (SEM, 3 separate experiments). *P <.01 versus baseline. (*Data from* Vergeer M, Stroes ES. The pharmacology and off-target effects of some cholesterol ester transfer protein inhibitors. Am J Cardiol 2009;104(Suppl):32E–8E.)

cell line as does torcetrapib. In comparison, anacetrapib is a more potent CETP inhibitor than dalcetrapib, and increases HDL-C by 50% to 75% and lowers LDL-C by approximately 30% at 100 mg/d. More data will be available from an ongoing clinical study, The Determining the EFficacy and Tolerability of CETP INhibition with AnacEtrapib (DEFINE) trial, which is evaluating the cardiovascular safety of anacetrapib, 100 mg/d in 1800 patients at high cardiovascular risk over the course of 18 months of therapy.[49]

Similarly, clinical trials evaluating the effects of dalcetrapib on cardiovascular outcome are presently under way. The investigators of the dal-OUTCOMES trial: efficacy and safety of dalcetrapib in patients with recent ACS, are evaluating 15,600 acute coronary syndrome patients with a minimum follow-up of at least 2 years.[50] The study is completing enrollment and will be reporting results in approximately 3 years. The DAL-vessel and the DAL-plaque study are evaluating the effects of dalcetrapib on endothelial function and atherosclerosis as measured by both IVUS and CIMT.[51,52] If successful in improving outcomes, dalcetrapib will become available for clinical use as a CETP inhibitor.

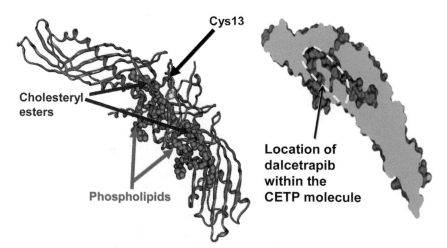

Fig. 14. Mechanism of action of dalcetrapib. Dalcetrapib forms a disulfide bond with the Cys13 residue of CETP. Dalcetrapib binding to CETP appears to induce a conformational change in the CETP molecule. (*Data from* Okamoto H, Yonemori F, Wakitani K, et al. A cholesteryl ester transfer protein inhibitor attenuates atherosclerosis in rabbits. Nature 2000;406:203–7.)

Promising Targets to Modify HDL

As outlined in **Box 1**, several promising targets exist to modify HDL, including targeting RCT. Data from studies on animal models and genetic disorders support that increases in Apo AI production would most likely result in the most favorable improvement in RCT. Synthetic forms of HDL, HDL mimetics, reconstituted HDL, and reinfusing delipidated HDL are all potential therapeutic approaches in human clinical trials. Enhancing LCAT activity will increase the esterification of cholesterol in HDL, resulting in HDL maturation. Inhibiting CETP will increase HDL particle size and delay catabolism of HDL. Modifying the holoparticle uptake of HDL (a possible action of niacin) will also delay catabolism by allowing the HDL particles to continue circulating and potentially increase RCT. Pharmacologic therapy to promote RCT would theoretically result in an increase in fecal cholesterol. Infusion of reconstituted HDL has resulted in an increase in fecal cholesterol. As only a very small fraction of HDL-C is derived from the macrophages in the atherosclerotic plaque, it is very difficult to measure changes in RCT with pharmacologic therapy.

As outlined in **Box 2**, several strategies to infuse synthetic or natural HDL into the plasma focus on enhancing RCT and induce atherosclerotic plaque regression. As Apo AI is active in stimulating RCT, these strategies involve infusions of reconstituted natural Apo AI or more active mutant forms of HDL such as Apo AI Milano, Apo AI peptides that have 18 to 21 amino acids that may be intestinally absorbed, or delipidating a person's HDL and reinfusing this HDL into the plasma.

Other emerging HDL-C therapies include infusion of mutant forms of Apo AI such as Apo AI Milano, and delipidated HDL-C, oral Apo AI

Box 2
HDL metabolism as a therapeutic target: potential strategies

Acute (parenteral therapies)

Apo AI Milano/phospholipids complexes

Apo AI mimetic peptides

Large unilamellar vesicles

Delipidated HDL

Apo AI isolated from human plasma and phosphatidylcholine derived from soybean

---

mimetics, and Apo AI Milano gene transfer. The Apo AI mimetic, D-4F, has been shown to enhance HDL-C's antioxidant and anti-inflammatory properties, as well as increasing RCT. Additional targets with the potential to raise HDL-C levels and/or increase RCT have been identified. Plasma concentrations of HDL-C are the net result of de novo production, catabolism, recycling of HDL-C particles, and the contribution to HDL-C from components of other lipoproteins. As a result, HDL-C levels can be modified by delaying the clearance of HDL-C from the plasma or by increasing production of Apo AI.

Enhance Transintestinal Cholesterol Efflux

The small intestine contains numerous transporter and nuclear receptors that modulate cholesterol homeostasis. As a result, the intestine remains an active target to potentially modify cardiovascular risk. The enterocyte, as the interface between the exogenous source of cholesterol and the lymphatics, plays a critical role in cholesterol efflux back into the lumen on incorporating the cholesterol into chylomicrons with secretion into the plasma. As up to one-third of RCT may involve the small intestine, therapeutic approaches that regulate LXR in the intestine may only reduce cholesterol absorption while enhancing RCT by increasing the expression of ABC A1. Intestinally specific LXR agonists may not have the adverse effect of increasing hepatic steatosis associated with up-regulation of LXR in the liver. Another alternative option to lower LDL-C or beneficially modify HDL metabolism is the use of drugs or nutritional products that affect only intestinal cells without systemic involvement. These agents potentially can be used in statin combination therapy or as monotherapy for patients with statin intolerance.

Box 1
Promising targets to modify HDL

Increase Apo AI production

Increase anti-inflammatory effect of HDL

Infuse Apo AI phospholipid complexes

PPAR-α, -δ, and -γ agonists

LXR agonists

Up-regulate ABC A1 or ABC G1

Enhance LCAT activity

Inhibit CETP

Modify hepatic holoparticle uptake of HDL (niacin receptor agonist)

SUMMARY

Targeting HDL-C is an integral component of the management of CHD and risk reduction. Clinical trial evidence demonstrates that low HDL-C is associated with increased risk for CHD-associated morbidity and mortality. It therefore becomes evident that targeting HDL-C in addition to LDL-C for the control of cardiovascular risk is beneficial. Several strategies can be used to increase HDL-C levels to target cardiovascular risk reduction, including pharmacologic management focused on the use of statin, statin-combination therapy, and investigational drugs targeting HDL-C metabolism and RCT. Although in vitro studies suggest that HDL has a wide range of antiatherogenic properties, research is needed to validate these functions in humans, in addition to studies examining the impact of HDL gene modulation on cardiovascular risk.[11,53] Additional research with newer combination therapies aimed at increasing HDL-C and targeting additional components of the dyslipidemic state may result in novel options for reducing residual cardiovascular risk for optimal CHD management.

REFERENCES

1. American Heart Association. Heart disease and stroke statistics—2009 update. Dallas (TX): American Heart Association; 2009.
2. Smith SC, Allen J, Blair SN, et al. AHA/ACC guidelines for secondary prevention for patients with coronary and other atherosclerotic vascular disease: 2006 update: endorsed by the National Heart, Lung, and Blood Institute. Circulation 2006;113: 2363–72.
3. Duffy D, Rader DJ. Update on strategies to increase HDL quantity and function. Nat Rev Cardiol 2009;6: 455–63.
4. Davidson MH, Toth PP. High-density lipoprotein metabolism: potential therapeutic targets. Am J Cardiol 2007;100(11A):n32–40.
5. Davidson MH. Focus on HDL as a therapeutic target for CAD risk reduction. Am J Cardiol 2009;104 (Suppl 10):1E–2E.
6. National Cholesterol Education Panel. Third Report of the National Cholesterol Education Program (NCEP) Expert Panel on Detection, Evaluation, and Treatment of High Blood Cholesterol in Adults (Adult Treatment Panel III) final report. Circulation 2002; 106:3143–421.
7. Castelli WP. Cholesterol and lipids in the risk of coronary heart disease: the Framingham Heart Study. Can J Cardiol 1988;4(Suppl A):5A–10A.
8. Castelli WP, Garrison RJ, Wilson PWF, et al. Incidence of coronary heart disease and lipoprotein cholesterol levels. The Framingham Study. JAMA 1986;256:2835–8.
9. Stampfer MJ, Sacks FM, Salvin S, et al. A prospective study of cholesterol, apolipoproteins, and the risk of myocardial infarction. N Engl J Med 1991;325:373–81.
10. Goldbourt U, Yaari JS, Medalie JH. Isolated low HDL cholesterol as a risk factor for coronary heart disease mortality: a 21-year follow-up of 8,000 men. Arterioscler Thromb Vasc Biol 1997;17:107–13.
11. Vergeer M, Holleboom AG, Kastelein JJ, et al. The HDL hypothesis: does high-density lipoprotein protect from atherosclerosis? J Lipid Res 2010; 51(8):2058–73.
12. Davidson MH. Targeting high-density lipoprotein cholesterol in the management of cardiovascular disease. Am Heart Hosp J 2007;5:210–6.
13. Birjmohun RS, Hutten BA, Kastelein JJ, et al. Efficacy and safety of high-density lipoprotein cholesterol-increasing compounds. J Am Coll Cardiol 2005;45: 185–97.
14. LaRosa JC, He J, Vuppiuturi S. Effect of statins on risk of coronary disease: a meta-analysis of randomized controlled trials. JAMA 1999;282: 2340–6.
15. Gordon DJ, Probstfield JL, Garrison RJ, et al. High-density lipoprotein cholesterol and cardiovascular disease: four prospective American studies. Circulation 1989;79:8–15.
16. Schwartz GG, Olsson AG, Szarek M, et al. Relation of characteristics of metabolic syndrome to short-term prognosis and effects of intensive statin therapy after acute coronary syndrome: an analysis of the Myocardial Ischemia Reduction with Aggressive Cholesterol Lowering (MIRACL) trial. Diabetes Care 2005;28:2508–13.
17. Wolfram RM, Brewer HB, Xue Z, et al. Impact of low high-density lipoproteins on in-hospital events and one-year clinical outcomes in patients with non-ST-elevation myocardial infarction acute coronary syndrome treated with drug-eluting stent implantation. Am J Cardiol 2006;98:711–7.
18. Shah PK, Kaul S, Nilsson J, et al. Exploiting the vascular protective effects of high-density lipoprotein and its apolipoproteins: an idea whose time for testing is coming, part I. Circulation 2001;104: 2376–83.
19. Barter PJ, Nicholls S, Rye KA, et al. Antiinflammatory properties of HDL. Circ Res 2004;95:764–72.
20. Singh IM, Shishehbor MH, Ansell BJ, et al. High density lipoprotein as a therapeutic target: a systematic review. JAMA 2007;298:786–98.
21. Cuchel M, Rader DJ. Genetics of increased HDL cholesterol levels: insights into the relationship between HDL metabolism and atherosclerosis. Arterioscler Thromb Vasc Biol 2003;23: 1710–2.

22. Toth PP. High density lipoprotein as a therapeutic target: clinical evidence and treatment strategies. Am J Cardiol 2005;96(9A):50K–8K.

23. Davidson MH, Rosenson RS. Novel targets that affect high-density lipoprotein metabolism: the next frontier. Am J Cardiol 2009;104(10 Suppl):52E–7E.

24. Study of Coronary Atheroma by Intravascular Ultrasound: effect of Rosuvastatin Versus Atorvastatin (SATURN). Available at: http://clinicaltrials.gov/ct2/show/NCT00620542. Accessed October 30, 2010.

25. Ridker PM, Buring JE, Cook NR, et al. C-reactive protein, the metabolic syndrome, and risk of incident cardiovasculr events. Circulation 2003;107:391–7.

26. Blake GJ, Otvos JD, Rifai N, et al. Low-density lipoprotein particle concentration and size as determined by nuclear magnetic resonance spectroscopy as predictors of cardiovascular disease in women. Circulation 2002;106:1930–7.

27. Mora S, Ridker PM. Justification for the use of statins in primary prevention: an intervention trial evaluating rosuvastatin (JUPITER)—can C-reactive protein be used to statin therapy in primary prevention? Am J Cardiol 2006;97(2A):33A–71A.

28. Berge KG, Canner PL. Coronary drug project: experience with niacin. Coronary Drug Project Research Group. Eur J Clin Pharmacol 1991;40(Suppl 1):S49–51.

29. Kamanna VS, Kashyap ML. Mechanism of action of niacin on lipoprotein metabolism. Curr Atheroscler Rep 2000;2:36–46.

30. Pike NB. Flushing out the role of GPR109A (HM74A) in the clinical efficacy of nicotinic acid. J Clin Invest 2005;115(12):3400–3.

31. Maciejewski-Lenoir D, Richman JG, Hakak Y, et al. Langerhans cells release prostaglandin D_2 in response to nicotinic acid. J Invest Dermatol 2006;126:2637–46.

32. Narumiya S, Sugimoto Y, Ushikubi F, et al. Prostanoid receptors: structures, properties, and functions. Physiol Rev 1999;79:1193–226.

33. Cheng K, Wu TJ, Wu KK, et al. Antagonism of the prostaglandin D_2 receptor 1 suppresses nicotinic acid-induced vasodilation in mice and humans. Proc Natl Acad Sci U S A 2006;103:6682–7.

34. Morrow JD, Parsons WG, Roberts LJ. Release of markedly increased quantities of prostaglandin D_2 in vivo in humans following the administration of nicotinic acid prostaglandins. J Invest Dermatol 1989;38:263–74.

35. Shepherd J, Betteridge J, Van Gaal L, European Consensus Panel. Nicotinic acid in the management of dyslipidaemia associated with diabetes and metabolic syndrome: a position paper developed by a European Consensus Panel. Curr Med Res Opin 2005;21:665–82.

36. Taylor AJ, Sullenberger LE, Lee HJ, et al. Arterial biology for the investigation of the treatment effects of reducing cholesterol (ARBITER) 2. Circulation 2004;110:3512–7.

37. Jones PH, Cusi K, Davidson MH, et al. Efficacy and safety of fenofibric acid co-administered with low- or moderate-dose statin in patients with mixed dyslipidemia and type 2 diabetes mellitus: results of a pooled subgroup analysis from three randomized, controlled, double-blind trials. Am J Cardiovasc Drugs 2010;10:73–84.

38. Davidson MH, Rooney MW, Drucker J, et al. Efficacy and tolerability of atorvastatin/fenofibrate fixed-dose combination tablet compared with atorvastatin and fenofibrate monotherapies in patients with dyslipidemia: a 12-week, multicenter, double-blind, randomized, parallel-group study. Clin Ther 2009;12:2824–38.

39. Davidson MH. Update on CETP inhibition. J Clin Lipidol 2010;4:394–8.

40. Tardiff JC, Gregoire J, L'Allier PL, et al. Effects of reconstituted high-density lipoprotein infusions on coronary atherosclerosis: a randomized controlled trial. JAMA 2007;297:1675–82.

41. DeGoma EM, Rader DJ. Novel HDL-directed pharmacotherapeutic strategies. Nat Rev Cardiol, in press.

42. Qiu X, Mistry A, Ammirati MJ, et al. Crystal structure of cholesteryl ester transfer protein reveals a long tunnel and four bound lipid molecules. Nat Struct Mol Biol 2007;14:106–13.

43. Tall AR. The effects of cholesterol ester transfer protein inhibition on cholesterol efflux. Am J Cardiol 2009;104(Suppl):39E–45E.

44. Nicholls SJ. High-density lipoprotein and progression rate of atherosclerosis in intravascular ultrasound trials. Am J Cardiol 2009;104(Suppl):16E–21E.

45. Kastelein JJ, van Leuven SI, Burgess L, et al, RADIANCE 1 Investigators. Effect of torcetrapib on carotid atherosclerosis in familial hypercholesterolemia. N Engl J Med 2007;356:1620–30.

46. Barter P. Lessons learned from the Investigation of Lipid Level Management to Understand its Impact in Atherosclerotic Events (ILLUMINATE) trial. Am J Cardiol 2009;104(Suppl):10E–5E.

47. Vergeer M, Stroes ES. The pharmacology and off-target effects of some cholesterol ester transfer protein inhibitors. Am J Cardiol 2009;104(Suppl):32E–8E.

48. Okamoto H, Yonemori F, Wakitani K, et al. A cholesteryl ester transfer protein inhibitor attenuates atherosclerosis in rabbits. Nature 2000;406:203–7.

49. Cannon CP, Dansky HM, Davidsom MH. Design of the DEFINE trial: Determining the EFficacy and Tolerability of CETP INhibition with AnacEtrapib. Am Heart J 2009;158:513–9.

50. Schwartz GG, Olsson AG, Ballantyne CM, et al, dal-OUTCOMES Committees and Investigators.

Rationale and design of the dal-OUTCOMES trial: efficacy and safety of dalcetrapib in patients with recent acute coronary syndrome. Am Heart J 2009;158:896–901.

51. DAL-vessel. A Study of the Effect of RO4607381 on atherosclerotic plaque in patients with coronary heart disease. Available at: http://www.clinicaltrials.gov/ct2/show/NCT00655473?term=dalcetrapib+AND+vessel&rank=1. Accessed October 10, 2010.

52. DAL-plaque. A Study of the Effect of RO4607381 on atherosclerotic plaque in patients with coronary heart disease. Available at: http://www.clinicaltrials.gov/ct2/show/NCT00655473?term=dalcetrapib+AND+plaque&rank=1. Accessed October 10, 2010.

53. Motazacker MM, Kastelein JJ, Kuivenhoven JA. Are high-density lipoprotein genes and their products targets for therapy? Curr Opin Lipidol 2010;21:157–8.

Emerging Therapies for Atherosclerosis Prevention and Management

Kuang-Yuh Chyu, MD, PhD, Prediman K. Shah, MD*

KEYWORDS

- Atherosclerosis • Low-density lipoprotein
- High-density lipoprotein • Immunomodulation
- Inflammation

Atherosclerotic arterial disease is the leading cause of mortality and morbidity throughout industrialized nations, and is expected to rival other diseases in developing nations as well.[1,2] Arterial occlusive disorders include atherosclerosis of native arteries, an accelerated variant of atherosclerosis involving vein grafts, transplant allograft vasculopathy, and restenosis resulting from neointima formation following angioplasty or stenting.

Atherosclerosis is a complex disease process that involves the build-up of a plaque composed of variable amounts of lipoproteins, extracellular matrix (collagen, proteoglycans, glycosaminoglycans), calcium, vascular smooth muscle cells, immunoinflammatory cells (chiefly monocyte-derived macrophages, T lymphocytes, mast cells, and dendritic cells), immunoglobulins, and new blood vessels (angiogenesis). A large body of evidence suggests that atherosclerosis represents a chronic immunoinflammatory response to vascular injury caused by a variety of agents that activate or injure endothelium and promote lipoprotein infiltration, retention, and modification, combined with immunoinflammatory cell entry, retention, and activation.[3–6]

Because retention and deposition of apoprotein B-100 (apoB-100)-containing atherogenic lipoproteins is essential for the development of plaque, lowering the circulating levels of these lipoproteins has been the major target for atherosclerosis management. In this regard statins, which lower circulating low-density lipoprotein cholesterol (LDL-C) levels by reducing hepatocyte sterol levels thereby up-regulating hepatic low-density lipoprotein (LDL) receptors, have emerged as the mainstay of atherosclerosis management with substantial body of evidence supporting their widespread use.[7,8] However, despite much progress, atherosclerotic cardiovascular disease continues to be highly prevalent. Multiple reasons account for the continuing epidemic of cardiovascular disease: underutilization of statins and less than optimal long-term compliance, intolerance of statins in some patients because of adverse effects, inability to achieve target cholesterol levels in many patients at tolerable doses, and relative ineffectiveness in patients such as those with homozygous familial hypercholesterolemia who lack the LDL receptor gene or carry a defective LDL receptor gene. Furthermore, because statins are often used later in life when atherosclerosis is already well established, their overall effectiveness may be compromised; this is supported by studies showing that lifelong low LDL-C levels beginning from birth, resulting from loss of function in genes such as PCSK-9 gene,[9] are associated with significantly greater protection against cardiovascular disease than would be predicted from equivalent degree of LDL-C lowering achieved with statins. Thus it should be recognized that statins reduce cardiovascular events by only about 20% to 30%, leaving at least 70%

Department of Medicine, UCLA, Los Angeles, CA, USA
* Corresponding author.
E-mail address: shahp@cshs.org

Cardiol Clin 29 (2011) 123–135
doi:10.1016/j.ccl.2010.10.003
0733-8651/11/$ — see front matter © 2011 Elsevier Inc. All rights reserved.

of the events to continue occurring (**Table 1**). These findings underscore the complexity and multifactorial nature of atherosclerosis and suggest the need for additional interventions, which are likely to include (1) nonstatin drugs to reduce LDL-C by mechanisms that do not involve HMG-CoA (3-hydroxy-3-methylglutaryl-coenzyme A) reductase inhibition; (2) a variety of regimens to augment high-density lipoprotein (HDL) levels and HDL function; (3) inflammation or immune-modulation strategies.

NEW NONSTATIN LDL-C–LOWERING AGENTS
Cholesterol Absorption Inhibitors

On average, 300 mg of cholesterol is absorbed daily from the gut and another 800 mg of cholesterol produced by the body is transported from the liver into the intestine. To maintain cholesterol homeostasis, about 1100 mg of cholesterol is excreted from the gut. Bile acid sequestering resins bind cholesterol-rich bile acids and prevent their enterohepatic recirculation, leading to loss of bile acids in the feces and subsequent reduction of intrahepatic cholesterol and increased hepatic conversion of cholesterol to bile acids, thereby resulting in a modest reduction in circulating total cholesterol and LDL-C levels. However, resins produce several annoying side effects that reduce their widespread applicability.

Other intestinally active agents include plant stanols. Oil-based products enriched with plant stanol esters can lower LDL-C concentrations by 10% to 14%.[10] Plant stanols are believed to act by preventing micellar cholesterol formation, thereby inhibiting intestinal absorption of cholesterol. Recent data also suggest that stanols may increase cholesterol efflux from intestinal cells into the intestinal lumen by activating intestinal activity of ABCA1 (adenosine triphosphate–binding cassette transporter) activity.[11] Newer agents

to block intestinal transport of cholesterol have been developed, including agents that inhibit the bile acid transporter or the putative intestinal cholesterol permease on the intestinal brush border, leading to selective inhibition of cholesterol absorption with little effect on fat-soluble vitamin absorption. One such agent, ezetimibe, was recently approved by the Food and Drug Administration for use in the United States. Niemann-Pick C1-like 1 (*NPC1L1*) is an intestinal cholesterol transporter and the molecular target of ezetimibe.[12] More recently, ezetimibe has also been shown to stimulate reverse cholesterol transport in a murine model.[13]

Ezetimibe has been shown to reduce total cholesterol levels by 15% to 20%, and its cholesterol-lowering effects are synergistic with those of statins.[14] In patients with familial hypercholesterolemia, ezetimibe produced a significant reduction in LDL-C when combined with 80 mg simvastatin, compared with simvastatin alone, and was well tolerated.[15] Ezetimibe is a welcome addition to our armamentarium as monotherapy for patients who need modest LDL lowering or as combination therapy with statins (or fibrates) for patients who need greater LDL lowering but are unable to tolerate high doses of statin or respond poorly to statins alone. A combination of low-dose statin (10 mg of atorvastatin) and 10 mg of ezetimibe has been shown to produce the same magnitude of LDL lowering as monotherapy with high-dose atorvastatin (80 mg).[16] Although ezetimibe reduces LDL-C levels, questions have been raised about its efficacy in reducing cardiovascular events. A combination of simvastatin and ezetimibe did not reduce the progression of carotid intima-medial thickness compared with simvastatin alone despite a greater reduction in LDL-C levels.[15] Another clinical trial (SEAS trial) in which ezetimibe was tested for aortic stenosis raised the possibility of increased cancer risk[17]; however,

Table 1
Residual cardiovascular risk (death or nonfatal myocardial infarction) after statin therapy in secondary prevention clinical trials

Clinical Trial	Statin Used	Event Rate in Statin Group	Event Rate in Placebo Group	Relative Residual CV Risk
Scandinavian Simvastatin Survival Study (4S)	Simvastatin 20 mg/d	19%	28%	68%
Cholesterol and Recurrent Events (CARE)	Pravastatin 40 mg/d	10.2%	13.2%	77%
Long-Term Intervention with Pravastatin in Ischemic Disease (LIPID)	Pravastatin 40 mg/d	12.3%	15.9%	77%

a composite analysis of several trials failed to confirm the cancer risk suggested by the SEAS trial.[18] The question of whether the combination of ezetimibe and statin provides additional reduction of cardiovascular events compared with statin alone after acute coronary syndrome remains to be answered at the completion of ongoing clinical trials.[19,20]

Acyl-Coenzyme A Cholesterol Acyl Transferase Inhibitors

Acyl-coenzyme A cholesterol acyltransferase (ACAT) is an enzyme that is responsible for cholesterol esterification in the macrophages, liver, and intestines. Two forms of ACAT, ACAT-1 and ACAT-2, have been described and are encoded by 2 different genes.[21] Macrophages express predominantly ACAT-1, whereas intestines express predominantly ACAT-2. Human liver expresses both ACAT-1 and ACAT-2, with a predominance of ACAT-1. Cholesterol ester formation by macrophages through the activity of ACAT-1 results in foam cell formation in atherosclerotic lesions, an event critical to formation and progression of atherosclerosis. Therefore, inhibition of cholesterol ester formation by ACAT-1 inhibition may produce antiatherogenic effects. In addition, inhibition of cholesterol ester formation in the intestine through inhibition of ACAT-2 may reduce cholesterol absorption, resulting in a reduction in circulating cholesterol levels. Complete elimination of ACAT-1 activity through gene targeting or transplantation of ACAT-1-null bone marrow has not been shown to reduce atherosclerosis in apoprotein E (apoE) or LDL-receptor–null mice.[22,23] In fact, increased lesion size and macrophage necrosis were observed, along with accumulation of cholesterol deposits, in the skin and brain. These observations have raised concerns about selective and complete inhibition of ACAT-1. On the other hand, partial inhibition of ACAT activity by using nonselective inhibitors of both ACAT-1 and ACAT-2 has shown promising results in murine hypercholesterolemia atherosclerosis models.[24] Similarly, inhibition of liver-specific ACAT-2 through gene targeting results in resistance to diet-induced hypercholesterolemia in mice,[25] suggesting that selective ACAT-2 inhibition may be another approach to reducing dietary absorption of cholesterol. A selective partial ACAT-1 inhibitor, K-604, developed by Kowa Research Institute, has demonstrated plaque stabilizing and antiatherogenic properties in preclinical models[26] and is currently undergoing a phase 2 clinical evaluation in the United States. Two nonspecific ACAT inhibitors have been tested in clinical trials (avasimibe and pactimibe) with negative results, raising serious questions about the usefulness of these agents for atherosclerosis management in humans.[27–29]

Microsomal Triglyceride Transfer Protein Inhibitors (Lomatipide)

Microsomal triglyceride transfer protein (MTP) is a heterodimeric lipid transfer protein present in the endoplasmic reticulum of hepatocytes and intestinal cells. A defect in MTP gene (producing a severe deficiency in MTP) causes marked reductions in plasma triglycerides, LDL, and very low-density lipoprotein (VLDL) cholesterol (abetalipoproteinemia). These findings suggest that synthetic inhibitors of MTP capable of producing a partial deficiency in MTP function might be therapeutically useful for inhibiting the production of VLDL and chylomicrons, thereby reducing the levels of atherogenic lipoprotein.

Bristol-Myers Squibb Company (Princeton, NJ, USA) has designed and tested small molecules capable of inhibiting MTP that can produce marked reductions in atherogenic lipoproteins in hyperlipidemic Watanabe rabbits that lack a functional LDL receptor.[30] Clinical applications of MTP inhibitors have been focused primarily on high-dose monotherapy to produce substantial reductions in LDL-C levels (particularly for patients with homozygous familial hypercholesterolemia). However, this strategy has been associated with a high rate of gastrointestinal and hepatic adverse events that has prohibited the use of these agents.

Data also suggest that the MTP inhibitor, lomitapide (AEGR-733; Aegerion Pharmaceuticals Inc, Bridgewater, NJ, USA), lowered LDL-C in patients with moderate hypercholesterolemia either as a single agent or in combination with ezetimibe.[31] MTP inhibition with lomitapide may offer a treatment option for patients who cannot tolerate statin therapy or who experience insufficient LDL-C reduction with available therapies. However, the safety concerns for MTP inhibitors for the treatment of hyperlipidemia must be fully addressed, and the assessment of the risk-to-benefit ratio for MTP inhibitors in patients at different levels of risk for cardiovascular disease is required before clinical use of this class of drugs may be recommended.

Antisense to ApoB-100 (Mipomersen)

Mipomersen is a second-generation antisense oligonucleotide developed to reduce the hepatic synthesis of apoB-100, a protein component of all atherogenic lipoproteins that is required for hepatic VLDL assembly and secretion. When given subcutaneously as an injection, mipomersen distributes predominantly into the liver and the kidney, and lowers LDL-C and apoB-100 levels by inhibiting the synthesis of apoB-100 when used as a single agent or in combination with other lipid-lowering drugs.[32] Two phase 3 human trials involving either homozygous familial hypercholesterolemia or heterozygous familial hypercholesterolemia patients have shown the efficacy of 200 mg/wk subcutaneous injection of mipomersen in LDL-C lowering by an average of 18% or greater (range of 2%–82%) in homozygous familial hypercholesterolemia patients,[33] and an average of 28% LDL-C lowering in heterozygous familial hypercholesterolemia patients (http://ir.isispharm.com; press release February 10, 2010). In several studies, Mipomersen has also reduced elevated lipoprotein(a) levels. Common adverse effects include a high frequency of local injection site reactions, flu-like symptoms, and elevation of hepatic enzymes. Preliminary studies have also suggested that mipomersen may increase hepatic triglyceride content and because hepatic steatosis is a potentially serious adverse effect, additional longer-term studies are needed to ensure long-term safety of this novel agent.[34] Mipomersen may emerge as a potentially valuable adjunct for patients unable to tolerate other approved lipid-modifying drugs, or when approved lipid-modifying drugs are ineffective or only partially effective.

PCSK-9 Inhibitors

Loss-of-function mutation in the PCSK-9 (proprotein convertase subtilisin kexin type 9) gene is associated with low LDL-C levels from birth and striking protection from coronary heart disease (CHD).[35] PCSK9 is responsible for degradation of LDL receptors, and its inhibition increases LDL receptor number on the cell surface.[9,36] Thus, inhibition of PCSK-9 is a potential strategy for LDL-C reduction and CHD prevention. Inhibition of PCSK9 and LDL-C lowering has been demonstrated following injection of an anti-PCSK9 antibody in mice and cynomolgus monkeys,[37] suggesting the feasibility and efficacy of this approach.

AMG 145 (Amgen Inc, Thousand Oaks, CA, USA) is a fully human monoclonal antibody to PCSK9 currently being investigated for the treatment of hypercholesterolemia as an add-on to stable statin therapy. The development program for AMG 145 builds on human genetic validation and compelling preclinical evidence. AMG 145 is in phase 1 clinical trials (ClinicalTrials.gov identifier: NCT01133522; http://www.clinicaltrials.gov/ct2/show/NCT01133522?term=A).

Thyroid Hormone Agonists

Increased thyroid hormone levels reduce LDL-C levels, and selective activation of thyroid β receptor, preferentially expressed in liver, by an experimental agonist KB2115 has been shown to reduce LDL-C levels in humans without cardiac side effects in a short-term study.[38] Another liver-selective thyromimetic, T-0681, was shown to reduce cholesterol levels and atherosclerosis in hyperlipidemic animals.[39,40] More data are needed to confirm long-term efficacy and safety of such agents in humans.

NEW HDL-BASED THERAPIES
HDL as a Target for Therapy

Several epidemiologic studies show that the HDL cholesterol (HDL-C) levels are inversely related to cardiovascular events, suggesting that HDL may be atheroprotective. These observations have been bolstered by the demonstration that HDL and its apolipoproteins, specifically apoA-1, exhibit several biologic actions that could favorably affect atherothrombosis. Furthermore, transgenic overexpression of apoA-1 gene (major protein component of HDL), direct infusion of plasma-derived or recombinant wild-type or mutant apoA-1, and gene transfer of HDL-associated proteins have been shown to be atheroprotective in various experimental and/or clinical settings, thereby justifying a renewed focus on HDL-based therapies.[41,42]

Biologic Basis for Beneficial Effects of HDL on Atherothrombosis

Stimulation of reverse cholesterol transport
Accumulation of cholesterol in the arterial wall is a major contributor to atherogenesis. One of the principal actions of HDL is to stimulate reverse cholesterol transport in which free cholesterol is mobilized from the peripheral tissues, including lipid-laden macrophages, and carried to the liver for uptake and elimination in feces through biliary sterols. Free cholesterol and phospholipid from the macrophage is transferred to lipid poor apoA-1 discoid particles by ABCA1 transporter and to larger spherical HDL particles by ABCG1 transporter in the initial steps of the reverse cholesterol transport; the free cholesterol is then esterified by lecithin cholesterol acyl transferase, leading to remodeling of HDL particles into spherical HDL2 and HDL3 particles. HDL then delivers cholesterol ester to the liver via SRB1 receptors or exchanges cholesterol ester for triglycerides from VLDL and LDL particles, an exchange facilitated by cholesteryl ester transfer protein (CETP).

The cholesterol ester transferred to LDL and VLDL is then targeted for hepatic uptake via the LDL receptor pathway or accumulates in the arterial wall via subendothelial retention. Thus, mobilization of free cholesterol from plaque macrophages by apoA-1 and HDL contributes to an antiatherogenic effect.[41]

Anti-inflammatory and immunomodulatory effects of ApoA-1 and HDL

Inflammation and immune activation play an important role in atherogenesis, and HDL inhibits inflammation and modulates the immune system by several mechanisms. The anti-inflammatory effects of HDL have been attributed to specific effects of apoA-1, inhibition of LDL oxidation, scavenging of proinflammatory lipids from oxidized LDL, sphingosine pathway activation, and activation of ABCA1-dependent JAK/STAT3 pathway attenuating TLR/MyD88-mediated proinflammatory responses.[41–44] HDL may also promote migration of dendritic cells out of vascular lesions into regional lymph nodes,[45] possibly by neutralizing the dendritic cell—immobilizing effects of phospholipids generated during LDL oxidation. HDL also attenuates the inhibitory effects of inflammation on reverse cholesterol transport. Recent experimental observations have shown that ABCA1 and ABCG1, critical players in the initial steps of reverse cholesterol transport from macrophages and critical regulators of HDL particle formation, play an important role in suppressing atherosclerosis-associated leukocytosis by inhibiting bone marrow derived progenitor cells.[44]

Antioxidant effects of ApoA-1 and HDL

LDL oxidation in the vessel wall likely plays a key role in atherogenesis. HDL inhibits LDL oxidation, scavenges toxic phospholipids from oxidized LDL, and protects vascular smooth muscle cells and endothelial cells from damaging effects of oxidized LDL. The antioxidant effects of HDL have been attributed to paraoxonase and platelet activating factor acetylhydrolase (PAF-AH) carried by HDL.[41,42]

Endothelial protective effects of HDL

Endothelial dysfunction and endothelial denudation are important contributors and consequences of atherosclerosis. HDL has been shown to attenuate endothelial dysfunction induced by dyslipidemia and atherosclerosis by SRB-1 dependent induction of endothelial nitric oxide synthase, to attenuate endothelial cell apoptosis, and to stimulate endothelial reparative capacity.[46–49]

Antithrombotic effects of ApoA-1 and HDL

HDL inhibits platelet aggregation, activates protein C, and inhibits assembly of the prothrombinase complex on anionic phospholipid surfaces.[50]

Pancreatic β-CELL PROTECTIVE EFFECTS OF HDL

Insulin resistance and type 2 diabetes are often associated with reduced levels of HDL-C. HDL infusion was shown to improve pancreatic β-cell function in type 2 diabetic patients. HDL may protect against diabetes by reducing stress-induced pancreatic β-cell apoptosis. Furthermore, ABCA1 and ABACG1 mediated anti-inflammatory effects of HDL may attenuate islet cell inflammation that is implicated in development of type 2 diabetes.[51–53]

HDL Functionality and the Concept of Dysfunctional HDL

Recent studies have shown that the reverse cholesterol-stimulating effects of HDL bear an inconsistent relationship to plasma HDL-C levels, suggesting that HDL-C levels may not be a reliable marker of HDL's antiatherogenic effects. High plasma HDL-C levels do not assure protection, in part because HDL may lose its beneficial effects by becoming proinflammatory and dysfunctional.[54] Conversely, certain low HDL-C states may not promote atherosclerosis because HDL function is intact or enhanced.[55,56] Dysfunctional HDL occurs in inflammatory states, and on exposure of HDL to oxidants such as malondialdehyde and inflammatory mediators such as myeloperoxidase and serum amyloid A.[54] The genesis of proinflammatory or dysfunctional HDL has been attributed, in part, to chlorination/nitration of apoA-1 at specific sites by exposure to oxidants, loss of apoA-1 and paraoxonase from HDL, and serum amyloid A enrichment.[54] Collectively, these observations have led to the notion that HDL functionality, rather than HDL-C level alone, may also be a critical determinant of its atheroprotective effects and that HDL composition may influence its atheroprotective effects. Detailed proteomic analysis of HDL could provide further new insights into the heterogeneity of HDL composition under various conditions.

Emerging New Therapies Targeting HDL and its Apoproteins

Based on epidemiologic observations, biologic plausibility, and experimental studies, it has been argued that improving HDL levels and/or functionality would reduce cardiovascular events. HDL levels tend to increase with adoption of a therapeutic lifestyle such as loss of excess weight, regular exercise, modest alcohol consumption, and smoking cessation. In addition, among the currently available drugs, statins increase HDL-C levels by about 5% to 15%, niacin by about 15% to 35%, and fibrates by about 10% to 15%.

Niacin-laropiprant combination

Niacin is the most effective HDL-raising drug currently available, and several small clinical trials have suggested that adding niacin to other lipid-lowering drugs reduces atherosclerosis progression, promotes regression, and has an overall favorable effect on outcome, but high rate of intolerance and adverse effects have precluded a more widespread use of niacin. The flushing-itching effect of niacin has been attributed to its interaction with niacin receptors on dermal Langerhans cells that activate a prostaglandin D2 pathway, leading to vasodilatation through activation of DP1 receptors on vascular smooth muscle cells. Laropiprant is a selective DP1 receptor inhibitor that attenuates niacin-induced flushing[57] and is currently being tested in combination with niacin in the Heart Protection-2 THRIVE clinical trial. This trial, along with the ongoing AIM-High Trial of niacin, is likely to provide definitive data regarding the clinical benefits and tolerability/safety of niacin and the niacin-laropiprant combination.

Fibrates

Fibrates act as agonists of peroxisome proliferator-activated receptor α, modestly increasing HDL-C and reducing triglycerides and LDL-C levels. Pooled results from randomized trials show no significant reduction in coronary mortality or all-cause mortality despite a significant reduction in nonfatal cardiovascular events.[58] Fibrates produce a high incidence of gastrointestinal side effects and, less frequently, cutaneous and musculoskeletal effects, especially when used in combination with other lipid-modifying drugs.

CETP inhibitors

Inhibition of CETP in order to increase circulating levels of HDL-C was stimulated by genetic studies showing that low-activity genetic variants of CETP were associated with elevated circulating levels of HDL-C, although the protective effect of such genetic variants on cardiovascular disease has been inconsistent. The first major clinical trials program involving an oral CETP inhibitor used torcetrapib, which advanced all the way to a phase 3 trial only to be discontinued because the group using torcetrapib plus atorvastatin experienced a significant excess in cardiovascular and noncardiovascular mortality, despite a marked increase in HDL-C and a significant additional lowering of LDL-C compared with recipients of atorvastatin alone.[59] Similarly, torcetrapib added to atorvastatin had no significant effect on the progression of atherosclerosis of carotid or coronary arteries compared with atorvastatin alone.[60,61] Although the failure of torcetrapib has been attributed to its molecule-specific and CETP-independent angiotensin-aldosterone activation and hypertensive effects, it has also been argued that CETP inhibition may disrupt the reverse cholesterol transport pathway and generate large HDL-C ester and apoE-enriched particles that are dysfunctional. Thus, at present the role of CETP inhibition in the management of atherosclerosis remains controversial. Two additional CETP inhibitors (dalcetrapib and anacetrapib) without angiotensin-aldosterone stimulating and hypertensive effects are currently in advanced clinical trials.[62,63] Results of these trials will likely provide definitive evidence in favor of or against CETP inhibition, and consequent increase in HDL-C as a strategy for cardiovascular protection.

Small-molecule stimulator of apoA-1 gene transcription

RVX-208 is an oral small molecule developed by Resverlogix (Calgary, AB, Canada) that increases endogenous production of apoA-1 by stimulating its gene transcription.[64] Experimental studies have shown that RVX-208 increases HDL-C and apoA-1 levels in monkeys and in humans, specifically increasing pre-β HDL particles believed to be highly effective stimulators of reverse cholesterol transport.[65] Phase 2 proof of concept clinical trials of this compound are currently under way.

Reinfusion of ex vivo delipidated endogenous HDL

Based on the hypothesis that lipid-poor apoA-1 particles are particularly effective in stimulating ABCA1-mediated reverse cholesterol transport, the idea of reinfusing ex vivo delipidated endogenous plasma HDL was tested in a small phase 1/2 human trial with a nonstatistically significant coronary plaque regression as measured by intravascular ultrasound[66]; however, larger studies are needed to validate this interesting but logistically complex approach.

ApoA-1 mimetic peptides

Several small peptides that simulate the lipid transport effects of apoA-1 have been synthesized and tested in experimental models of atherosclerosis, with promising results. One such peptide, D-4F (18mer peptide with 4 phenylalanine residues, made from dextro-isomers of amino acids to improve oral bioavailability, Novartis APP018; Novartis, Basel, Switzerland) was shown to be highly atheroprotective in murine models,[67] but further clinical development remains uncertain in view of modest oral bioavailability and anti-inflammatory efficacy observed in a phase 1/2 human trial.[68] Another peptide, ATI 5261, from Artery Therapeutics (Danville, CA, USA) is on its way to clinical development after it was shown to increase fecal sterol excretion and reduce atherosclerosis on intraperitoneal delivery in mice.[69] Human studies of these peptides have thus far been limited, and their utility remains as yet unproven.

Intravenous infusion of apoA-1$_{Milano}$ or wild-type apoA-1 (synthetic HDL)

ApoA-1$_{Milano}$ is a naturally occurring mutant (A173C) of apoA-1, carried by a small number of inhabitants of Limone sul Garda who, despite high triglycerides and very low HDL-C and apoA-1 levels, have low incidence of cardiovascular disease, suggesting that apoA-1$_{Milano}$ may be a gain-of-function mutation.[55] Several experimental studies from the authors' laboratories and those of others have shown that infusion of recombinant apoA-1$_{Milano}$-phospholipid complex (synthetic HDL) rapidly and favorably remodels atherosclerotic plaques with reduced plaque lipid and inflammation, inhibits progression of lesions, reverses endothelial dysfunction, and promotes rapid regression in various experimental models.[70–73] These observations were subsequently confirmed in a small phase 2 proof of concept clinical trial in which sequential intravascular ultrasound studies done before and after 5 weekly infusions of r-apoA-I$_{Milano}$-phospholipid complex (ETC216) showed rapid coronary plaque regression.[74] Obstacles in developing this therapy further included the need for intravenous infusion, the expensive production process for large-scale manufacturing, and challenges involved in preventing bacterial host-derived protein contamination in the recombinant product produced by *Escherichia coli*. However, recent progress in plant biotechnology by SemBiosys Genetics (Calgary, AB, Canada) whereby apoA-I$_{Milano}$ can be expressed in safflower seed has given renewed impetus to developing this therapy. This plant-engineered protein appears to be functionally similar to *E coli*–derived recombinant protein despite lacking 2 amino acids (Des1,2 apoA-I$_{Milano}$), can be produced at low cost, is scalable, and free of bacterial host-derived protein. Preclinical experiments in the authors' laboratory using plant-derived Des1,2 apoA-I$_{Milano}$ have shown promising results. Some, but not all, experimental studies have suggested that apoA-I$_{Milano}$ has more potent atheroprotective effects than wild-type apoA-1, although the precise reasons for this possible gain-of-function effect remain to be fully defined.[75]

Intravenous infusion of human plasma derived wild-type apoA-1

Human plasma derived wild-type apoA-1 linked to soybean phospholipid (CSL111) was infused at 40 mg/kg per infusion in humans in a small proof of concept trial. Five weekly infusions did not show a significant benefit on coronary plaque in comparison with placebo (primary end point); however, when compared with pretreatment baseline, apoA-1 recipients showed regression in contradistinction to the placebo arm.[76] The 80 mg/kg per infusion regimen was abandoned because of hepatic toxicity even though a single infusion of 80 mg/kg, in an unrelated study, was shown to favorably change femoral artery plaque composition.[77]

Overall, short-term infusion of synthetic HDL (containing apoA-I$_{Milano}$ or wild-type apoA-1) holds considerable promise as a potential strategy for rapid plaque remodeling and stabilization that could later be sustained with the use of orally LDL-lowering and HDL-raising agents, or even possibly repeated infusions.

Endothelial lipase inhibition to raise HDL levels

Endothelial lipase is a recently identified enzyme that modulates HDL metabolism. Overexpression of endothelial lipase in animals reduces plasma HDL-C levels whereas endothelial lipase gene knockout[78] or inhibition by an antibody increases plasma HDL-C levels, suggesting that its inhibition may be a viable strategy for increasing HDL in humans.[79]

Gene transfer of HDL-associated proteins (apoA-1, paraoxonase, and PAF-AH)

Several preclinical studies have demonstrated that effective transfer of genes encoding apoA-1 or apoA-1 mutants and other protective proteins associated with HDL, using viral vectors, produces significant reduction and/or promote regression of atherosclerosis[75,80]; however, clinical translation of such studies has not been reported to date. There are many challenges that must be overcome before clinical translation of gene transfer for atherosclerosis can become a reality: these have largely to do with the development of high-efficiency, safe, nonimmunogenic, scalable vectors that can lead to stable and long-term transgene expression in the host without provoking adverse immunologic or nonimmunologic complications. Various isoforms of adeno-associated viral vectors hold considerable promise for human gene transfer and are under active investigation.[80]

INFLAMMATION- OR IMMUNE-MODULATION THERAPIES

Lipoprotein-Associated Phospholipase Inhibitor (Darapladib)

Lipoprotein-associated phospholipase 2 is a circulating lipid-associated phospholipase that has been shown to be a marker for increased cardiovascular risk in numerous human studies, and has also been implicated as a proinflammatory risk factor that might contribute to plaque formation and plaque inflammation.[81] A synthetic inhibitor, darapladib, has been shown to have atheroprotective effects in preclinical models,[82] but has failed to reduce atherosclerosis progression, high-sensitivity C-reactive protein levels, or arterial stiffness in a phase 2 human clinical trial (Integrated Biomarker and Imaging Study-2 [IBIS-2]) involving sequential coronary plaque assessment using intravascular ultrasound and palpography; however, darapladib-treated subjects showed no increase in necrotic lipid core size whereas placebo-treated subjects showed a significant increase in necrotic lipid core size on secondary analysis.[83] Two recently commenced phase 3 clinical trials (STABILITY trial and SOLID TIMI 52 trial) will investigate the efficacy and safety of darapladib in nearly 13,000 individuals with CHD. When completed, these trials should provide important insights into the utility of darapladib to reduce myocardial infarction, stroke, and cardiovascular death.

Inhibitors of Soluble Phospholipase A2 (Varespladib)

Several circulating secretory phospholipases have also been implicated in atherogenesis and inflammation, and inhibitors of these secretory phospholipases have been developed as potential therapy for inflammatory disorders including atherosclerosis.[84,85] One such inhibitor, varespladib, has been investigated in human studies by Anthera Pharmaceuticals (San Mateo, CA, USA) in phase 1 and 2 studies. In the first phase 2 trial of varespladib, substantial dose-dependent reductions in plasma soluble phospholipase A2-IIA concentration were observed, interestingly along with reduction in LDL-C levels, using 4 doses over 8 weeks.[86] A further phase 2 study of varespladib in patients with acute coronary syndrome is now ongoing (FRANCIS-ACS trial: a study of the safety and efficacy of A 002 in subjects with acute coronary syndromes. http://clinicaltrials.gov/ct2/show/NCT00743925?term=varespladib&rank=1).

Liver X Receptor Agonists

The liver X receptors (LXRs) are nuclear receptors that are activated by endogenous oxysterols derived from oxidized lipids. There are 2 isoforms of LXR, LXRα and LXRβ, both of which regulate gene expression by binding to DNA sequences associated with target genes as heterodimers with isoforms of the retinoid X receptor, RXRα and RXRβ as well as RXRγ. LXRs act as cholesterol sensors: when cellular oxysterols accumulate as a result of increasing concentrations of cholesterol, LXR induces the transcription of genes that protect cells from cholesterol overload. The 2 isoforms of LXRs (α and β) function as sterol sensors with important roles in regulating lipid homeostasis and inflammation, prompting interest in the development of synthetic LXR ligands as therapeutic agents for cardiovascular disease, specifically atherosclerosis.[87] The abundant expression of the LXRα protein in macrophages in human atherosclerotic plaques supports the hypothesis that LXRα agonists could have a beneficial effect on atherosclerosis.[88]

Recently, synthetic LXR ligands have been characterized in several animal models for the treatment of atherosclerosis. A nonsteroidal LXR agonist, GW3965, has been shown to reduce plaques in a murine model of atherosclerosis, providing direct evidence for an atheroprotective effect of LXR agonists.[89] Terasaka and colleagues[90] subsequently showed reduction of atherosclerosis by T0901317, a synthetic LXR ligand, in *LDLR*−/− mice, without affecting total plasma cholesterol levels. Moreover, an agonist for RXR, the obligate heterodimeric partner of LXRs, has also been shown to reduce experimental atherosclerosis.[91] These results suggest that LXR ligands may be useful therapeutic agents for the treatment of atherosclerosis. However, this therapeutic benefit has to be balanced by the adverse effects of LXR agonists whereby LXR activation is associated with stimulation of lipogenesis, resulting in increased plasma triglyceride levels and hepatic fat accumulation.[92–94] Recently, another potent synthetic steroidal LXR activator, *N,N*-dimethyl-3β-hydroxy-cholenamide (DMHCA), has been shown to reduce atherosclerosis in apoE-deficient mice, without elevating hepatic and plasma triglyceride levels. Based on these observations, DMHCA could be a candidate for further development as a therapeutic agent for atherosclerosis.[95]

Immune Modulation of Atherosclerosis with a Peptide-Based Vaccine (CVX210) or Monoclonal Anti-LDL Epitope Antibody (BI204)

Several experimental studies have shown that both the adaptive and innate immune systems modulate atherosclerosis in a complex manner, with evidence for proatherogenic as well as atheroprotective actions.[96–99] One of the major autoantigens against which evidence of both a humoral and cellular immune response exists in preclinical and clinical atherosclerosis is oxidized LDL. Experimental studies from the authors' laboratories as well as the laboratory of a collaborator, Professor Jan Nilsson at Lund University, have shown that immunization of hyperlipidemic rabbits and mice using various forms of LDL (oxidized or native) as an immunogen reduces atherosclerosis without a significant change in circulating cholesterol levels.[100–102] Using human apoB-100 as a target, several antigenic sequences have been identified within this molecule, and synthetic mimics of these sequences consisting of a 20-amino-acid peptide have been tested as vaccines in mice.[103–105] The authors have shown that several of these apoB-100–related peptide vaccines reduce atherosclerosis and plaque inflammation in hyperlipidemic mice.[103–105] Human trials of the lead candidate peptide vaccine are anticipated in the foreseeable future. In addition to active immunotherapy with a vaccine, the authors have also evaluated the effect of a monoclonal antibody BI-204 against one of the apoB-100–related antigenic peptides in experimental animals, and have shown it to induce rapid plaque regression and anti-inflammatory response in hyperlipidemic mice.[106,107] A phase 1 human trial of this antibody has been completed, with plans under way for a phase 2 human trial (Nilsson J, personal communication, 2010).

SUMMARY

Many new potential therapeutic strategies, including (1) nonstatin drugs to reduce LDL-C, (2) various regimens to augment HDL levels and HDL function, and (3) inflammation- or immune-modulation therapies, are now being developed and tested in different phases of preclinical or clinical trials (**Box 1**). Once they are proved to be effective and safe in humans, they will be valuable additions to our current pharmacologic armamentarium for the treatment of atherosclerotic arterial disease and its associated complications. The authors are now cautiously but optimistically awaiting these exciting new developments.

Box 1
Novel interventions being tested in preclinical or clinical studies for the prevention and management of atherosclerosis

Nonstatin LDL-C–Lowering Therapies

1. Cholesterol absorption inhibitors
2. ACAT inhibitors
3. MTP inhibitors
4. Antisense to apoB-100
5. PCSK-9 inhibitors
6. Thyroid hormone agonists

New HDL-Based Therapies

1. Niacin-laropiprant combination
2. Fibrates
3. CETP inhibitors
4. Small-molecule stimulator of apoA-1 gene transcription
5. Reinfusion of ex vivo delipidated endogenous HDL
6. ApoA-1 mimetic peptides
7. Intravenous infusion of apoA-1$_{Milano}$ or wild-type apoA-1 (synthetic HDL)
8. Intravenous infusion of human plasma derived wild-type apoA-1
9. Endothelial lipase inhibition
10. Gene transfer of HDL-associated proteins (apoA-1, paraoxonase, and PAF-AH)

Inflammation- or Immune-Modulation Therapies

1. Lipoprotein-associated phospholipase 2 inhibitor
2. Inhibitors of soluble phospholipase A2
3. Liver X receptor agonists
4. Immune modulation of atherosclerosis with a peptide-based vaccine or monoclonal anti-LDL epitope antibody

REFERENCES

1. Yusuf S, Reddy S, Ounpuu S, et al. Global burden of cardiovascular diseases: part I: general considerations, the epidemiologic transition, risk factors, and impact of urbanization. Circulation 2001; 104(22):2746–53.
2. Yusuf S, Reddy S, Ounpuu S, et al. Global burden of cardiovascular diseases: part II: variations in cardiovascular disease by specific ethnic groups and geographic regions and prevention strategies. Circulation 2001;104(23):2855–64.
3. Shah PK. Molecular mechanisms of plaque instability. Curr Opin Lipidol 2007;18(5):492–9.
4. Chyu KY, Shah PK. The role of inflammation in plaque disruption and thrombosis. Rev Cardiovasc Med 2001;2(2):82–91.
5. Andersson J, Libby P, Hansson GK. Adaptive immunity and atherosclerosis. Clin Immunol 2010; 134(1):33–46.
6. Hansson GK. Inflammatory mechanisms in atherosclerosis. J Thromb Haemost 2009;(7 Suppl 1): 328–31.

7. Third report of the National Cholesterol Education Program (NCEP) expert panel on detection, evaluation, and treatment of high blood cholesterol in adults (Adult Treatment Panel III) final report. Circulation 2002;106(25):3143–421.

8. Grundy SM, Cleeman JI, Merz CN, et al. Implications of recent clinical trials for the National Cholesterol Education Program Adult Treatment Panel III guidelines. J Am Coll Cardiol 2004;44(3):720–32.

9. Soutar AK, Naoumova RP. Mechanisms of disease: genetic causes of familial hypercholesterolemia. Nat Clin Pract Cardiovasc Med 2007;4(4):214–25.

10. Plat J, Mensink RP. Plant stanol and sterol esters in the control of blood cholesterol levels: mechanism and safety aspects. Am J Cardiol 2005;96(1A): 15D–22D.

11. Plat J, Mensink RP. Increased intestinal ABCA1 expression contributes to the decrease in cholesterol absorption after plant stanol consumption. FASEB J 2002;16(10):1248–53.

12. Garcia-Calvo M, Lisnock J, Bull HG, et al. The target of ezetimibe is Niemann-Pick C1-Like 1 (NPC1L1). Proc Natl Acad Sci U S A 2005; 102(23):8132–7.

13. Becker JC, Kolanus W, Lonnemann C, et al. Human natural killer clones enhance in vitro antibody production by tumour necrosis factor alpha and gamma interferon. Scand J Immunol 1990;32: 153–62.

14. Kerzner B, Corbelli J, Sharp S, et al. Efficacy and safety of ezetimibe coadministered with lovastatin in primary hypercholesterolemia. Am J Cardiol 2003;91(4):418–24.

15. Kastelein JJ, Akdim F, Stroes ES, et al. Simvastatin with or without ezetimibe in familial hypercholesterolemia. N Engl J Med 2008;358(14):1431–43.

16. Ballantyne CM, Houri J, Notarbartolo A, et al. Effect of ezetimibe coadministered with atorvastatin in 628 patients with primary hypercholesterolemia: a prospective, randomized, double-blind trial. Circulation 2003;107(19):2409–15.

17. Rossebo AB, Pedersen TR, Boman K, et al. Intensive lipid lowering with simvastatin and ezetimibe in aortic stenosis. N Engl J Med 2008;359(13): 1343–56.

18. Peto R, Emberson J, Landray M, et al. Analyses of cancer data from three ezetimibe trials. N Engl J Med 2008;359(13):1357–66.

19. Cannon CP, Giugliano RP, Blazing MA, et al. Rationale and design of IMPROVE-IT (IMProved Reduction of Outcomes: Vytorin Efficacy International Trial): comparison of ezetimbe/simvastatin versus simvastatin monotherapy on cardiovascular outcomes in patients with acute coronary syndromes. Am Heart J 2008;156(5):826–32.

20. Califf RM, Lokhnygina Y, Cannon CP, et al. An update on the IMProved reduction of outcomes: Vytorin Efficacy International Trial (IMPROVE-IT) design. Am Heart J 2010;159(5):705–9.

21. Chang TY, Li BL, Chang CC, et al. Acyl-coenzyme A:cholesterol acyltransferases. Am J Physiol Endocrinol Metab 2009;297(1):E1–9.

22. Accad M, Smith SJ, Newland DL, et al. Massive xanthomatosis and altered composition of atherosclerotic lesions in hyperlipidemic mice lacking acyl CoA: cholesterol acyltransferase 1 [see comments]. J Clin Invest 2000;105(6):711–9.

23. Fazio S, Major AS, Swift LL, et al. Increased atherosclerosis in LDL receptor-null mice lacking ACAT1 in macrophages. J Clin Invest 2001;107(2): 163–71.

24. Kusunoki J, Hansoty DK, Aragane K, et al. Acyl-CoA:cholesterol acyltransferase inhibition reduces atherosclerosis in apolipoprotein E-deficient mice. Circulation 2001;103(21):2604–9.

25. Bell TA III, Brown JM, Graham MJ, et al. Liver-specific inhibition of acyl-coenzyme a:cholesterol acyltransferase 2 with antisense oligonucleotides limits atherosclerosis development in apolipoprotein B100-only low-density lipoprotein receptor -/- mice. Arterioscler Thromb Vasc Biol 2006;26(8): 1814–20.

26. Ikenoya M, Yoshinaka Y, Kobayashi H, et al. A selective ACAT-1 inhibitor, K-604, suppresses fatty streak lesions in fat-fed hamsters without affecting plasma cholesterol levels. Atherosclerosis 2007;191(2):290–7.

27. Tardif JC, Gregoire J, L'Allier PL, et al. Effects of the acyl coenzyme A: cholesterol acyltransferase inhibitor avasimibe on human atherosclerotic lesions. Circulation 2004;110(21):3372–7.

28. Nissen SE, Tuzcu EM, Brewer HB, et al. Effect of ACAT inhibition on the progression of coronary atherosclerosis. N Engl J Med 2006;354(12): 1253–63.

29. Meuwese MC, de GE, Duivenvoorden R, et al. ACAT inhibition and progression of carotid atherosclerosis in patients with familial hypercholesterolemia: the CAPTIVATE randomized trial. JAMA 2009;301(11):1131–9.

30. Wetterau JR, Gregg RE, Harrity TW, et al. An MTP inhibitor that normalizes atherogenic lipoprotein levels in WHHL rabbits. Science 1998;282(5389): 751–4.

31. Samaha FF, McKenney J, Bloedon LT, et al. Inhibition of microsomal triglyceride transfer protein alone or with ezetimibe in patients with moderate hypercholesterolemia. Nat Clin Pract Cardiovasc Med 2008;5(8):497–505.

32. Visser ME, Kastelein JJ, Stroes ES. Apolipoprotein B synthesis inhibition: results from clinical trials. Curr Opin Lipidol 2010;21(4):319–23.

33. Raal FJ, Santos RD, Blom DJ, et al. Mipomersen, an apolipoprotein B synthesis inhibitor, for lowering

of LDL cholesterol concentrations in patients with homozygous familial hypercholesterolaemia: a randomised, double-blind, placebo-controlled trial. Lancet 2010;375(9719):998–1006.

34. Kling J. Safety signal dampens reception for mipomersen antisense. Nat Biotechnol 2010;28(4):295–7.

35. Cohen JC, Boerwinkle E, Mosley TH Jr, et al. Sequence variations in PCSK9, low LDL, and protection against coronary heart disease. N Engl J Med 2006;354(12):1264–72.

36. Lambert G, Charlton F, Rye KA, et al. Molecular basis of PCSK9 function. Atherosclerosis 2009;203(1):1–7.

37. Chan JC, Piper DE, Cao Q, et al. A proprotein convertase subtilisin/kexin type 9 neutralizing antibody reduces serum cholesterol in mice and nonhuman primates. Proc Natl Acad Sci U S A 2009;106(24):9820–5.

38. Berkenstam A, Kristensen J, Mellstrom K, et al. The thyroid hormone mimetic compound KB2115 lowers plasma LDL cholesterol and stimulates bile acid synthesis without cardiac effects in humans. Proc Natl Acad Sci U S A 2008;105(2):663–7.

39. Tancevski I, Wehinger A, Demetz E, et al. The thyromimetic T-0681 protects from atherosclerosis. J Lipid Res 2009;50(5):938–44.

40. Tancevski I, Demetz E, Eller P, et al. The liver-selective thyromimetic T-0681 influences reverse cholesterol transport and atherosclerosis development in mice. PLoS One 2010;5(1).e8722.

41. Shah PK, Kaul S, Nilsson J, et al. Exploiting the vascular protective effects of high-density lipoprotein and its apolipoproteins: an idea whose time for testing is coming, part I. Circulation 2001;104(19):2376–83.

42. Shah PK, Kaul S, Nilsson J, et al. Exploiting the vascular protective effects of high-density lipoprotein and its apolipoproteins: an idea whose time for testing is coming, part II. Circulation 2001;104(20):2498–502.

43. Yin K, Liao DF, Tang CK. ATP-Binding Membrane Cassette Transporter A1 (ABCA1): a possible link between Inflammation and reverse cholesterol transport. Mol Med 2010;16(9–10):438–49.

44. Yvan-Charvet L, Wang N, Tall AR. Role of HDL, ABCA1, and ABCG1 transporters in cholesterol efflux and immune responses. Arterioscler Thromb Vasc Biol 2010;30(2):139–43.

45. Angeli V, Llodra J, Rong JX, et al. Dyslipidemia associated with atherosclerotic disease systemically alters dendritic cell mobilization. Immunity 2004;21(4):561–74.

46. Pu DR, Liu L. HDL slowing down endothelial progenitor cells senescence: a novel anti-atherogenic property of HDL. Med Hypotheses 2008;70(2):338–42.

47. Mineo C, Shaul PW. Role of high-density lipoprotein and scavenger receptor B type I in the promotion of endothelial repair. Trends Cardiovasc Med 2007;17(5):156–61.

48. Kimura T, Tomura H, Mogi C, et al. Role of scavenger receptor class B type I and sphingosine 1-phosphate receptors in high density lipoprotein-induced inhibition of adhesion molecule expression in endothelial cells. J Biol Chem 2006;281(49):37457–67.

49. Seetharam D, Mineo C, Gormley AK, et al. High-density lipoprotein promotes endothelial cell migration and reendothelialization via scavenger receptor-B type I. Circ Res 2006;98(1):63–72.

50. Oslakovic C, Krisinger MJ, Andersson A, et al. Anionic phospholipids lose their procoagulant properties when incorporated into high density lipoproteins. J Biol Chem 2009;284(9):5896–904.

51. Fryirs M, Barter PJ, Rye KA. Cholesterol metabolism and pancreatic beta-cell function. Curr Opin Lipidol 2009;20(3):159–64.

52. Fryirs MA, Barter PJ, Appavoo M, et al. Effects of high-density lipoproteins on pancreatic beta-cell insulin secretion. Arterioscler Thromb Vasc Biol 2010;30(8):1642–8.

53. Kruit JK, Brunham LR, Verchere CB, et al. HDL and LDL cholesterol significantly influence beta-cell function in type 2 diabetes mellitus. Curr Opin Lipidol 2010;21(3):178–85.

54. Smith JD. Dysfunctional HDL as a diagnostic and therapeutic target. Arterioscler Thromb Vasc Biol 2010;30(2):151–5.

55. Sirtori CR, Calabresi L, Franceschini G, et al. Cardiovascular status of carriers of the apolipoprotein A-I(Milano) mutant: the Limone sul Garda study. Circulation 2001;103(15):1949–54.

56. Franceschini G, Calabresi L, Chiesa G, et al. Increased cholesterol efflux potential of sera from ApoA-IMilano carriers and transgenic mice. Arterioscler Thromb Vasc Biol 1999;19:1257–62.

57. Sanyal S, Kuvin JT, Karas RH. Niacin and laropiprant. Drugs Today (Barc) 2010;46(6):371–8.

58. Jun M, Foote C, Lv J, et al. Effects of fibrates on cardiovascular outcomes: a systematic review and meta-analysis. Lancet 2010;375(9729):1875–84.

59. Barter PJ, Caulfield M, Eriksson M, et al. Effects of torcetrapib in patients at high risk for coronary events. N Engl J Med 2007;357(21):2109–22.

60. Nicholls SJ, Tuzcu EM, Brennan DM, et al. Cholesteryl ester transfer protein inhibition, high-density lipoprotein raising, and progression of coronary atherosclerosis: insights from ILLUSTRATE (Investigation of Lipid Level Management Using Coronary Ultrasound to Assess Reduction of Atherosclerosis by CETP Inhibition and HDL Elevation). Circulation 2008;118(24):2506–14.

61. Bots ML, Visseren FL, Evans GW, et al. Torcetrapib and carotid intima-media thickness in mixed dyslipidaemia (RADIANCE 2 study): a randomised, double-blind trial. Lancet 2007;370(9582):153–60.

62. Schwartz GG, Olsson AG, Ballantyne CM, et al. Rationale and design of the dal-OUTCOMES trial: efficacy and safety of dalcetrapib in patients with recent acute coronary syndrome. Am Heart J 2009;158(6):896–901.

63. Cannon CP, Dansky HM, Davidson M, et al. Design of the DEFINE trial: determining the EFficacy and tolerability of CETP INhibition with AnacEtrapib. Am Heart J 2009;158(4):513–9.

64. McNeill E. RVX-208, a stimulator of apolipoprotein AI gene expression for the treatment of cardiovascular diseases. Curr Opin Investig Drugs 2010; 11(3):357–64.

65. Bailey D, Jahagirdar R, Gordon A, et al. RVX-208: a small molecule that increases apolipoprotein A-I and high-density lipoprotein cholesterol in vitro and in vivo. J Am Coll Cardiol 2010;55(23):2580–9.

66. Waksman R, Torguson R, Kent KM, et al. A first-in-man, randomized, placebo-controlled study to evaluate the safety and feasibility of autologous delipidated high-density lipoprotein plasma infusions in patients with acute coronary syndrome. J Am Coll Cardiol 2010;55(24):2727–35.

67. Sherman CB, Peterson SJ, Frishman WH. Apolipoprotein A-I mimetic peptides: a potential new therapy for the prevention of atherosclerosis. Cardiol Rev 2010;18(3):141–7.

68. Bloedon LT, Dunbar R, Duffy D, et al. Safety, pharmacokinetics, and pharmacodynamics of oral apoA-I mimetic peptide D-4F in high-risk cardiovascular patients. J Lipid Res 2008;49(6): 1344–52.

69. Bielicki JK, Zhang H, Cortez Y, et al. A new HDL mimetic peptide that stimulates cellular cholesterol efflux with high efficiency greatly reduces atherosclerosis in mice. J Lipid Res 2010;51(6): 1496–503.

70. Kaul S, Coin B, Hedayiti A, et al. Rapid reversal of endothelial dysfunction in hypercholesterolemic apolipoprotein E-null mice by recombinant apolipoprotein A-I(Milano)-phospholipid complex. J Am Coll Cardiol 2004;44(6):1311–9.

71. Kaul S, Rukshin V, Santos R, et al. Intramural delivery of recombinant apolipoprotein A-IMilano/phospholipid complex (ETC-216) inhibits in-stent stenosis in porcine coronary arteries. Circulation 2003;107(20):2551–4.

72. Shah PK, Yano J, Reyes O, et al. High-dose recombinant apolipoprotein A-I(milano) mobilizes tissue cholesterol and rapidly reduces plaque lipid and macrophage content in apolipoprotein e-deficient mice. Potential implications for acute plaque stabilization. Circulation 2001;103(25):3047–50.

73. Shah PK, Nilsson J, Kaul S, et al. Effects of recombinant apolipoprotein A-I(Milano) on aortic atherosclerosis in apolipoprotein E-deficient mice. Circulation 1998;97(8):780–5.

74. Nissen SE, Tsunoda T, Tuzcu EM, et al. Effect of recombinant ApoA-I Milano on coronary atherosclerosis in patients with acute coronary syndromes: a randomized controlled trial. JAMA 2003; 290(17):2292–300.

75. Wang L, Sharifi BG, Pan T, et al. Bone marrow transplantation shows superior atheroprotective effects of gene therapy with apolipoprotein A-I Milano compared with wild-type apolipoprotein A-I in hyperlipidemic mice. J Am Coll Cardiol 2006;48(7): 1459–68.

76. Tardif JC, Gregoire J, L'Allier PL, et al. Effects of reconstituted high-density lipoprotein infusions on coronary atherosclerosis: a randomized controlled trial. JAMA 2007;297(15):1675–82.

77. Shaw JA, Bobik A, Murphy A, et al. Infusion of reconstituted high-density lipoprotein leads to acute changes in human atherosclerotic plaque. Circ Res 2008;103(10):1084–91.

78. Santamarina-Fojo S, Haudenschild C. Role of hepatic and lipoprotein lipase in lipoprotein metabolism and atherosclerosis: studies in transgenic and knockout animal models and somatic gene transfer. Int J Tissue React 2000;22(2–3):39–47.

79. Badellino KO, Rader DJ. The role of endothelial lipase in high-density lipoprotein metabolism. Curr Opin Cardiol 2004;19(4):392–5.

80. Sharifi BG, Wu K, Wang L, et al. AAV serotype-dependent apolipoprotein A-I(Milano) gene expression. Atherosclerosis 2005;181(2):261–9.

81. Corson MA. Emerging inflammatory markers for assessing coronary heart disease risk. Curr Cardiol Rep 2009;11(6):452–9.

82. Wilensky RL, Shi Y, Mohler ER III, et al. Inhibition of lipoprotein-associated phospholipase A2 reduces complex coronary atherosclerotic plaque development. Nat Med 2008;14(10):1059–66.

83. Serruys PW, Garcia-Garcia HM, Buszman P, et al. Effects of the direct lipoprotein-associated phospholipase A(2) inhibitor darapladib on human coronary atherosclerotic plaque. Circulation 2008; 118(11):1172–82.

84. Suckling K. Phospholipase A(2)s: developing drug targets for atherosclerosis. Atherosclerosis 2010; 212(2):357–66.

85. Ebara T, Ramakrishnan R, Steiner G, et al. Chylomicronemia due to apolipoprotein CIII overexpression in apolipoprotein E-null mice. Apolipoprotein CIII-induced hypertriglyceridemia is not mediated by effects on apolipoprotein E. J Clin Invest 1997;99: 2672–81.

86. Rosenson RS, Hislop C, McConnell D, et al. Effects of 1-H-indole-3-glyoxamide (A-002) on concentration

of secretory phospholipase A2 (PLASMA study): a phase II double-blind, randomised, placebo-controlled trial. Lancet 2009;373(9664):649—58.

87. Zhao C, Dahlman-Wright K. Liver X receptor in cholesterol metabolism. J Endocrinol 2010;204(3): 233—40.

88. Watanabe Y, Jiang S, Takabe W, et al. Expression of the LXRalpha protein in human atherosclerotic lesions. Arterioscler Thromb Vasc Biol 2005;25(3): 622—7.

89. Joseph SB, McKilligin E, Pei L, et al. Synthetic LXR ligand inhibits the development of atherosclerosis in mice. Proc Natl Acad Sci U S A 2002;99(11): 7604—9.

90. Terasaka N, Hiroshima A, Koieyama T, et al. T-0901317, a synthetic liver X receptor ligand, inhibits development of atherosclerosis in LDL receptor-deficient mice. FEBS Lett 2003; 536(1—3):6—11.

91. Claudel T, Leibowitz MD, Fievet C, et al. Reduction of atherosclerosis in apolipoprotein E knockout mice by activation of the retinoid X receptor. Proc Natl Acad Sci U S A 2001;98(5):2610—5.

92. Repa JJ, Liang G, Ou J, et al. Regulation of mouse sterol regulatory element-binding protein-1c gene (SREBP-1c) by oxysterol receptors, LXRalpha and LXRbeta. Genes Dev 2000;14(22):2819—30.

93. Schultz JR, Tu H, Luk A, et al. Role of LXRs in control of lipogenesis. Genes Dev 2000;14(22): 2831—8.

94. Grefhorst A, Elzinga BM, Voshol PJ, et al. Stimulation of lipogenesis by pharmacological activation of the liver X receptor leads to production of large, triglyceride-rich very low density lipoprotein particles. J Biol Chem 2002;277(37):34182—90.

95. Kratzer A, Buchebner M, Pfeifer T, et al. Synthetic LXR agonist attenuates plaque formation in apoE-/- mice without inducing liver steatosis and hypertriglyceridemia. J Lipid Res 2009;50(2): 312—26.

96. Shah PK, Chyu KY, Fredrikson GN, et al. Immunomodulation of atherosclerosis with a vaccine. Nat Clin Pract Cardiovasc Med 2005;2(12):639—46.

97. Nilsson J, Hansson GK. Autoimmunity in atherosclerosis: a protective response losing control? J Intern Med 2008;263(5):464—78.

98. Hansson GK, Libby P. The immune response in atherosclerosis: a double-edged sword. Nat Rev Immunol 2006;6(7):508—19.

99. Nilsson J, Hansson GK, Shah PK. Immunomodulation of atherosclerosis: implications for vaccine development. Arterioscler Thromb Vasc Biol 2005; 25(1):18—28.

100. Ameli S, Hultgardh-Nilsson A, Regnstrom J, et al. Effect of immunization with homologous LDL and oxidized LDL on early atherosclerosis in hypercholesterolemic rabbits. Arterioscler Thromb Vasc Biol 1996;16:1074—9.

101. Chyu KY, Reyes OS, Zhao X, et al. Timing affects the efficacy of LDL immunization on atherosclerotic lesions in apo E (-/-) mice. Atherosclerosis 2004; 176(1):27—35.

102. Nilsson J, Calara F, Regnstrom J, et al. Immunization with homologous oxidized low density lipoprotein reduces neointimal formation after balloon injury in hypercholesterolemic rabbits. J Am Coll Cardiol 1997;30:1886 91.

103. Chyu KY, Zhao X, Reyes OS, et al. Immunization using an Apo B-100 related epitope reduces atherosclerosis and plaque inflammation in hypercholesterolemic apo E (-/-) mice. Biochem Biophys Res Commun 2005;338(4):1982—9.

104. Fredrikson GN, Soderberg I, Lindholm M, et al. Inhibition of atherosclerosis in ApoE-Null mice by immunization with ApoB-100 peptide sequences. Arterioscler Thromb Vasc Biol 2003;23(5):879—84.

105. Fredrikson GN, Hedblad B, Berglund G, et al. Identification of immune responses against aldehyde-modified peptide sequences in ApoB associated with cardiovascular disease. Arterioscler Thromb Vasc Biol 2003;23(5):872—8.

106. Schiopu A, Bengtsson J, Soderberg I, et al. Recombinant human antibodies against aldehyde-modified apolipoprotein B-100 peptide sequences inhibit atherosclerosis. Circulation 2004;110: 2047—52.

107. Schiopu A, Frendeus B, Jansson B, et al. Recombinant antibodies to an oxidized low-density lipoprotein epitope induce rapid regression of atherosclerosis in apobec-1(-/-)/low-density lipoprotein receptor(-/-) mice. J Am Coll Cardiol 2007;50(24):2313—8.

Renin-Angiotensin-Aldosterone Blockade for Cardiovascular Disease Prevention

Krishnaswami Vijayaraghavan, MD, MS[a,b,*],
Prakash Deedwania, MD[c]

KEYWORDS

- Renin-angiotensin-aldosterone system
- Angiotensin-converting enzyme inhibitors
- Angiotensin receptor blockers • Cardiovascular disease

The renin-angiotensin-aldosterone system (RAAS) plays a significant role in the pathophysiology of multiple disease states. Its activation leads to vasoconstriction, vascular smooth muscle and cardiac hypertrophy, and fibrosis. Subsequent cardiac, vascular, and renal complications are secondary to vascular stiffness arising from cellular signaling, leading to negative remodeling. RAAS blockade has been shown to be beneficial in patients with hypertension, acute myocardial infarction, chronic heart failure, stroke, and diabetic renal disease. Extensive RAAS blockade with a combination of 2 commonly used RAAS blockers (angiotensin-converting enzyme inhibitors [ACEIs] and angiotensin receptor blockers [ARBs]) have demonstrated conflicting results in recent clinical trials. The RAAS has been known for more than a century.[1] It took 40 years for scientists to realize the existence of angiotensinogen since Tigesedt first demonstrated that an extract from renal cortex of rabbits increased blood pressure.[2–6] Further work by Skeggs and colleagues[7,8] demonstrated that angiotensin existed in 2 distinct forms, angiotensin I (A-I) and angiotensin II (A-II), whereby A-I was cleaved by ACE to generate the biologically active A-II. The hypothesized relationship between A-II and aldosterone was confirmed by Davis.[9] These original works have increased our understanding of the RAAS and has led to some outstanding research.[10] This article summarizes all the important clinical trials and facilitated knowledge of the role of RAAS in the prevention of cardiovascular disease.

ROLE OF RAAS ACTIVATION

The conventional and archetypal RAAS cascade begins with production of renin (**Fig. 1**). Renin, an aspartyl protease produced by the juxtaglomerular cells of the kidney, regulates the initial and rate-limiting step of the RAAS by catalyzing the conversion of angiotensinogen to A-I, which is subsequently hydrolyzed by angiotensin-converting enzymes (ACEs) to form A-II.[11,12] Alternative pathways exist that convert angiotensinogen directly to A-II, such as tissue plasminogen activator, cathepsin G, and tonin, whereas A-I is also catalyzed to A-II by chymase and cathepsin G,[13,14] which form the basis of "A-II escape." A-II acts on the adrenal cortex and causes the release of aldosterone.[15] The net effects of the activation of the RAAS include

[a] Cardiovascular Research and Education, Scottsdale Healthcare, Scottsdale, AZ, USA
[b] Department of Medicine, Midwestern University, Glendale, AZ, USA
[c] Division of Cardiology, Department of Medicine, Veterans Affairs Central California Health Care System/ University of California, San Francisco, Fresno Program, 2615 East Clinton Avenue, Fresno, CA 93703, USA
* Corresponding author. Cardiovascular Research and Education, Scottsdale Healthcare, Scottsdale, AZ.
E-mail address: kvijaymd@gmail.com

Cardiol Clin 29 (2011) 137–156
doi:10.1016/j.ccl.2010.11.003
0733-8651/11/$ − see front matter © 2011 Elsevier Inc. All rights reserved.

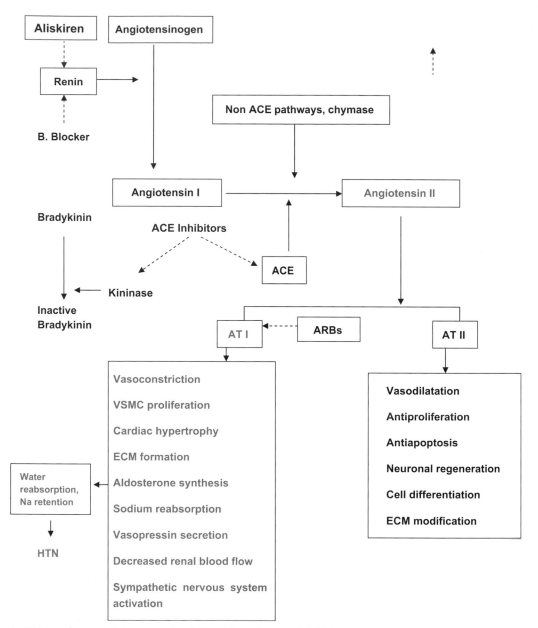

Fig. 1. RAAS pathway. Solid arrow, stimulation; dotted arrow, inhibition. AT I, angiotensin receptor type I; AT II, angiotensin receptor type II; ACE, angiotensin-converting enzyme; ARBs, angiotensin receptor blockers; ECM, extracellular matrix; HTN, hypertension; VSMC, vascular smooth muscle cell.

vasoconstriction, sodium and water retention, increased arterial blood pressure, and increased myocardial contractility, which in combination increase the effective circulating volume. A-II receptor type II expression is less well studied, but appears to mediate beneficial effects that include vasodilatation, inhibition of cell growth and proliferation, and cell differentiation.[16,17] The differential effects are shown in **Fig. 2**. An increase in perfusion of the juxtaglomerular apparatus inhibits the release

of renin through a negative feedback mechanism. Apart from the classic endocrine pathway in the circulation, there is increasing evidence that the renin-angiotensin system (RAS) functions at the tissue level in a paracrine or autocrine manner.[18] For the most part, it is thought that the tissue or local RAS works with the classic circulating RAAS in a complementary manner.

The sequential progression of cardiovascular disease begins with the risk factors of hypertension,

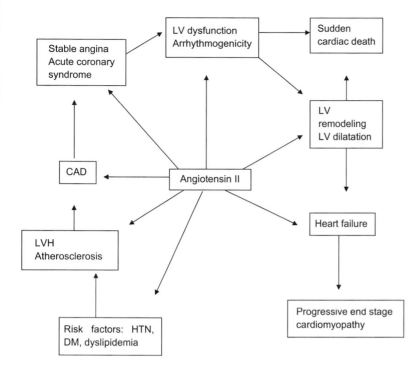

Fig. 2. Angiotensin II and the sequential progression of cardiovascular disease. CAD, coronary artery disease; DM, diabetes mellitus; LV, left ventricular; LVH, left ventricular hypertrophy. Solid arrow, activation.

diabetes, smoking, metabolic syndrome, and dyslipidemia. These risk factors are independently associated with levels of A-II, which in turn triggers the cascade of events. RAAS is involved in certain forms of secondary hypertension, including renin-secreting neoplasms, renovascular hypertension (eg, renal artery stenosis), malignant hypertension, pheochromocytoma, and primary hyperaldosteronism. In patients with primary (essential) hypertension, the plasma renin activity (PRA) can be high, normal, or low.[19] "Low-renin" hypertension is more commonly seen in the elderly, diabetic patients, and those with chronic renal parenchymal disease. Studies have shown that the PRA may not necessarily reflect tissue activities (such as the vascular endothelium, kidneys, brain, and the adrenal glands),[20] which was evidenced by experimental transgenic rat models into which a mouse renin gene was inserted to produce angiotensin-mediated hypertension. The PRA, plasma A-II level and renal renin content were all below normal, whereas adrenal renin content, vascular A-II formation, and plasma level of prorenin (the precursor of active renin) were all markedly elevated.[21] These findings suggest a possible link between primary hypertension and abnormal activation of local RAS.

RAAS activation after acute myocardial infarction has been considered as a compensatory and adaptive response to maintain blood pressure and systemic perfusion. However, sustained activation of the RAAS with A-II production increases myocardial oxygen demand,[22–24] but causes vasoconstriction of the coronary vasculatures. This process further worsens oxygen imbalance and myocardial ischemia after myocardial infarction, and may result in irreversible myocardial damage.[25] A-II has a toxic effect on myocytes, stimulating fibroblast and smooth muscle hypertrophy,[26] with abnormal deposition of fibrillar collagen,[27] leading to progressive ventricular dysfunction after myocardial infarction.

Neurohormonal mechanisms play a central role in the progression of systolic heart failure, whereby activation of the sympathetic nervous system and RAAS have a direct deleterious effect on the heart that is independent of the hemodynamic perturbations produced by these endogenous systems.[28] The main neurohormonal systems involved are the sympathetic nervous system, RAAS, and antidiuretic hormone.[29,30] Other vasoactive substances including endothelin, atrial natriuretic peptide, and nitric oxide are also mediators of cardiac remodeling. Along with A-II, they stimulate fibroblasts to produce collagen, cause myocyte hypertrophy, and promote fibrosis. Secondary hyperaldosteronism is commonly seen in patients with chronic heart failure, and aldosterone-induced cardiac fibrosis[31] results in maladaptive cardiac remodeling, which causes relentless progression of cardiac dysfunction.[32]

ROLE OF RAAS IN VASCULAR ENDOTHELIAL FUNCTION AND ATHEROSCLEROSIS

Endothelium has fivefold functions. First, it acts as a permeability barrier blocking exocytosis of macrophage and small dense low-density lipoprotein (LDL) entering the subendothelial layer to initiate genesis of the fatty streak, an initial step in formation of atheroma. Second, it plays an important role in maintaining vascular tone by releasing A-II and endothelin, powerful vasoconstrictors, and balancing it by release of nitric oxide for a vasodilatory effect. Third, it balances hemostasis through mediating coagulation by inhibiting platelet aggregation and expressing adhesion molecules as well as by releasing von Willebrand factor, tissue plasminogen activator, and plasminogen activator inhibitor-1 (PAI-1), all of which maintains a balance between bleeding and clotting. Fourth, it releases inflammatory cytokines such as interleukin-6, tumor necrosis factor (TNF)-α, and others that are involved in compensatory mechanisms in atherogenesis. Finally, it acts as a transducer of biomechanical forces and prevents sheer stress from denudation of the endothelial layer to allow plaque accumulation (**Fig. 3**).[33,34] A-II contributes to endothelial dysfunction by increasing oxidative stress, attenuating chemoattractants, and adhesion molecule expression, leading to inflammation. In addition, A-II can also exert proliferative and prothrombotic actions to produce superoxide radicals, scavenging nitric oxide and reducing vasodilatation. There is evidence that an increased expression

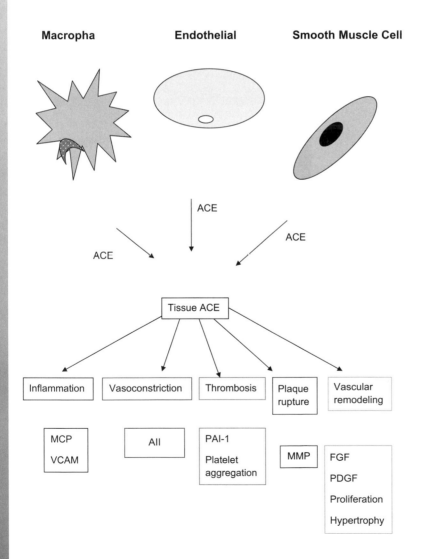

Fig. 3. Role of ACE in vascular function. FGF, fibroblast growth factor; MCP, monocyte chemotactic protein; MMP, matrix metalloproteinase; PAI-1, plasminogen activator inhibitor-1; PDGF, platelet derived growth factor; VCAM, vascular cell adhesion molecule.

of ACE is present in endothelial growth arrest. ACE is induced by glucocorticoids in vascular smooth muscle[35] while activation of ACE induces PAI-1 levels, which are contributors of atherothrombosis. Bradykinin, which is unopposed with blockade of ACE, has significant beneficial effects on endothelium, primarily due to its powerful vasodilating properties. Thus, there is evidence that A-II accumulation impairs endothelial function and enhances atherogenic process.

CROSS-TALK BETWEEN ANGIOTENSIN, ENDOTHELIUM, AND INSULIN RESISTANCE, AND ROLE OF RAAS IN DEVELOPMENT OF DIABETES AND ITS COMPLICATIONS

Insulin resistance is associated with metabolic syndrome, which increases the risk of adverse cardiovascular outcomes. There is definitive evidence of a parallel progression between insulin resistance and endothelial dysfunction. As insulin resistance progresses to clinical metabolic syndrome, impaired glucose tolerance, and development of diabetes, there is a parallel track that leads from endothelial dysfunction to inflammation, thrombosis, and oxidation to overt atherosclerotic disease. Insulin resistance has been shown to interact with this parallel track of endothelial dysfunction by accumulation of free fatty acids, proinflammatory adipokines, and TNF-α.[36] In addition, increased oxidative stress and oxidized LDL with reduction of high-density lipoprotein, and development of hypertension, hyperuricemia, and hyperglycemia contribute to the underlying mechanisms of endothelial dysfunction in insulin resistance.

Because A-II plays a significant role in endothelial dysfunction, interplay of A-II in glucose homeostasis has been of significant interest to biochemical and molecular biologists. The relationship between A-II and insulin signaling pathways is becoming evident in preclinical studies. Insulin binds to the cell surface receptor, tyrosine kinase, which leads to autophosphorylation of tyrosine residue turning on the insulin signaling pathways. The initial step is activation of phosphatidylinositol kinase pathway (PI-3K), which is important for glucose transport in skeletal muscle. In addition, this pathway enhances nitric oxide production and insulin-induced vasodilatory response.[37,38] The second pathway that is activated that of the mitogen-activated protein kinase (MAPK). This pathway promotes vascular smooth muscle cell proliferation and migration induced by insulin, thrombin, and platelet-derived growth factors. In addition, a third pathway is triggered

that leads to activation of P70 S6 kinase, a regulator of protein synthesis.[39,40]

A-II plays an important role in signaling pathways for maintaining structure and function of the heart. AT_1 stimulation results in activation of the MAPK, PI-3K, and tyrosine phosphorylation, both in vivo and in vitro. In the heart, A-II blocks the insulin-induced PI-3K but stimulates MAPK, thus inhibiting the metabolic effects of insulin, but not the proliferative ones.[41] This cross-talk between the 2 signaling pathways may play a pivotal role in understanding how cardiovascular and neuroendocrine physiology relate to each other and thus may explain the role of A-II blockade in insulin resistance and prevention of diabetes.

RAAS AS A THERAPEUTIC TARGET

There are 4 groups of RAAS blockers, namely, direct renin inhibitor (DRI), ACEI, ARB, and aldosterone antagonist. Aliskiren was the first DRI and was approved by the United States Food and Drug Administration in 2007 for the treatment of primary hypertension. Remikiren is another DRI currently under development. ACEIs inhibit ACE and can be divided into 3 groups based on their chemical structures, namely, dicarboxylate containing (eg, benazepril, enalapril, lisinopril, perindopril, ramipril, and quinapril), sulfhydryl containing (eg, captopril, zofenopril), and phosphate containing (fosinopril). ARBs block the activation of A-II type 1 receptors. Examples include candesartan, eprosartan, irbesartan, losartan, olmesartan, and telmisartan. Aldosterone antagonists block the action of aldosterone on mineralocorticoid receptors. Spironolactone was the first member of this class. Other examples include eplerenone and canrenone.

ACE INHIBITORS IN CLINICAL STUDIES
ACE Inhibitors in Hypertension

ACEIs were initially developed in the late 1970s for the treatment of hypertension. Their use has since been expanded to heart failure, postmyocardial infarction, and renal disease. ACEIs, by blocking the conversion of A-I to A-II, as well as by catalyzing the breakdown of bradykinin, exert numerous beneficial effects that maintain blood pressure and salt and water homeostasis. In addition, salutary effects are seen with ACEIs due to their vasodilating, anti-inflammatory, plaque-stabilizing, antithrombotic, and antiproliferative properties. Numerous studies in literature have demonstrated a significant benefit with use of ACE inhibition (**Table 1**). Despite the negative

Table 1
Summary of ACEI clinical trials

Trial	ACEI/Study Meds	Patient Group	Outcome
CAPP (N = 10,985)	Captopril vs diuretics or β-blockers	Hypertension	No difference in major CV events
STOP 2 (N = 6614)	β-Blocker or diuretic vs ACEI or CCB	HTN	No difference in major CV events
HYVET-Pilot (N = 1283)	Diuretic vs ACEI vs no treatment	HTN	ACEI reduced stroke by 53% and stroke mortality by 43%
HYVET (N = 3845)	Indapamide +/− perindopril vs placebo	HTN	ACEI reduced mortality by 21% and CHF by 64%
ACCOMPLISH (N = 11,506)	Benazepril + amlodipine vs benazepril + HCTZ	HTN	Benazepril + amlodipine showed a 20% reduction in CV events
CONSENSUS (N = 253)	Enalapril vs placebo	NYHA IV, CHF	40% and 31% reduction in mortality in 6 mo and 1 y, respectively
SOLVD, treatment arm (N = 2569)	Enalapril vs placebo	NYHA II & III, CHF	16% reduction in mortality and 26% reduction in death and hospitalization combined
V-HeFT II (N = 804)	Enalapril vs hydralazine-isosorbide	NYHA II & III, CHF	28% reduction in 2-year mortality
SAVE (N = 2231)	Captopril vs placebo	Recent MI with asymptomatic LVD	32% reduction in mortality
SOLVD, prevention arm (N = 4228)	Enalapril vs placebo	Asymptomatic LVD	29% reduction in death and hospitalization due to CHF
AIRE (N = 2006)	Ramipril vs placebo	Recent MI with overt CHF	30% reduction in sudden cardiac death and 23% reduction in CHF progression
ISIS-4 (N >58,050)	Captopril vs placebo	Acute MI	7% reduction in mortality
GISSI-3 (N = 19,394)	Lisinopril vs open control	Acute MI	12% reduction in mortality in 6 wk and 6% in 6 mo
TRACE (N = 1749)	Trandolapril vs placebo	Recent MI with LVD	25% reduction in mortality
SMILE (N = 1556)	Zofenopril vs placebo	Acute MI	34% reduction in mortality in 6 wk and 29% in 1 y
PROGRESS (N = 6105)	Perindopril +/− indapamide vs placebo	Stroke	28% reduction in stroke and 26% in CV events
HOPE (N = 9297)	Ramipril vs placebo	Vascular disease or diabetes plus one risk factor	26%, 20%, 32%, and 33% reduction in CV death, MI, stroke, and CHF, respectively
PEACE (N = 6904)	Perindopril vs placebo	HTN	23% reduction in CHF. No mortality benefit

Abbreviations: CHF, congestive heart failure; CV, cardiovascular; HCTZ, hydrochlorothiazide; HTN, hypertension; LVD, left ventricular dysfunction; MI, myocardial infarction; NYHA, New York Heart Association class.
Data from Refs.[43–70]

result of the Captopril Prevention Project,[42] subsequent large trials involving other ACEIs (eg, ramipril, perindopril, lisinopril, enalapril) such as STOP-2, HOPE, and ACCOMPLISH,[43–45] demonstrated that antihypertensive treatment with ACEIs improved clinical outcomes. Previous meta-analysis raised the concern that controlling hypertension (with thiazide or β-blocker as first-line treatment, resulting in a mean reduction of systolic blood pressure by 15.0 mm Hg and diastolic blood pressure by 6.1 mm Hg) in the elderly may increase the risk of death.[46] In the HYVET-Pilot study, which involved hypertensive patients older than 80 years, use of ACEI (lisinopril and enalapril) reduced the risk of stroke by 40%, but was associated with a trend toward increased risk of total deaths (relative risk [RR] 1.14, 95% confidence interval [CI] 0.65–2.02) and cardiac deaths (RR 1.40, 95% CI 0.50–3.92). The later HYVET study,[47] in which indapamide was used as the first line therapy and perindopril as add-on therapy, however, showed improvement in cardiovascular outcomes with no increase in adverse events.[48] In the PEACE study,[49] use of perindopril was associated with a 23% reduction in stroke without any mortality benefit.

ACE Inhibitors in Postmyocardial Infarction

Multiple prospective randomized trials have assessed the use of ACEIs following acute myocardial infarction (AMI). These trials could be divided into: (1) those in which ACEI were given to all AMI patients in a randomized fashion (ISIS-4, GISSI-3, and CONSENSUS II)[50–53]; and (2) those that required evidence of asymptomatic or symptomatic left ventricular dysfunction before randomization (SAVE, TRACE, AIRE, and SMILE).[54–58] In the ISIS-4 and GISSI-3 studies, oral use of captopril and lisinopril when compared with placebo resulted in a 7% (at 5 weeks) and 12% (12% at 6 weeks; 6.2% at 6 months) reduction in mortality, respectively. This outcome was accomplished above and beyond thrombolytic therapy. The negative result shown by the CONSENSUS II study was thought to be secondary to significant hypotension caused by intravenous enalaprilat given in the first 24 h after AMI. In patients with AMI and left ventricular systolic dysfunction, captopril in the SAVE study and trandolapril in the TRACE study resulted in 32% and 25% reduction in mortality, respectively, compared with placebo. In patients with AMI and clinically evident congestive heart failure, ramipril reduced mortality and heart failure progression as compared with placebo. The AIRE results suggested that halting heart failure progression in AMI

patients could improve survival with benefits sustained for many years. The SMILE study showed that in patients with anterior AMI without thrombolysis, zofenopril reduced mortality and incidence of severe heart failure when the drug was started within 24 h after the onset of AMI. Studies regarding ACEI in low-risk patients such as PEACE and QUIET[59] with stable coronary heart disease were more conflicting. Several meta-analyses of ACEI trials have consistently demonstrated a favorable effect on survival after AMI. Meta-analysis of pooled data showed that use of ACEI was associated with a reduction in cardiovascular mortality (RR 0.83, 95% CI 0.72–0.96, $P = .01$), nonfatal myocardial infarction (MI) (RR 0.84, 95% CI 0.75–0.94, $P = .003$), all-cause mortality (RR 0.87, 95% CI 0.81–0.94, $P = .0003$) and revascularization rates (RR 0.93, 95% CI 0.87–1.00, $P = .04$).[60–64]

ACE Inhibitors in Congestive Heart Failure

Enalapril in CONSENSUS, SOLVD treatment and prevention, and VHeft II demonstrated significant overall mortality reduction in patients with congestive heart failure.[65–67] Compared with hydralazine and isosorbide dinitrate combination, enalapril was superior in terms of reducing mortality, as shown in the V-HeFT II study, although subsequent analysis showed that the mortality benefit was only seen in white patients with hypertension and higher PRA.[68] Previous meta-analysis showed that ACEI therapy increased survival, reduced heart failure-related hospitalizations, and improved symptoms in patients with left ventricular dysfunction or heart failure.[61]

ACE Inhibitors in Stroke

Two large trials with ACEI, PROGRESS and HOPE, have been performed. In the PROGRESS study, subjects with a history of cerebrovascular disease were randomly assigned to receive perindopril with or without addition of indapamide or placebo. At 4-year follow up, perindopril alone reduced the incidence of recurrent stroke by 28%, whereas the combination with indapamide reduced stroke risk by 43%. Treatment effects were consistent across different patient subgroups, including those with and without hypertension, and for both ischemic and hemorrhagic strokes.[69] Similarly, in the HOPE study, ramipril reduced the RR of any stroke by 32% and the risk of fatal stroke by 61%. ACEIs seem to lower stroke risk by mechanisms other than lowering of blood pressure.[70]

ARBS IN CLINICAL STUDIES
ARBs in Hypertension

In the LIFE study, losartan was superior to atenolol in decreasing the risk of cardiovascular death, stroke or MI, and new-onset diabetes, while accomplishing clinical equipoise in blood pressure reduction in patients with essential hypertension and left ventricular hypertrophy.[71] In the VALUE study, in hypertensive patients at high cardiovascular risk, valsartan was equivalent to amlodipine in cardiac mortality and morbidity.[72] Although the amlodipine group had a significantly lower incidence of myocardial infarction than the valsartan group, the amlodipine group attained a lower blood pressure, which may have made the difference. Similar to the LIFE study, patients on valsartan had a lower incidence of new-onset diabetes.

ARBs After AMI

ARBs have had a favorable impact on survival in AMI patients. In the OPTIMAAL study, AMI patients with congestive heart failure randomized to losartan or captopril had similar outcomes after a mean follow-up of 2.7 years. However, losartan was better tolerated than captopril, with fewer patients withdrawing from treatment (17% vs 23%, RR 0.70, 95% CI 0.62–0.79, $P<.0001$).[73] Similarly, in the VALIANT study, valsartan was shown to be equally effective as captopril in reducing mortality in AMI patients.[74]

ARBs in Congestive Heart Failure

In the ELITE and ELITE II studies, the role of losartan in heart failure was evaluated as primary therapy compared with ACEI or placebo.[75,76] In addition, Candesartan was evaluated as an alternative in patients intolerant of ACEIs (CHARM-alternative) and as add-on therapy (CHARM-added) in patients already treated with an ACEI.[77] The ELITE I study showed losartan to provide a similar benefit when compared with captopril, and had a similar risk of renal dysfunction. There was a trend toward better clinical outcome for death and/or hospital admission for heart failure in the losartan group (9.4% in losartan group vs 13.2% in captopril group) ($P = .075$), primarily due to a decrease in all-cause mortality (4.8% vs 8.7%; $P = .035$). However, such mortality benefit was not seen in the ELITE II study, which showed a similar all-cause mortality (11.7% vs 10.4% average annual mortality rate), sudden death, or resuscitated cardiac arrests (9.0% vs 7.3%) between the losartan and captopril groups. The ELITE I result was thought to be a chance finding, as the event rate was small compared with the event rate in ELITE II. In the CHARM-alternative study, candesartan was shown to reduce cardiovascular deaths or hospital admissions for heart failure by 30% ($P<.0001$) in patients intolerant to ACEI. The recent HEAAL study suggested that in patients with heart failure (New York Heart Association [NYHA] class II–IV), left ventricular ejection fraction (LVEF) 40% or less, and intolerant to ACEI, losartan 150 mg daily was superior to 50 mg daily in reducing the mortality or admissions for heart failure, suggesting that increased doses of an ARB would be needed to achieve the maximal benefit.[78] While the HEAAL study certainly added information that losartan at 150 mg daily seemed to be more effective and generally tolerated, it did not provide any information about whether a high-dose ARB is better than ACEI monotherapy. Neither did it offer insights about whether maximizing the dose of one RAAS blocker would be better than the use of combination therapy (eg, comparing high-dose ARB with low-dose ARB plus low-dose ACEI). A meta-analysis[79] showed that ARB reduced all-cause mortality and heart failure hospitalizations as compared with placebo, and had similar efficacy when compared with ACEI in patients with chronic heart failure.

ARBs in Stroke

Candesartan, losartan, telmisartan, and eprosartan have been examined in large clinical trials, both for primary prevention (LIFE, SCOPE,[80] TRANSCEND, and ONTARGET[81,82]) and secondary prevention (MOSES and PRoFESS[83,84]) in the treatment of stroke (**Table 2**). In the LIFE study, losartan was shown to be superior to atenolol in stroke prevention, where losartan reduced the risk of fatal or nonfatal stroke by 25%. Similarly, in the SCOPE study, candesartan reduced the risk of nonfatal stroke by 27.8% and all stroke by 23.6%. In the TRANSCEND study, there was a 13% reduction in the risk of the secondary composite outcome of cardiovascular death, myocardial infarction, or stroke by using telmisartan ($P = .048$), yet the reduction of stroke risk in isolation was not statistically significant (3.8% vs 4.6%; $P = .136$). The stroke subgroup of the ONTARGET study also showed telmisartan treatment to be no better than ramipril regarding risk of recurrent stroke (hazard ratio [HR] 0.91; $P = .85$). In the MOSES study, eprosartan was superior to nitrendipine in reducing the risk of combined cardiovascular events by 21% ($P = .014$) and cerebrovascular events by 25% ($P = .03$) despite a similar degree of blood pressure reduction. However, the PRoFESS trial, which was the largest

Table 2
Summary of ARBs in clinical trials

Trial	Patient Group	Study Meds	Outcome	Result
LIFE[71] (N = 9193)	HTN	Losartan 50–100 mg vs atenolol 50–100 mg	Composite CV mortality, MI, stroke	Losartan showed 13% RR (P = .021) in composite end point and 25% reduction in stroke
VALUE[72] (N = 15,245)	HTN	Valsartan, up to 160 mg vs amlodipine, up to 10 mg	Composite end point of mortality and morbidity	No difference between valsartan and amlodipine in composite CV end points and mortality
OPTIMAAL[73] (N = 5477)	AMI with heart failure	Losartan 50 mg/d or captopril 50 mg 3 times a day	All-cause mortality, SCD, and total and NFMI	No difference between captopril and losartan, 13.3% death captopril vs 15.3% death losartan (P = .03)
ELITE II[75] (N = 3152)	CHF	Losartan 50 mg/d, captopril 50 mg 3 times a day	All-cause mortality	No difference
CHARM, alternate[77] (N = 2028)	CHF	Candesartan 32 mg/d, placebo	Composite of CV death at hospital	23% reduction, statistically significant
HEAAL[78] (N = 3846)	CHF	Losartan 50 mg/d vs losartan 150 mg/d	Death or CHF admissions	High-dose losartan (46% reduction) better than low-dose losartan (43% reduction)
MOSES (N = 1405)	HTN, high vascular risk, previous stroke	Eprosartan vs nitrendipine	CV events and stroke	Eprosartan reduced CV events by 21% and stroke by 25%
PRoFESS (N = 20,332)	Ischemic stroke	Telmisartan vs placebo	Stroke and major CV events	No difference
TRANSCEND (N = 5926)	CV disease or diabetes with end organ damage and ACE intolerant	Telmisartan vs placebo	Stroke	No difference
SCOPE (N = 4964)	HTN	Candesartan vs placebo	Stroke	Candesartan reduced stroke by 28%

Abbreviations: AMI, acute myocardial infarction; NFMI, nonfatal myocardial infarction; RR, relative risk; SCD, sudden cardiac death.
Data from Refs.[71–84]

stroke trial, failed to demonstrate such benefit. The PRoFESS study was designed to compare the effects of telmisartan against placebo, in addition to standard stroke prevention therapy including other antihypertensive drugs, on the further reduction of recurrent stroke. In this study 20,332 patients with ischemic stroke were randomized to telmisartan versus placebo and to 2 antiplatelets (aspirin and dipyridamole) in a 2 × 2 factorial design. After a mean follow-up of 2.5 years, telmisartan showed an insignificant lower rate of recurrent stroke (HR 0.95, 95% CI 0.86–1.04, P = .23). The findings of the PRoFESS study suggest that ARBs do not offer additional benefits beyond an ACEI. ARBs remain an appropriate alternative in patients who are intolerant to ACEI, but not as first line for stroke prevention.

COMBINATION OF ACE INHIBITORS AND ARBS

Following the recent publication of large clinical trials involving combination therapy for ACEI and ARB (**Table 3**), the Canadian Hypertension Education Program (CHEP) recommended that the combination not be used. However, the European Society of Cardiology (ESC) still recommended ACEI/ARB combination in their heart failure guidelines as a reasonable option. There are data that suggest standard doses of ACEI offer only a limited blockade of ACE and that the ACE escape phenomenon with generation of enzymes such as chymase, cathepsin G, and chymostatin-sensitive angiotensin-generating enzyme can form A-II from angiotensinogen and other peptide substrates.[85,86] A more complete blockade of A-II produced by the alternative pathway can be accomplished by targeting both the ACE and the angiotensin receptors. Whether the mechanism of telmisartan's selective peroxisome proliferator-activated receptor modulation (PPAR-γ) has an impact on the metabolism, proliferation, and inflammation of cardiovascular cells needs further clarification.[87]

In a meta-analysis of combination therapy for hypertension that included 14 trials,[88] ACEI/ARB combination reduced 24-h ambulatory blood pressure by 4.7/3.0 mm Hg compared with ACEI monotherapy, and 3.8/2.9 mm Hg compared with ARB monotherapy. Proteinuria was also reduced by 30% and 39% when compared with ACEI monotherapy and ARB monotherapy, respectively. However, one caveat of this meta-analysis was that the majority of studies used submaximal doses or once-daily dosing of shorter-acting ACEIs, and had a short duration of follow-up (4–8 weeks). Hence, the long-term effect of

adding ARB to chronic ACEI therapy could not be concluded. The study with the longest duration of follow-up (2.9 years) included in this meta-analysis was the COOPERATE study,[89] which used the longest acting ACEI trandolapril and showed no additional reduction in trough blood pressure with combination therapy (trandolapril plus losartan) compared with monotherapy. However, the COOPERATE study was recently withdrawn because of problems with authenticity of the data. Hence, most of the evidence on the effect of ACEI/ARB combination on hypertension has come from the ONTARGET study. The ONTARGET study is a large morbidity and mortality trial involving ARB and ACEI/ARB combination, which compared ramipril, telmisartan, and their combination in patients with vascular disease or high-risk diabetes. The study was designed to determine whether telmisartan, an ARB, is as effective as ramipril in high-risk patients and whether combination therapy of ramipril and telmisartan could further improve clinical outcomes. A total of 25,620 patients were randomized to ramipril 10 mg daily, telmisartan 80 mg daily, or a combination of both. Both telmisartan and ramipril reduced blood pressure to a similar extent (about 6 mm Hg reduction for systolic and 5 mm Hg for diastolic blood pressure). However, there was no significant difference in the incidence of the primary outcome (death from cardiovascular causes, myocardial infarction, stroke, or hospitalization for heart failure). The JNC-7 and the European Society of Hypertension and ESC, published before the ONTARGET study, did not specifically mention the role of ACEI/ARB combination in the management of hypertension. However, the latest 2009 CHEP recommendations specifically stated that regarding treatment of adults with hypertension without compelling indications for specific agents, "the combination of ACEI and ARB is not recommended (grade A)," and therapy using the combination of an ACEI and an ARB should only be considered in selected and closely monitored patients with advanced heart failure or proteinuric nephropathy.[90]

The VALIANT study addressed the role of ACEI/ARB combination in patients with myocardial infarction. A total of 14,703 patients with less than 10 day history of myocardial infarction and heart failure were randomized into captopril, 50 mg daily (n = 4909), valsartan, 160 mg twice daily (n = 4909), or a combination of 2 drugs (n = 4885). The mortality rate was 19.5% in the captopril group, 19.9% in the valsartan group, and 19.3% in the combination group after a median follow-up of 24.7 months. The secondary end point of death from cardiovascular causes, recurrent

Table 3
Summary of clinical trials with a combination of ACEI and ARBs

Trial	Patient Groups	Study Meds	Outcome	Results
CHARM,[77] overall (N-7601)	CHF	Candesartan 32 mg/d vs placebo (both groups on ACEI)	All-cause mortality	17% reduction with candesartan
CHARM, added[77] (N = 2548)	CHF	Candesartan 32 mg/d, placebo (both groups on ACEI)	Composite	15% reduction, statistically significant
CHARM, preserved[77] (N = 3023)	CHF diastolic dysfunction	Candesartan 32 mg/d, placebo (both groups on ACEI)	CV death or hospitalization	11% reduction, statistically significant
VALIANT[74] (N = 14,703)	AMI with CHF	Valsartan 160 mg twice a day, captopril 50 mg 3 times a day, or combinations of valsartan 80 mg twice a day and captopril 50 mg 3 times a day	All-cause mortality, CV death, MI, hospitalization to CHF	No difference between groups. Valsartan as effective as captopril
ValHeft[76] (N = 5010)	CHF	Valsartan 160 mg, placebo	Mortality and composite end point of mortality and morbidity	No difference in mortality, improvement in hospitalization with valsartan
ONTARGET (N = 25,620)	ASHD or diabetes with end organ damage	Ramipril vs telmisartan vs combination	CV death, MI, stroke, or hospitalization for CHF	No difference. Combination associated with more hypotension, renal impairment, and hyperkalemia

Abbreviation: ASHD, arteriosclerotic heart disease.

myocardial infarction, or hospitalizations for heart failure was also similar in the 3 groups. However, patients receiving combination therapy had a significantly higher rate of hypotension and renal impairment. The incidence of hyperkalemia was similar among the 3 groups. Combining valsartan with captopril in patients with myocardial infarction and heart failure increased the rate of adverse events without improving survival. In the ONTARGET study population, the combination of ramipril and telmisartan did not reduce the risk of death from cardiovascular causes, myocardial infarction, or stroke when compared with ramipril alone. The current evidence does not support ACEI/ARB combination therapy in the setting of AMI. For patients with coronary artery disease, the CHEP recommendation suggested "the combination of an ACEI and ARB is not recommended in patients without coexisting systolic heart failure."

A significant reduction in neurohormonal and hemodynamic perturbations was noted in patients with chronic systolic heart failure. There was also a suggestion of improvement of symptoms, exercise capacity, and quality of life. In the Val-HeFT study, 5010 patients with heart failure of NYHA class II to IV were randomized to receive 160 mg of valsartan or placebo twice daily. At the time of randomization, 93% of the patients were being treated with ACEIs. Overall mortality was similar in the 2 groups. The incidence of the combined end point of mortality and morbidity (defined as the incidence of cardiac arrest with resuscitation, hospitalizations for heart failure, or receipt of intravenous inotropic or vasodilator therapy for at least 4 h) was 13.2% lower with valsartan than with placebo ($P = .009$). Treatment with valsartan also resulted in significant improvements in NYHA class, LVEF, and quality of life as compared with placebo. In the subgroup analysis, valsartan had an adverse effect on mortality, and was associated with a trend toward an increase in the combined end point of mortality and morbidity among those who were receiving both ACEI and β-blocker at base line. However, further analysis of subjects in Val-HeFT receiving ACEI, but not β-blocker at baseline, showed that mortality was not affected by valsartan, but morbidity end points were significantly reduced. In the CHARM-Added study, 2548 patients with heart failure (NYHA class II–IV) and being treated with ACEI were randomized to candesartan or placebo. The primary outcome (composite of cardiovascular death or hospital admission for heart failure) was significantly lower in the candesartan group (38% vs 42% in placebo group, HR 0.85, 95% CI 0.75–0.96, $P = .011$). The benefits of candesartan were similar in patients receiving baseline β-blocker treatment. Incorporating the positive findings of the Val-HeFT and CHARM-Added studies, the latest American Heart Association/American College of Cardiology guidelines suggest that addition of an ARB may be considered in persistently symptomatic patients with reduced LVEF who are already being treated with conventional therapy. This proposal was supported by the latest guidelines by the Canadian Cardiovascular Society and ESC. It should be noted that the Val-HeFT investigators have subsequently pointed out that in those patients on optimal or maximally tolerated doses of ACEI, there was no benefit of adding valsartan. A recent meta-analysis[91] also suggested that overall combination therapy did not reduce mortality in patients with heart failure, although it may reduce hospitalizations for heart failure. Close monitoring for hypotension and hyperkalemia is warranted in such patients.

ACEI/ARB COMBINATION AND DIABETIC NEPHROPATHY

Several early studies suggested that the ACEI/ARB combination provided additive benefit in diabetic nephropathy (DN). However, most of these studies were small in size and had a short duration of follow-up. In one meta-analysis which included 10 trials, 156 patients received ACEI/ARB combination therapy and 159 received ACEI only .The duration of follow-up for most studies was between 8 and 12 weeks. ACEI/ARB combination was shown to reduce proteinuria, at the expense of a statistically and clinically significant reduction in glomerular filtration rate (GFR) and an increase in serum creatinine. The investigators suggested that this decrease could be secondary to the observed reductions in both systolic and diastolic blood pressure, which could have resulted in diminished renal perfusion.[92] In the ONTARGET study, analysis of the renal outcome showed that the primary renal outcome (composite of dialysis, doubling of serum creatinine, and death) was similar for telmisartan (13.4%) and ramipril (13.5%), but was increased with combination therapy (14.5%, $P = .037$). The secondary renal outcome of dialysis or doubling of serum creatinine was more frequent with combination therapy (HR 1.24, 95% CI 1.01–1.51, $P = .038$). Although combination therapy was associated with reduced albuminuria, it caused the greatest decline in the estimated GFR. These findings suggested that ACEI/ARB combination reduced proteinuria to a greater extent than monotherapy with ACEI, but overall it worsened major renal outcomes.[93] More information will be forthcoming on this topic in the ongoing trial of The Combination

Angiotensin Receptor Blocker and Angiotensin-converting Enzyme Inhibitor for Treatment of Diabetic Nephropathy (VA NEPHRON-D) which will assess the effect of combination losartan and lisinopril, compared with losartan alone, on the progression of kidney disease in 1850 patients with diabetes and overt proteinuria.[94] The CHEP 2009 recommendation advised against combination of an ACEI and ARB for patients with nonproteinuric chronic kidney disease or in patients with diabetes and normal urinary albumin levels.[90] In summary, although evidence from previous short-term studies indicates that combined therapy with ACEI/ARB reduced proteinuria, there was no evidence of a beneficial effect of ACEI/ARB on progression of DN, and combination therapy resulted in a clinically significant decrease in GFR in some studies.

The NAVIGATOR trial was a double-blind, randomized clinical trial on 9306 patients with impaired glucose tolerance and established cardiovascular disease or cardiovascular risk factors, who received valsartan (up to 160 mg daily) or placebo (and nateglinide or placebo) in addition to lifestyle modification. The patients were followed for a median of 5.0 years for the development of diabetes . The effects of valsartan were studied on the occurrence of 3 coprimary outcomes: the development of diabetes, an extended composite outcome of death from cardiovascular causes, nonfatal myocardial infarction, nonfatal stroke, hospitalization for heart failure, arterial revascularization, or hospitalization for unstable angina; and a core composite outcome that excluded unstable angina and revascularization. The cumulative incidence of diabetes was 33.1% in the valsartan group, as compared with 36.8% in the placebo group (HR in the valsartan group, 0.86; 95% CI, 0.80–0.92; P<.001). Valsartan, as compared with placebo, did not significantly reduce the incidence of either the extended cardiovascular outcome (14.5% vs 14.8%; HR 0.96; 95% CI, 0.86–1.07; P = .43) or the core cardiovascular outcome (8.1% vs 8.1%; HR 0.99; 95% CI, 0.86–1.14; P = .85).[95]

OTHER TYPES OF COMBINED RAAS BLOCKADE
Aldosterone Antagonists

Short-term therapy with both ACEIs and ARBs lower circulating levels of aldosterone. However, such suppression may not be sustained during long-term treatment. Experimental data suggest that aldosterone exerts adverse effects on the structure and function of the heart in addition to the detrimental effects produced by A-II.

Spironolactone is the most widely used aldosterone antagonist. In a large heart failure study, low doses of spironolactone (starting at 12.5 mg daily) were added to ACEI therapy for patients with NYHA functional class IV heart failure symptoms or class III symptoms and recent hospitalization. The risk of death was reduced from 46% to 35% (30% RR reduction) over 2 years, with a 35% reduction in hospitalization for heart failure and an improvement in functional class. A recent trial investigated the newer aldosterone antagonist, eplerenone, in patients with LVEF less than or equal to 40% and clinical evidence of heart failure or diabetes mellitus within 14 days of MI. Mortality was decreased from 13.6% to 11.8% at 1 year. Hyperkalemia occurred in 5.5% of patients treated with eplerenone compared with 3.9% of those given placebo overall, and in up to 10.1% versus 4.6% of patients with estimated creatinine clearance less than 50 mL per minute. . Decisions regarding the selection of patients for aldosterone antagonists reflect the balance between potential benefit to decrease death and hospitalization for heart failure and potential risks of life-threatening hyperkalemia. Following a population-based analysis of 30,000 patients taking ACEIs after hospitalization for heart failure, prescriptions for spironolactone in this geographic area more than tripled; this led to an increase in the rate of hospitalization for hyperkalemia from 2.4 to 11 patients per thousand, and the associated mortality increased from 0.3 to 2 per thousand.[96–98] It is strongly recommended that caution be used in the selection of patients to be given aldosterone antagonists, and frequent monitoring of potassium and renal function is warranted. The routine triple combination of ACEIs, ARBs, and an aldosterone antagonist should be avoided.

Direct Renin Inhibitors

Renin catalyzes the first and rate-limiting step of the RAAS and has high specificity for its substrate angiotensinogen. Hence, DRIs offer the potential for blocking this complex hormonal system at its initial point of activation. Renin inhibitors prevent the formation of both A-I and A-II; hence, they may offer a therapeutic profile distinct from that of both ACEIs and ARBs. Inhibition of ACE causes an increase in A-I, which is then available for conversion to A-II by ACE-independent pathways not blocked by ACEIs. ARBs increase levels of A-II, an effect that does not occur with renin inhibitors. A wide variety of potential renin inhibitors have been developed over the past 20 years, but low potency, poor bioavailability, and short duration of action after oral administration in humans meant that these compounds were not clinically useful drugs.[99–102] Clinical trials with DRIs are summarized in **Table 4**.

Aliskiren is the first in a new class of orally effective, nonpeptide, low-molecular-weight renin inhibitors for the treatment of hypertension. Designed through a combination of molecular modeling techniques and crystal structure elucidation, aliskiren is a potent and specific inhibitor of human renin in vitro (IC_{50} = 0.6 nmol/L). Oral administration of aliskiren to sodium-depleted marmosets caused complete inhibition of renin and sustained reductions in arterial blood pressure. In humans, once-daily oral doses of aliskiren of up to 640 mg were well tolerated and caused dose-dependent and sustained RAS inhibition in healthy volunteers. Moreover, a recent study in 226 patients with mild to moderate hypertension showed that aliskiren, 300 mg daily, lowered blood pressure with efficacy and tolerability similar to those of the ARB losartan at twice the recommended daily dose.[103–106]

In a double-blind study, 1797 hypertensive patients were randomly assigned to receive aliskiren 150 mg/d alone, valsartan 160 mg/d alone, a combination of aliskiren and valsartan, or placebo for 4 weeks. Then the dose in each arm was doubled to the maximum recommended dose for another 4 weeks. At 8 weeks, the combination of aliskiren and valsartan lowered diastolic blood pressure from baseline by 12.2 mm Hg, more

than monotherapy with aliskiren (−9.0 mm Hg), valsartan (29.7 mm Hg), or placebo (24.1 mm Hg). This study concludes that the combination of aliskiren and valsartan provides greater reductions in blood pressure than monotherapy with either agent, with a tolerability profile not dissimilar to that of monotherapies.[107] The clinical results obtained thus far on blood pressure with the combination of aliskiren and valsartan and aliskiren and ramipril are in agreement with this pharmacologic concept, which attributes to the reactive increase in renin release and synthesis associated with all RAAS inhibitors.[108] This process leads to a self-limiting efficacy as a result of the reappearance of A-I and/or A-II, in addition to A-II producing enzymes other that ACE, such as chymase. The Aliskiren Observation of Heart Failure Treatment trial (ALOFT) was a randomized between-patient comparison of aliskiren 150 mg/d and placebo in patients with heart failure. The primary end point was change in the plasma concentration of N-terminal pro-brain natriuretic peptide (NT-proBNP). Plasma levels of NT-proBNP increased by approximately 762 pg/mL with placebo and decreased by 244 pg/mL with aliskiren.[109] Thus, the ALOFT study demonstrated that the addition of aliskiren to an optimal therapy in patients with heart failure has favorable neurohormonal effects and is well tolerated.

The Aliskiren in the Evaluation of Proteinuria in Diabetes trial (AVOID) was a randomized study

Table 4
Summary of clinical trials with direct renin inhibitors

Trial	Patient Groups	Study Meds	Results
AVOID (N = 599)	Diabetes, HTN, and proteinuria	Losartan alone vs losartan and aliskiren	Combination reduced urinary ACR by 20%
HTN (N = 1797)	Mild to moderate HTN	Aliskiren vs losartan vs combination	Combination lowered SBP more than either one alone
ALTITUDE substudy (N = 837)	HTN plus diabetes	Aliskiren vs ramipril vs combination	SBP lowered more in combination treatment than either one alone
ALOFT (N = 302)	CHF	Aliskiren vs placebo	Aliskiren reduced plasma NT-proBNP, BNP, and urinary aldosterone more than placebo
ALLAY (N = 465)	Overweight HTN with LVH	Aliskiren vs losartan vs combination	No difference in LV mass between groups
AGELESS (N = 912)	Elderly with Systolic HTN	Aliskiren vs ramipril	Aliskiren lowered SBP more than ramipril in 12 wk. In 36 wk, no difference noted

Abbreviations: ACR, albumin/creatinine ratio; BNP, B-type natriuretic peptide; NT-proBNP, N-terminal pro-BNP; SBP, systolic blood pressure.
    Data from Refs.[110–114]

comparing aliskiren and placebo in addition to losartan in diabetic patients. Treatment of aliskiren reduced the mean urinary albumin-to-creatinine ratio by 20%. A reduction by 50% or more was noted in 24.7% of patients under aliskiren and 12.5% of patients under placebo. Blood pressure was 2/1 mm Hg lower with aliskiren than with placebo and tolerability was the same in the 2 groups.[110,111] The investigators concluded that the renoprotective effects of aliskiren are independent of its antihypertensive effect in patients with hypertension, type 2 diabetes, and nephropathy who are being treated with an ARB. Another trial ALTITUDE,[112] an international, randomized, double-blind, placebo-controlled, parallel-group study, is performed in about 8600 patients with type 2 diabetes associated with persistent macroalbuminuria, persistent microalbuminuria, or a history of cardiovascular disease with reduced renal function. ALTITUDE is an event-driven study that will be concluded when 1628 patients will experience the primary end point (composite of cardiovascular and renal events). The study will determine whether dual RAAS blockade with the DRI aliskiren in combination with an ACEI or ARB will reduce major morbidity and mortality in a broad range of high-risk patients with type 2 diabetes. The dual therapy in the AVOID trial achieved the goal of reducing albuminuria; however, it is not known what the result would have been had the patients taken the medications for a longer period of time. Another study demonstrates that the aliskiren provides additional, significant blood pressure reduction when administered in combination with the highest commonly used dosage of ramipril (10 mg) in patients with hypertension and diabetes. Aliskiren treatment was well tolerated and had no adverse effects on glycemic control when administered alone or in combination with ramipril. ALLAY was a study to assess the impact of aliskiren compared with losartan and the combination of aliskiren and losartan on left ventricular mass in obese hypertensives with left ventricular hypertrophy.[113] ALLAY showed no difference in left ventricular mass between the 2 groups. AGELESS was a study to assess the effect of aliskiren compared with ramipril on the elderly with systolic hypertension. AGELESS revealed that aliskiren significantly lowered systolic blood pressure more than ramipril did in 12 weeks, but after 36 weeks no difference was noted between the 2 groups.[114]

The ATMOSPHERE (Aliskiren Trial to Mediate Outcome Prevention in Heart FailuRE) will address patients with heart failure similar to those included in ALOFT. Cardiovascular death and rehospitalization for heart failure will be the components of the primary end point. The APOLLO (Aliskiren in Prevention Of Later Life Outcomes) in elderly subjects with normal blood pressure, no overt cardiovascular disease, and a high cardiovascular risk profile will address the efficacy of the drug in reducing the risk of major cardiovascular end points. ASPIRE and ASPIRE HIGHER will assess major cardiovascular events in subjects with heart failure. Furthermore, because aliskiren inhibits the initial and rate-limiting step of the RAAS, it might become a reasonable therapeutic choice also in a broad number of clinical conditions, sharing an increased cardiovascular risk, in which the inhibition of the RAAS has been shown to be beneficial. These conditions include stable coronary artery disease, cerebrovascular disease, diabetes, and peripheral arterial disease. Further light will be shed by these outcome trials.

SUMMARY

There is ample evidence that RAAS plays an important role in the pathophysiology of many cardiovascular diseases. RAAS blockade by ACEI or ARB has greatly improved clinical outcomes in a wide range of patients. RAAS blockers have a beneficial effect in the prevention of cardiovascular disease in high-risk individuals and protection from progression to end-stage heart failure and death in high-risk individuals with cardiovascular disease. ARBs have evolved to become an effective alternative to ACEI in patients with ACE intolerance and may even be used as first-line treatment in selected cases. The aim of ACEI/ARB combination therapy is to overcome the phenomenon of "angiotensin escape" and provide more complete blockade of the RAAS. However, despite a theoretical advantage, ACEI/ARB combination therapy has not been shown to provide additional benefits in most patients, with the exception of systolic heart failure and possibly overt proteinuria due to DN. It should not be routinely prescribed and, if indicated, a close monitoring of renal function and potassium level will be warranted. Aldosterone inhibitors play a major role in NYHA class III and IV patients. The only caveat of using aldosterone antagonists includes watching potassium and renal function closely and frequently. DRIs in initial surrogate end-point studies appear promising in a wide array of disease states due to its effect on renin, the rate-limiting step of RAAS activation. Further studies are warranted to look for the optimal strategy to modify the multifaceted RAAS to attain favorable cardiovascular and renal outcomes.

REFERENCES

1. Tigerstedt R, Bergman P. Niere und Kreislauf. Skand Arch Physiol 1898;8:223–71.
2. Braun-Menendez E, Page IH. Suggested revision of nomenclature—angiotensin. Science 1958;127:242.
3. Page IH, Helmer OM. A crystalline pressor substance (angiotonin) resulting from the reaction between renin and renin-activator. J Exp Med 1940;71:29–42.
4. Skeggs LT Jr, Lentz KE, Kahn JR, et al. The amino acid sequence of hypertensin. II. J Exp Med 1956;104:193–7.
5. Kageyama R, Ohkubo H, Nakanishi S. Primary structure of human preangiotensinogen deduced from the cloned cDNA sequence. Biochemistry 1984;23:3603–9.
6. Braun-Menendez E, Fasciolo JC, Leloir LF, et al. The substance causing renal hypertension. J Physiol 1940;98:283–98.
7. Skeggs LT Jr, Kahn JR, Lentz K, et al. The existence of two forms of hypertensin. J Exp Med 1957;99:275–82.
8. Skeggs LT Jr, Kahn JR, Lentz K, et al. The preparation, purification, and amino acid sequence of a polypeptide renin substrate. J Exp Med 1957;106:439–53.
9. Davis JO. Mechanisms regulating the secretion and metabolism of aldosterone in experimental secondary hyperaldosteronism. Recent Prog Horm Res 1959;17:293–352.
10. Hedner T, Hansson L, Himmelmann A. The renin-angiotensin system—a century of progress. Blood Press 1998;7:68–70.
11. Hackenthal E, Paul M, Ganten D, et al. Morphology, physiology, and molecular biology of renin secretion. Physiol Rev 1990;70:1067–116.
12. Persson PB, Skalweit A, Thiele BJ. Controlling the release and production of renin. Acta Physiol Scand 2004;181:375–81.
13. Johnston CI, Risvanis J. Preclinical pharmacology of angiotensin II receptor antagonists: update and outstanding issues. Am J Hypertens 1997;10:306S–10S.
14. Chung O, Stoll M, Unger T. Physiologic and pharmacologic implications of AT_1 versus AT_2 receptors. Blood Press 1996;5(Suppl 2):47–52.
15. Quinn SJ, Williams GH. Regulation of aldosterone secretion. Annu Rev Physiol 1988;50:409–26.
16. Timmermans PB, Wong PC, Chiu AT, et al. Angiotensin II receptors and angiotensin II receptor antagonists. Pharmacol Rev 1993;45:205–51.
17. Unger T, Culman J, Gohlke P. Angiotensin II receptor blockade and end-organ protection: pharmacological rationale and evidence. J Hypertens 1998;16(Suppl 7):S3–9.
18. Paul M, Poyan Mehr A, Kreutz R. Physiology of local renin-angiotensin systems. Physiol Rev 2006;86:747–803.
19. Bühler FR, Bolli P, Kiowski W, et al. Renin profiling to select antihypertensive baseline drugs. Renin inhibitors for high-renin and calcium entry blockers for low-renin patients. Am J Med 1984;77:36–42.
20. Redgrave J, Rabinowe S, Hollenberg NK, et al. Correction of abnormal renal blood flow response to angiotensin II by converting enzyme inhibition in essential hypertensives. J Clin Invest 1985;75:1285–90.
21. Bachmann S, Peters J, Engler E, et al. Transgenic rats carrying the mouse renin gene—morphological characterization of a low-renin hypertension model. Kidney Int 1992;41:24–36.
22. Vaney C, Waeber B, Turini G, et al. Renin and the complications of acute myocardial infarction. Chest 1984;86:40–3.
23. Remes J. Neuroendocrine activation after myocardial infarction. Br Heart J 1994;72:S65–9.
24. Isnard R, Pousset F, Trochu J, et al. Prognostic value of neurohormonal activation and cardiopulmonary exercise testing in patients with chronic heart failure. Am J Cardiol 2000;86:417–21.
25. Perondi R, Saino A, Tio RA, et al. ACE inhibition attenuates sympathetic coronary vasoconstriction in patients with coronary artery disease. Circulation 1992;85:2004–13.
26. Lonn EM, Yusuf S, Jha P, et al. Emerging role of angiotensin-converting enzyme inhibitors in cardiac and vascular protection. Circulation 1994;90:2056–69.
27. Weber KT, Brilla CG. Pathological hypertrophy and cardiac interstitium. Fibrosis and renin-angiotensin-aldosterone system. Circulation 1991;83:1849–65.
28. Packer M. The neurohormonal hypothesis: a theory to explain the mechanism of disease progression in heart failure. J Am Coll Cardiol 1992;20:248–54.
29. Francis GS, Goldsmith SR, Levine TB, et al. The neurohumoral axis in congestive heart failure. Ann Intern Med 1984;101:370–7.
30. Dzau VJ. Renal and circulatory mechanisms in congestive heart failure. Kidney Int 1987;31:1402.
31. Kawano H, Do YS, Kawano Y, et al. Angiotensin II has multiple profibrotic effects in human cardiac fibroblasts. Circulation 2000;101:1130–7.
32. Lijnen P, Petrov V. Induction of cardiac fibrosis by aldosterone. J Mol Cell Cardiol 2000;32:865–79.
33. Britten MB, Zeiher AM, Schachinger V. Clinical importance of coronary endothelial vasodilator dysfunction and therapeutic options. J Intern Med 1999;245:315–27.
34. Diet F, Pratt RE, Berry GJ, et al. Increased accumulation of tissue ACE in human atherosclerotic coronary artery disease. Circulation 1996;94:2756–67.

35. Brown NJ, Agirbasli MA, Williams GH, et al. Effect of activation and inhibition of the rennin-angiotensin system on plasma PAI-1. Hypertension 1998;32:965–71.

36. Moule KS, Denton RM. Multiple signaling pathways involved in the metabolic effects of insulin. Am J Cardiol 1997;80(3):41A–9A.

37. Nascimben L, Bothwell JH, Dominguez DY, et al. Angiotensin II stimulates insulin-independent glucose uptake in hypertrophied rat hearts [abstract]. J Hypertens 1997;15(Suppl 4):S84.

38. Schorb W, Peeler TC, Madigan NN, et al. Angiotensin II-induced protein tyrosine phosphorylation in neonatal rat. J Biol Chem 1994;269:19626–32.

39. Wan J, Kurosaki T, Huant XY, et al. Tyrosine kinases in activation of the MAP-kinase cascade by G protein-coupled receptors. Nature 1996;380:541–4.

40. Saad MJA, Velloso LA, Carvalho CR. Angiotensin II induces tyrosine phosphorylation of insulin receptor substrate 1 and its association with phosphatidylinositol 3-kinase in rat heart. Biochem J 1995;310:741–4.

41. Bernobich E, de Angelis L, Lerin C, et al. The role of the angiotensin system in cardiac glucose homeostasis: therapeutic implications. Drugs 2002;62(9):1295–314.

42. Hansson L, Lindholm LH, Niskanen L, et al. Effect of angiotensin-converting-enzyme inhibition compared with conventional therapy on cardiovascular morbidity and mortality in hypertension: the Captopril Prevention Project (CAPPP) randomised trial. Lancet 1999;353:611–6.

43. Hansson L, Lindholm LH, Ekbom T, et al. Randomised trial of old and new antihypertensive drugs in elderly patients: cardiovascular mortality and morbidity the Swedish Trial in Old Patients with Hypertension-2 Study. Lancet 1999;354:1751–6.

44. Yusuf S, Sleight P, Pogue J, et al. Effects of an angiotensin-converting-enzyme inhibitor, ramipril, on cardiovascular events in high-risk patients. The Heart Outcomes Prevention Evaluation Study investigators. N Engl J Med 2000;342:145–53.

45. Jamerson K, Weber MA, Bakris GL, et al. Benazepril plus amlodipine or hydrochlorothiazide for hypertension in high-risk patients. N Engl J Med 2008;359:2417–28.

46. Gueyffier F, Bulpitt C, Boissel JP, et al. Antihypertensive drugs in very old people: a subgroup meta-analysis of randomised controlled trials. IN-DANA group. Lancet 1999;353:793–6.

47. Bulpitt CJ, Beckett NS, Cooke J, et al. Results of the pilot study for the Hypertension in the Very Elderly Trial. J Hypertens 2003;21:2409–17.

48. Beckett NS, Peters R, Fletcher AE, et al. Treatment of hypertension in patients 80 years of age or older. N Engl J Med 2008;358:1887–98.

49. Braunwald E, Domanski MJ, Fowler SE, et al. PEACE Trial Investigators. Angiotensin-converting-enzyme inhibition in stable coronary artery disease. N Engl J Med 2004;351:2058–68.

50. ISIS-4 (Fourth International Study of Infarct Survival) Collaborative Group. ISIS-4: a randomised factorial trial assessing early oral captopril, oral mononitrate, and intravenous magnesium sulphate in 58, 050 patients with suspected acute myocardial infarction. ISIS-4 (Fourth International Study of Infarct Survival) Collaborative Group. Lancet 1995;345:669–85.

51. Gruppo Italiano per lo Studio della Sopravvivenza nell'Infarto Miocardico. Six-month effects of early treatment with lisinopril and transdermal glyceryl trinitrate singly and together withdrawn six weeks after acute myocardial infarction: the GISSI-3 trial. J Am Coll Cardiol 1996;27:337–44.

52. The CONSENSUS Trial Study Group. Effects of enalapril on mortality in severe congestive heart failure. Results of the Cooperative North Scandinavian Enalapril Survival Study (CONSENSUS). N Engl J Med 1987;316:1429–35.

53. Swedberg K, Held P, Kjekshus J, et al. Effects of the early administration of enalapril on mortality in patients with acute myocardial infarction. Results of the Cooperative New Scandinavian Enalapril Survival Study II (CONSENSUS II). N Engl J Med 1992;327:678–84.

54. Rutherford JD, Pfeffer MA, Moye LA, et al. Effects of captopril on ischemic events after myocardial infarction. Results of the Survival and Ventricular Enlargement trial. SAVE investigators. Circulation 1994;90:1731–8.

55. Kober L, Torp-Pedersen C, Carlsen JE, et al. A clinical trial of the angiotensin-converting-enzyme inhibitor trandolapril in patients with left ventricular dysfunction after myocardial infarction. Trandolapril Cardiac Evaluation (TRACE) Study group. N Engl J Med 1995;333:1670–6.

56. Torp-Pedersen C, Kober L. Effect of ACE inhibitor trandolapril on life expectancy of patients with reduced left-ventricular function after acute myocardial infarction. TRACE Study Group. Trandolapril cardiac evaluation. Lancet 1995;354:9–12.

57. Cleland JG, Erhardt L, Murray G, et al. Effect of ramipril on morbidity and mode of death among survivors of acute myocardial infarction with clinical evidence of heart failure. A report from the AIRE Study investigators. Eur Heart J 1997;18:41–51.

58. Ambrosioni E, Borghi C, Magnani B. The effect of the angiotensin-converting-enzyme inhibitor zofenopril on mortality and morbidity after anterior myocardial infarction. The Survival of Myocardial Infarction Long-term Evaluation (SMILE) study investigators. N Engl J Med 1995;332:80–5.

59. Pitt B, O'Neill B, Feldman R, et al, QUIET Study Group. The QUinapril Ischemic Event Trial (QUIET): evaluation of chronic ACE inhibitor therapy in patients with ischemic heart disease and preserved left ventricular function. Am J Cardiol 2001;87:1058–63.

60. ACE Inhibitor Myocardial Infarction Collaborative Group. Indications for ACE inhibitors in the early treatment of acute myocardial infarction: systematic overview of individual data from 100,000 patients in randomized trials. Circulation 1998;97:2202–12.

61. Flather MD, Yusuf S, Kober L, et al. Long-term ACE-inhibitor therapy in patients with heart failure or left-ventricular dysfunction: a systematic overview of data from individual patients. ACE-Inhibitor Myocardial Infarction Collaborative Group. Lancet 2000;355:1575–81.

62. Latini R, Tognoni G, Maggioni AP, et al. Clinical effects of early angiotensin-converting enzyme inhibitor treatment for acute myocardial infarction are similar in the presence and absence of aspirin: systematic overview of individual data from 96,712 randomized patients. Angiotensin-Converting Enzyme Inhibitor Myocardial Infarction Collaborative Group. J Am Coll Cardiol 2000;35:1801–7.

63. Rodrigues EJ, Eisenberg MJ, Pilote L. Effects of early and late administration of angiotensin-converting enzyme inhibitors on mortality after myocardial infarction. Am J Med 2003;115:473–9.

64. Al-Mallah MH, Tleyjeh IM, Abdel-Latif AA, et al. Angiotensin-converting enzyme inhibitors in coronary artery disease and preserved left ventricular systolic function: a systematic review and meta-analysis of randomized controlled trials. J Am Coll Cardiol 2006;47:1576–83.

65. The SOLVD Investigators. Effect of enalapril on survival in patients with reduced left ventricular ejection fractions and congestive heart failure. The SOLVD investigators. N Engl J Med 1991;325:293–302.

66. The SOLVD Investigators. Effect of enalapril on mortality and the development of heart failure in asymptomatic patients with reduced left ventricular ejection fractions. N Engl J Med 1992;327:685–91.

67. Cohn JN, Johnson G, Ziesche S, et al. A comparison of enalapril with hydralazine-isosorbide dinitrate in the treatment of chronic congestive heart failure. N Engl J Med 1991;325:303–10.

68. Carson P, Ziesche S, Johnson G, et al. Racial differences in response to therapy for heart failure: analysis of the vasodilator-heart failure trials. Vasodilator-Heart Failure Trial Study Group. J Card Fail 1999;5:178–87.

69. PROGRESS Collaborative Group. Randomised trial of a perindopril-based blood-pressure-lowering regimen among 6,105 individuals with previous stroke or transient ischaemic attack. Lancet 2001;358:1033–41.

70. Bosch J, Yusuf S, Pogue J, et al. Heart outcomes prevention evaluation. Use of ramipril in preventing stroke: double blind randomised trial. BMJ 2002;324:699–702.

71. Dahlöf B, Devereux RB, Kjeldsen SE, et al. Cardiovascular morbidity and mortality in the Losartan Intervention for Endpoint Reduction in Hypertension Study (LIFE): a randomised trial against atenolol. Lancet 2002;359:995–1003.

72. Julius S, Kjeldsen SE, Weber M, et al. Outcomes in hypertensive patients at high cardiovascular risk treated with regimens based on valsartan or amlodipine: the VALUE randomised trial. Lancet 2004;363:2022–31.

73. Dickstein K, Kjekshus J, OPTIMAAL Steering Committee of the OPTIMAAL Study Group. Effects of losartan and captopril on mortality and morbidity in high-risk patients after acute myocardial infarction: the OPTIMAAL randomised trial. Optimal trial in myocardial infarction with angiotensin II antagonist losartan. Lancet 2002;360:752–60.

74. Pfeffer MA, McMurray JJ, Velazquez EJ, et al. Valsartan, captopril, or both in myocardial infarction complicated by heart failure, left ventricular dysfunction, or both. N Engl J Med 2003;349:1893–906.

75. Pitt B, Segal R, Martinez FA, et al. Randomised trial of losartan versus captopril in patients over 65 with heart failure (Evaluation of Losartan in the Elderly Study, ELITE). Lancet 1997;349:747–52.

76. Pitt B, Poole-Wilson PA, Segal R, et al. Effect of losartan compared with captopril on mortality in patients with symptomatic heart failure: randomised trial-the Losartan Heart Failure Survival Study ELITE II. Lancet 2000;355:1582–7.

77. Granger CB, Ertl G, Kuch J, et al. Randomized trial of candesartan cilexetil in the treatment of patients with congestive heart failure and a history of intolerance to angiotensin-converting enzyme inhibitors. Am Heart J 2000;139:609–17.

78. Konstam MA, Neaton JD, Dickstein K, et al. Effects of high-dose versus low-dose losartan on clinical outcomes in patients with heart failure (HEAAL study): a randomised, double-blind trial. Lancet 2009;374:1840–8.

79. Lee VC, Rhew DC, Dylan M, et al. Meta-analysis: angiotensin-receptor blockers in chronic heart failure and high-risk acute myocardial infarction. Ann Intern Med 2004;141:693–704.

80. Lithell H, Hansson L, Skoog I, et al. The Study on Cognition and Prognosis in the Elderly (SCOPE): principal results of a randomized double-blind intervention trial. J Hypertens 2003;21:875–86.

81. Yusuf S, Teo K, Anderson C, et al. Effects of the angiotensin-receptor blocker telmisartan on

cardiovascular events in high-risk patients intolerant to angiotensin-converting enzyme inhibitors: a randomised controlled trial. Lancet 2008;372:1174–83.

82. Yusuf S, Teo KK, Pogue J, et al. Telmisartan, ramipril, or both in patients at high risk for vascular events. N Engl J Med 2008;358:1547–59.

83. Schrader J, Lüders S, Kulschewski A, et al. Morbidity and mortality after stroke, eprosartan compared with nitrendipine for secondary prevention: principal results of a prospective randomized controlled study (MOSES). Stroke 2005;6:1218–26.

84. Yusuf S, Diener HC, Sacco RL, et al. Telmisartan to prevent recurrent stroke and cardiovascular events. N Engl J Med 2008;359:1225–37.

85. Ennezat PV, Berlowitz M, Sonnenblick EH, et al. Therapeutic implications of escape from angiotensin-converting enzyme inhibition in patients with chronic heart failure. Curr Cardiol Rep 2000;2:258–62.

86. Balcells E, Meng QC, Johnson WH Jr, et al. Angiotensin II formation from ACE and chymase in human and animal hearts: methods and species considerations. Am J Physiol 1997;273:H1769–74.

87. Brown JD, Plutzky J. Peroxisome proliferator-activated receptors as transcriptional nodal points and therapeutic targets. Circulation 2007;115:518–33.

88. Doulton TW, He FJ, MacGregor GA. Systematic review of combined angiotensin converting enzyme inhibition and angiotensin receptor blockade in hypertension. Hypertension 2005;45:880–6.

89. Nakao N, Yoshimura A, Morita H, et al. Combination treatment of angiotensin-II receptor blocker and angiotensin-converting-enzyme inhibitor in non-diabetic renal disease (COOPERATE): a randomised controlled trial. Lancet 2003;361:117–24.

90. Campbell NR, Khan NA, Hill MD, et al. 2009 Canadian Hypertension Education Program recommendations: the scientific summary—an annual update. Can J Cardiol 2009;25:271–7.

91. Phillips CO, Kashani A, Ko DK, et al. Adverse effects of combination angiotensin II receptor blockers plus angiotensin-converting enzyme inhibitors for left ventricular dysfunction: a quantitative review of data from randomized clinical trials. Arch Intern Med 2007;167:1930–6.

92. Jennings DL, Kalus JS, Coleman CI, et al. Combination therapy with an ACE inhibitor and an angiotensin receptor blocker for diabetic nephropathy: a meta-analysis. Diabet Med 2007;24:486–93.

93. Mann JF, Schmieder RE, McQueen M, et al. Renal outcomes with telmisartan, ramipril, or both, in people at high vascular risk (the ONTARGET study): a multicentre, randomised, double-blind, controlled trial. Lancet 2008;372:547–53.

94. Fried LF, Duckworth W, Zhang JH, et al. Design of combination angiotensin receptor blocker and angiotensin-converting enzyme inhibitor for treatment of diabetic nephropathy (VA NEPHRON-D). Clin J Am Soc Nephrol 2009;4:361–8.

95. McMurray JJ, Holman RR, Haffner SM, et al. Effect of valsartan on the incidence of diabetes and cardiovascular events. NAVIGATOR Study Group. N Engl J Med 2010;362(16):1477–90.

96. Dickstein K, Cohen-Solal A, Filippatos G, et al. ESC guidelines for the diagnosis and treatment of acute and chronic heart failure 2008: the Task Force for the Diagnosis and Treatment of Acute and Chronic Heart Failure 2008 of the European Society of Cardiology. Developed in collaboration with the Heart Failure Association of the ESC (HFA) and endorsed by the European Society of Intensive Care Medicine (ESICM). Eur Heart J 2008;19:2388–442.

97. Ezekowitz JA, McAlister FA. Aldosterone blockade and left ventricular dysfunction: a systematic review of randomized clinical trials. Eur Heart J 2009;30:469–77.

98. Hunt SA, Abraham WT, Chin MH, et al. 2009 Focused update incorporated into the ACC/AHA 2005 Guidelines for the Diagnosis and Management of Heart Failure in Adults: a report of the American College of Cardiology Foundation/American Heart Association Task Force on Practice Guidelines: developed in collaboration with the International Society for Heart and Lung Transplantation. Circulation 2009;119:e391–479.

99. Atlas SA. The Renin-Angiotensin Aldosterone System: Pathophysiological role and pharmacologic inhibition. J Manag Care Pharm 2007;13:S9–20.

100. Piepho RW, Beal J. An overview of antihypertensive therapy in the 20th century. J Clin Pharmacol 2000;40:967–77.

101. Pool JL. Direct renin inhibition: focus on aliskiren. J Manag Care Pharm 2007;13:21–33.

102. Buczko W, Hermanowicz JM. Pharmacokinetics and pharmacodynamics of aliskiren, an oral direct renin inhibitor. Pharmacol Rep 2008;60:623–31.

103. Kelly DJ, Wilkinson-Berka JL, Gilbert RE. Renin inhibition: new potential for an old therapeutic target. Hypertension 2005;46:569–76.

104. Staessen JA, Li Y, Richart T. Oral renin inhibitors. Lancet 2006;368:1449–56.

105. Wood JM, Schnell CR, Cumin F, et al. Aliskiren: a novel, orally effective renin inhibitor, lowers blood pressure in marmosets and spontaneously hypertensive rats. J Hypertens 2005;23:417–26.

106. Gradman AH, Schmieder RE, Lins RL, et al. Aliskiren, a novel orally effective renin inhibitor, provides dose-dependent antihypertensive efficacy and placebo-like tolerability in hypertensive patients. Circulation 2005;111:1012–8.

107. Oparil S, Yarows SA, Patel S, et al. Dual inhibition of the renin system by aliskiren and valsartan. Lancet 2007;370:1126–7.

108. Andersen K, Weinberger MH, Egan B, et al. Comparative efficacy and safety of aliskiren, an oral direct renin inhibitor, and ramipril in hypertension: a 6-month, randomized, double-blind trial. J Hypertens 2008;26:589–99.

109. McMurray JJV, Pitt B, Latini R, et al, Aliskiren Observation of Heart Failure Treatment, I. effects of the oral direct renin inhibitor aliskiren in patients with symptomatic heart failure. Circ Heart Fail 2008;1:17–24.

110. Ingelfinger JR. Aliskiren and dual therapy in type 2 diabetes mellitus. N Engl J Med 2008;358:2503–5.

111. Parving HH, Persson F, Lewis JB, et al. Aliskiren combined with losartan in type 2 diabetes and nephropathy. Nat Clin Pract Nephrol 2008;4: 656–7.

112. Parving HH, Brenner BM, McMurray JJ, et al. Aliskiren Trial in Type 2 Diabetes Using Cardio-Renal Endpoints (ALTITUDE): Rationale and study design. Nephrol Dial Transplant 2009;24:1663–71.

113. Solomon SD, Appelbaum E, Manning WJ, et al. Effect of the direct renin inhibitor aliskiren, the angiotensin receptor blocker losartan, or both on left ventricular mass in patients with hypertension and left ventricular hypertrophy. Circulation 2009; 119:530–7.

114. Daniel AD, Pamela D, Jaco B. The AGELESS Study: The effect of aliskiren vs ramipril alone or in combination with hydrochlorothiazide and amlodipine in patients ≥65 years of age with systolic hypertension. Circulation 2008;118:S886–7.

Role of Medical Versus Interventional Strategies to Prevent Coronary Events in Patients with Stable Coronary Artery Disease

Enrique V. Carbajal, MD, Prakash Deedwania, MD*

KEYWORDS

- Stable CAD • Chronic angina • Risk factors
- Myocardial revascularization • Coronary outcomes

Chronic coronary artery disease (CAD) is a highly prevalent and complex health problem in the United States. Most patients with stable CAD experience stable CAD, and this group includes those who have experienced and who have recovered from an acute coronary syndrome (unstable CAD or myocardial infarction [MI]).[1] Although the risk of death associated with heart disease has decreased over the decades, heart disease remains the leading cause of death in the United States. It has been estimated that approximately 2500 Americans die of cardiovascular (CV) disease (CVD) each day. In the United States, coronary heart disease (CHD) accounts for the largest proportion of CVD. In one year, an estimated 700,000 Americans experience a coronary event and approximately 500,000 have a recurrent event. Identification of individuals at risk for CAD leads to implementation of therapies aimed at reduction in the incidence of CAD and a reduction in the incidence of complications (MI, death) from CAD. Although it is not realistic to identify in an accurate manner individuals who may develop CAD and potential complications of CAD, assessment of risk factors can be used to estimate a person's risk of developing major clinical events associated with CAD. The article by Wilson in this issue provides a detailed discussion about the clinical utility of various risk-scoring methods and tools available to predict future risk of coronary events. However, it is well known that the presence of CAD and/or history of prior coronary events are one of the most powerful predictors of future risk of coronary events and CV deaths. In this article the authors review the evidence regarding the role of medical versus interventional strategies in reducing the risk of future coronary events in patients with stable CAD.

The goals of treatment in patients with stable CAD are to reduce symptoms and thus improve quality of life, reduce myocardial ischemia, and, more importantly, reduce the risk of MI and death.[2] Although there are several available pharmacologic agents as well as various revascularization modalities for treatment of patients with stable CAD, few studies have shown that anti-ischemic drugs or routine revascularization either by percutaneous intervention (PCI) or by coronary artery bypass graft surgery (CABGS) reduce the risk of MI or improve

The authors have nothing to disclose.

Division of Cardiology, Department of Medicine, Veterans Affairs Central California Health Care System/University of California, San Francisco, Fresno Program, 2615 East Clinton Avenue, Fresno, CA 93703, USA
* Corresponding author.
E-mail address: deed@fresno.ucsf.edu

Cardiol Clin 29 (2011) 157–165
doi:10.1016/j.ccl.2010.11.001
0733-8651/11/$ – see front matter. Published by Elsevier Inc.

survival in patients with stable CAD. It is vital to emphasize that, in addition to anti-ischemic therapy, concomitant aggressive intervention aimed at modification of the risk factor burden is essential because such strategy is more likely to reduce risk of coronary events and death.[3,4]

The treatment of patients with stable CAD consists of a multiprong approach that includes the use of appropriate aggressive risk factor modification, antiplatelet therapy, anti-ischemic drugs, and revascularization procedures with the goal of controlling symptoms and reducing the risk of future CV events while improving survival. As several other articles in this issue have already discussed the role of antiplatelet drugs (see the article by Kolandaivelu and Bhatt elsewhere in this issue for further exploration of this topic), lipid-lowering therapy (see the article by Lardizabal and Deedwania elsewhere in this issue for further exploration of this topic), and management of diabetes for primary and secondary prevention (see the article by Srikanth and Deedwania elsewhere in this issue for further exploration of this topic), the authors focus their discussion on the role of anti-ischemic therapy and interventional strategies for myocardial revascularization for prevention of coronary events and CV death in patients with stable CAD.

PHARMACOLOGIC APPROACH WITH ANTIANGINAL/ANTI-ISCHEMIC DRUGS

The pharmacologic agents used in the treatment of patients with stable CAD and chronic angina include nitrates, β-blockers, and calcium channel blockers (CCBs). These drugs exert their antianginal effect by reduction in the parameters of cardiac workload, such as heart rate, blood pressure, and myocardial contractility (**Table 1**).

β-Blockers

β-Blockers have been considered as the core of pharmacologic therapy for most patients with stable CAD, especially those with a prior MI.[2] β-Blockers exert their anti-ischemic effect through a reduction of hemodynamic determinants of cardiac work that include heart rate, blood pressure, and myocardial inotropy. Although the ischemic threshold is not increased by treatment with a β-blocker, the time to reach the ischemic threshold is prolonged, thus allowing the patient to engage in longer-lasting physical activities before developing ischemia and experiencing anginal discomfort.

There is a dearth of data available from randomized controlled trials (RCTs) assessing the role of β-blocker therapy in improving long-term outcome in patients with stable CAD, which is in contrast to the greater amount of data available from studies that have evaluated the clinical benefit of β-blocker treatment in patients who have had an MI. Treatment with a β-blocker has been associated with a significant risk reduction in mortality in patients who have survived an MI. This survival benefit with β-blockers in the post-MI period is observed both in the acute hospitalization phase as well as in the postdischarge period up to 4 to 5 years after MI. However, such benefit has not been demonstrated in a conclusive manner in patients with stable CAD. Limited data from the Atenolol Silent Ischemia Study (ASIST) are available, evaluating the effects of β-blocker on clinical outcomes.[5] The ASIST primarily assessed the effects of atenolol on clinical outcomes in patients with evidence of CAD who were mildly symptomatic (Canadian Cancer Society class I and II) or asymptomatic and who had demonstrated asymptomatic ischemia during ambulatory electrocardiogram monitoring. Treatment with atenolol, compared with placebo, resulted in a significant reduction in the heart rate, frequency of ischemic episodes, average duration of ischemia, and proportion of patients who experienced ischemia. In addition, atenolol therapy, compared with placebo, resulted in a significantly lower risk (11.1% vs 25.3%,

Table 1
Pharmacologic properties of commonly used anti-ischemic agents

Class	Heart Rate	Arterial Pressure	Venous Return	Myocardial Contractility	Coronary Flow
β-blockers	↓	↓	↔	↓	↔
DHP CCB	↑[a]	↓	↔	↓	↑
Non–DHP CCB	↓	↓	↔	↓	↑
Long-Acting Nitrates	↑ ↔	↓	↓	↔	↑

Abbreviations: ↓, decrease; ↔, no effect; ↑, increase; DHP CCB, dihydropyridine CCB.
[a] Except amlodipine.

respectively; $P = .001$) of the primary composite clinical end point that included death, resuscitation from ventricular tachycardia or ventricular fibrillation, nonfatal MI, hospitalization for unstable CAD, aggravation of angina requiring known antianginal therapy, or need for myocardial revascularization during the follow-up period of 12 months. Nevertheless, the groups experienced a similar risk of death and nonfatal MI. The ASIST is the only study that compared the effects of treatment using a β-blocker with placebo on clinical outcomes in patients with stable CAD.[5–7]

β-Blockers have limited utility in patients with resting bradycardia and are poorly tolerated by patients with peripheral arterial disease or chronic obstructive pulmonary disease.

Nitrates

Although nitrates are useful as antianginal agents in the treatment of stable CAD,[2] these drugs have not undergone evaluation in prospective trials to determine their effects on the risk of hard clinical outcomes (MI, death) in patients with stable CAD. The antianginal effect of nitrates is attributed to vasodilatation, primarily through venodilation, that results in a reduced chamber dimension and decreased cardiac work. A drawback of prophylactic long-acting nitrate therapy is the tendency to develop tolerance with regular long-term use. The development of tolerance to nitrates can be avoided by scheduling a nitrate-free period of 10 to 12 hours. Because of the lack of data demonstrating effectiveness of nitrate therapy in the prevention of coronary events in patients with stable CAD, this therapy should not be routinely used in patients with stable CAD, except when necessary for relief of symptoms in those patients who have anginal episodes.

CCBs

CCBs are recommended as a second-line antianginal drug only when initial treatment with a β-blocker is contraindicated, the β-blocker was found not effective in controlling angina, or the β-blocker triggered unacceptable side effects. Similar to β-blockers and nitrates, CCBs exert their antianginal effect through reduction in parameters of cardiac workload (heart rate, blood pressure, and myocardial contractility) and additional coronary vasodilatory properties (see **Table 1**). Because of their potent vasodilator activity, CCBs are particularly effective for angina associated with coronary artery vasospasm. However, similar to nitrates, there is also lack of data from prospective controlled trials that have evaluated the effects of CCBs on clinical outcomes in

patients with stable CAD and angina. The ACTION (A Coronary disease Trial Investigating Outcome with Nifedipine) gastrointestinal therapeutic system (GITS) study in patients with stable CAD evaluated the clinical benefit of treatment with nifedipine GITS.[8] In this trial, compared with placebo, treatment with the long-acting nifedipine GITS was associated with similar rates of the primary composite end point as well as individual end points of death, MI, and stroke.

RISK FACTOR INTERVENTION AND OTHER PHARMACOLOGIC APPROACHES TO PREVENT MI AND DEATH IN PATIENTS WITH STABLE CAD

The American College of Cardiology/American Heart Association guidelines[2] for patients with stable CAD and angina have emphasized the importance of identification and management of coronary disease factors to reduce the risk of future coronary events. Specifically, these guidelines have emphasized that class 1 risk factors, which include hypertension, diabetes, hypercholesterolemia, smoking, and obesity, must be aggressively managed with both lifestyle changes as well as pharmacologic interventions as necessary. In contrast to lack of documentation of improvement in hard events with anti-ischemic drugs, risk factor modification (especially lipid-lowering therapy with statins) and treatment of hypertension in patients with stable CAD have been convincingly shown to reduce the risk of coronary events and cardiac mortality. The benefits of lipid-lowering therapy, antiplatelet drugs, and management of diabetes have been discussed elsewhere in this article, and as such, in the following section, the authors briefly discuss the role of other risk factor management and pharmacologic agents in the prevention of CV events in patients with stable CAD.

Treatment of Hypertension

Data from numerous observational studies indicate a continuous and graded relation between blood pressure and CVD risk. A meta-analysis by MacMahon and colleagues[9] of 9 prospective observational studies involving more than 400,000 subjects showed a strongly positive relationship between both systolic and diastolic blood pressure and CHD; the relationship was linear, was without a threshold effect, and showed a relative risk that approached 3.0 at the highest pressures. Hypertension probably predisposes patients to coronary events both as a result of the direct vascular injury caused by increases in blood pressure and because of its effects on the myocardium, including increased wall stress and myocardial oxygen demand. Hypertensive patients with stable CAD and chronic angina are at a high risk of coronary events and cardiac mortality. The benefits and safety of hypertension treatment in such patients have been established. The treatment of hypertension should consist of lifestyle modifications, dietary alterations, and pharmacologic intervention as necessary. The modest benefit of antihypertensive therapy for coronary event reduction in hypertension trials may underestimate the efficacy of such therapy in hypertensive patients with established CAD. In general, blood pressure should be lowered to less than 140/90 mm Hg; however, even lower blood pressure goals (less than 130/85 mm Hg) maybe beneficial in those with CAD and left ventricular (LV) dysfunction. In patients with stable CAD who have angina as well as in those who have had a prior MI, β-blockers without intrinsic sympathomimetic activity should be used as a preferential antihypertensive agent. Use of angiotensin-converting enzyme (ACE) inhibitors should also be considered in hypertensive patients with stable CAD who have LV systolic dysfunction to prevent subsequent heart failure and mortality. Also, in patients with stable CAD who have diabetes and/or chronic kidney disease (CKD), antihypertensive therapy with a renin-angiotensin system (RAS) blocker, such as ACE inhibitor, or an angiotensin receptor blocker (ARB), is recommended because such therapy is beneficial in reducing the risk of future coronary events as well as the progression of nephropathy. It is important to emphasize that the risk of CV events in hypertensive patients is dependent on levels of blood pressure and also related to the frequently associated coexisting risk factors such as obesity, diabetes, hyperlipidemia, and CKD.

Smoking Cessation

It is well established that cigarette smoking increases the risk for coronary events and sudden cardiac death. The 1990 Surgeon General's report summarized clinical data that strongly suggested that smoking cessation reduces the risk of CV events.[10] Prospective cohort studies show that the risk of MI declines rapidly in the first several months after smoking cessation. Randomized clinical trials of smoking cessation have not been performed in patients with stable CAD and chronic angina. In the primary prevention trials, smoking cessation was associated with a reduction of 7% to 47% in cardiac events.[11–13] The reduction in cardiac events after smoking cessation was seen within a short period of time and is consistent with the immediate known adverse effects of

smoking on vasomotor tone, blood pressure, and increased thrombogenicity because of increased levels of fibrinogen levels and enhanced platelet aggregation.

Patients with symptomatic CAD are generally receptive to smoking cessation recommendations. There are now several behavioral and pharmacologic approaches for smoking cessation, which are available for use by trained health care professionals. For a successful smoking cessation program, identification of experienced allied health care professionals is essential and should be a priority when dealing with patients with CAD. The importance of a structured program cannot be overemphasized.

RAS Blocker Therapy

Treatment with RAS blockers, especially ACE inhibitors (ACEIs), is recommended in patients with stable CAD, especially those who have LV dysfunction, diabetes, systemic hypertension, and CKD.[14] The article by Vijayaraghavan and Deedwania in this issue provides a detailed review of ACEI as a cardioprotective agent. In this section, the authors briefly describe the role of ACEI in patients with stable CAD. ACEIs have demonstrated vasculoprotective effects and, because of this property, are an attractive treatment in patients with stable CAD. Two relatively large randomized controlled studies, the Heart Outcomes Prevention Evaluation (HOPE) trial[15] and the EUropean trial on Reduction Of cardiac events with Perindopril in stable CAD (EUROPA)[16] study, evaluated the clinical effects of ACE inhibition in patients with stable CAD.

The HOPE trial showed that, compared with placebo, the group treated with the ACEI ramipril experienced a significantly lower risk (17.8% vs 14%, respectively; P<.001) of the primary clinical composite end point that included CV death, MI, or stroke.[15]

The EUROPA study evaluated the effect of another ACEI, perindopril, on clinical outcomes in patients with stable CAD and angina. In this study, compared with placebo, the group that received perindopril experienced a small but significantly lower risk (9.9% vs 8%, respectively; P = .0003) of the composite end point that included nonfatal MI, CV death, or resuscitated arrest.[16]

Because some patients are unable to tolerate ACEI therapy (primarily because of recurrent cough), the ONTARGET (ONgoing Telmisartan Alone and in Combination With Ramipril Global Endpoint Trial) study[17] evaluated whether treatment with the ARB telmisartan was noninferior to ramipril and whether the combination of the 2 drugs results in any additional benefit. The results of this large study revealed that treatment with telmisartan was indeed noninferior to ramipril and also that there was no benefit of combining the 2 drugs.[17]

INTERVENTIONAL STRATEGIES TO PREVENT CORONARY EVENTS IN PATIENTS WITH STABLE CAD

Coronary intervention with CABGS and PCI are commonly used in clinical practice for patients with stable CAD. Although these interventions are established revascularization modalities in the treatment of patients with stable CAD and chronic angina, there is little evidence that their routine use in patients with stable CAD is beneficial in reducing future risk of coronary events and CV deaths. Both modalities are, however, effective in decreasing the frequency and severity of angina episodes, particularly in patients who show progression of angina despite treatment with a combination of antianginal drugs.

In most trials to date, when compared with medical treatment, revascularization by CABGS or PCI in patients with stable CAD has improved angina to a greater degree,[18-21] but revascularization has not reduced the risk of death or the risk of subsequent MI in patients with stable CAD (**Table 2**).[18-22] In addition, revascularization by CABGS or PCI in patients with stable CAD, compared with medical treatment, has not improved LV function as assessed by calculated

---

Table 2
Findings from revascularization trials: stable CAD and chronic angina

Trials	Mortality	MI
VACSS	↔	↔
ECSS	↔ ↓	↔
CASS	↔	↔
MASS I (p-LAD)	↔	↔
MASS II	↔	↓
CARP	↔	↔
COURAGE	↔	↔
BARI 2D	↔	↔

Abbreviations: ↔, no effect; ↓, decrease; BARI 2D, Bypass Angioplasty Revascularization Investigation 2 Diabetes Trial; CARP, Coronary Artery Revascularization Prophylaxis; CASS, Coronary Artery Surgery Study; COURAGE, Clinical Outcomes Using Revascularization and Aggressive Drug Evaluation Trial; ECSS, European coronary surgery study; MASS I (p-LAD), Medicine, Angioplasty, or Surgery Study 1 (proximal left anterior descending); MASS II, Medicine, Angioplasty, or Surgery Study II; VACSS, Veterans Administration Cooperative Study of Surgery.

LV ejection fraction (LVEF).[19,23] Furthermore, although revascularization results in symptomatic improvement, this beneficial effect does not lead to better employment rates or status.[19]

Several relatively recent randomized studies in patients with stable CAD have evaluated the effects of revascularization by CABGS or PCI, compared with optimal medical treatment on multiple clinical and nonclinical outcomes.[19-22] In the following section the authors briefly discuss the findings from some of the important randomized clinical trials in this regard.

Some of the earlier intervention trials with revascularization have attempted to identify the high-risk cohort of patients with stable CAD who might conceivably receive greater benefit from intervention with PCI or CABGS. The post hoc analyses of some of the earlier randomized CABGS trials have unveiled several high-risk clinical profiles derived from angiographic findings.[18] The high-risk angiographic profiles include patients with 3-vessel CAD and evidence of impaired LV contractility, left main coronary artery involvement with more than 75% luminal stenosis, and involvement of the proximal left anterior descending (p-LAD) coronary artery with more than 75% stenosis as part of 2-vessel CAD.[18] Of these high-risk angiographic profiles, only the subgroup of patients with involvement of the p-LAD coronary artery has been evaluated in a prospective manner in the randomized trial, the prospective medical therapy, balloon angioplasty, or bypass surgery study (MASS-1).[18,19,24] The MASS-1 trial, in patients with single p-LAD stenosis (≥80% stenosis), assessed the clinical effects of revascularization by CABGS or PCI (primarily percutaneous transluminal coronary angioplasty) and medical therapy on various outcomes. In this study, compared with medical treatment and PCI, treatment with CABGS was associated with a significantly lower risk (23.6% vs 40.3% vs 8.6%, respectively; $P = .001$) of the combined outcome (cardiac death, MI, or angina requiring revascularization) driven primarily by a lower incidence (16.7% vs 29.2% vs 0.0%, respectively) of subsequent revascularization during the 5-year follow-up period.[19] However, there was no significant difference among the treatment groups on the risk (8.3% vs 8.3% vs 2.9%, respectively) of all-cause death, the risk of cardiac-related death (2.8% vs 5.6% vs 2.9%, respectively), the risk of MI (4.2% vs 5.6% vs 4.3%, respectively), employment status (84.8% vs 69.7% vs 82.3%, respectively), or the calculated LVEF percentage (71% ± 7% vs 68% ± 10% vs 72% ± 6%, respectively). At the 5-years follow-up, a significantly smaller proportion (25.8% vs 64.7% vs 72.7%, respectively; *P*<.001) of patients remained free of angina in the medical treatment group compared with either revascularization group.

Further insight is provided by the results of the Medicine, Angioplasty, or Surgery Study II (MASS II), which was conducted in patients with stable CAD.[20] In the MASS II trial, all patients were placed on an optimal open-label medical regimen that included the use of nitrates, aspirin, β-blockers, CCBs, ACEI, or a combination regimen of these drugs before randomization was performed. Dietary intervention and lipid-lowering therapy were provided individually. Patients were subsequently randomized to continue medical treatment only or to undergo revascularization by CABGS or PCI. Medical treatment was provided concomitantly with each revascularization arm.[20] During revascularization with PCI, the devices and procedures available to the interventionist included balloon angioplasty, coronary stents, and laser/directional atherectomy. During the 5-years follow-up period, compared with medical treatment and PCI, only with CABGS did a significantly lower risk (43.41% vs 55.12% vs 14.63%, respectively, *P* = .0026) of the primary composite end point that included all-cause mortality, MI, or need for revascularization because of angina result. The lower risk of the primary end point was largely because of a significantly lower proportion of patients in the CABGS group, compared with medical therapy and PCI, that required subsequent revascularization for angina (3.5% vs 24.2% vs 32.2%, respectively; *P*<.0001). Also, compared with medical therapy, revascularization by PCI or CABGS resulted in a significantly greater proportion of patients free of angina (54.8% vs 77.3% vs 74.2%, respectively, both *P*<.001 vs medical therapy). However, evaluation of individual end points revealed that, compared with medical therapy, revascularization by PCI or CABGS resulted in a similar risk (16.2% vs 15.5% vs 12.8%, respectively) of overall mortality, of cardiac death (12.3% vs 11.6% vs 7.9%, respectively), of acute MI (15.3% vs 11.2% vs 8.3%, respectively), and of cerebrovascular accident (3.5% vs 3.4% vs 5.9%, respectively).[20]

Perhaps the best set of data that are currently available comparing the effects of optimal medical therapy (OMT) with interventional strategy by PCI on CV outcome comes from the Clinical Outcomes Using Revascularization and Aggressive Drug Evaluation (COURAGE) trial.[21] The COURAGE trial compared the clinical efficacy of PCI plus OMT versus OMT alone in patients with stable CAD. OMT consisted of therapy with a β-blocker and, when needed, diltiazem and aggressive management of risk factors for CAD. During the median follow-up of 55 months, the group with OMT as well as the group with OMT plus PCI had similar rates of the primary composite (death and nonfatal MI) outcome (18.5% vs 19.0%, respectively) (**Fig. 1**). As expected, significantly greater proportion of patients in the group undergoing PCI were angina free at 12 months (58% vs 66%, respectively; *P*<.001) and at 3 years (67% vs 72%, respectively; *P* = .02) (**Fig. 2**). However, this benefit was lost at 5 years (72% vs 74%, respectively).[21]

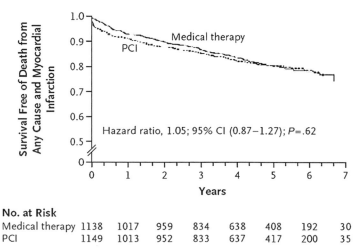

No. at Risk

Medical therapy	1138	1017	959	834	638	408	192	30
PCI		1149	1013	952	833	637	417	200	35

Fig. 1. The estimated 4.6-year rate of the composite primary outcome of death from any cause and nonfatal myocardial infarction was 19.0% in the PCI group and 18.5% in the medical therapy group. (*Adapted from* Boden W, O'Rourke R, Teo K, et al. Optimal medical therapy with or without PCI for stable coronary disease. COURAGE Trial Research Group. N Engl J Med 2007;356:1512; with permission.)

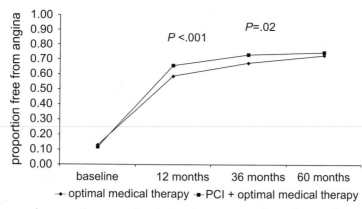

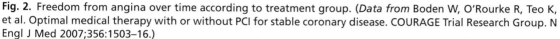

Fig. 2. Freedom from angina over time according to treatment group. (*Data from* Boden W, O'Rourke R, Teo K, et al. Optimal medical therapy with or without PCI for stable coronary disease. COURAGE Trial Research Group. N Engl J Med 2007;356:1503–16.)

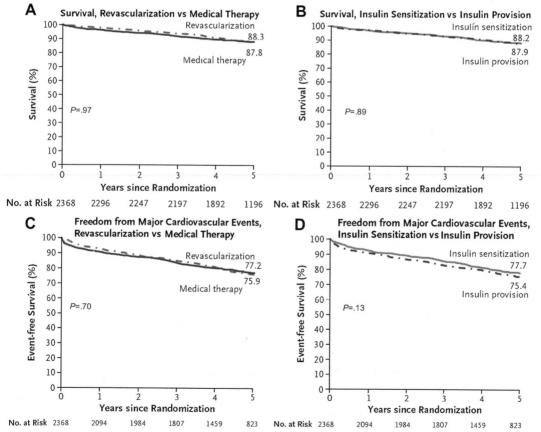

Fig. 3. Rates of survival and freedom from major CV events. There was no significant difference in the rates of survival between the revascularization group and the medical therapy group (*Panel A*) and between the insulin-sensitization group and the insulin-provision group (*Panel B*). The rates of major CV events (death, myocardial infarction, or stroke) also did not differ significantly between the revascularization group and the medical therapy group (*Panel C*) or between the insulin-sensitization group and the insulin-provision group (*Panel D*). (*From* Frye R, August P, Brooks M, et al. A randomized trial of therapies for type 2 diabetes and coronary artery disease. BARI 2D Study Group. N Engl J Med 2009;360:2510; with permission.)

The other important and recently completed randomized clinical trial in this regard is the Bypass Angioplasty Revascularization Investigation 2 Diabetes (BARI 2D) trial in patients with diabetes, CAD, and classic angina.[22] In the BARI 2D study, the effects of prompt revascularization by discretionary CABGS or PCI or medical therapy alone were compared regarding the efficacy of each strategy on clinical outcomes that only included hard end points (death, MI, and stroke).[22] During the 5-year follow-up, there was no difference between the groups undergoing medical therapy and revascularization on the risk (13.5% vs 13.2%, respectively) of the primary outcome (all-cause death), the risk of MI (11.6% vs 10.0%, respectively), or the risk of stroke (2.8% vs 2.6%, respectively) (**Fig. 3**).

These recent well-done randomized controlled studies have provided data that confirm the impression from previous CABGS trials in patients with stable CAD, which suggested that, compared with medical treatment, revascularization has resulted in similar rates of hard clinical outcomes in the main groups studied. The only benefit of revascularization compared with medical treatment appears to be the pronounced, albeit temporary, improvement in angina.

The findings from the studies discussed earlier indicate that in patients with stable CAD and chronic angina, pharmacologic therapy as well as aggressive risk-factor modification are reasonable first-line treatments. In most patients with stable CAD and chronic angina, revascularization should be considered as a complementary strategy after a long-term management with optimized medical strategy has failed to control the patient's anginal symptoms. The available data do not support routine use of coronary intervention to reduce the risk of MI and cardiac death in patients with stable CAD.

SUMMARY

Stable CAD is a highly prevalent medical condition in the United States. The management of patients with stable CAD should consist of evidence-based therapy. Goals of therapy should not only include control of symptoms but also focus on reducing the risk of future coronary events and cardiac death. The findings from several earlier as well as more recent randomized clinical trials comparing the role of aggressive and OMT with various interventional strategies (either by PCI or CABGS) in patients with stable CAD have failed to show any superiority of interventional approach over medical therapy in reducing the risk of future MI or cardiac death.[18–22]

It is important to emphasize that OMT consists of appropriate use of anti-ischemic drugs and should also include aggressive modification of all risk factors.[21,22] Interventional approach might indeed be appropriate in an occasional patient who continues to experience significant anginal symptoms despite OMT.

The available evidence from several recent large RCTs indicate that routine interventional approach by either PCI or CABGS in patients with stable CAD is not necessary because it is neither cost-effective nor protective against future risk of MI or cardiac death.

REFERENCES

1. McGill HC Jr, McMahan CA, Gidding SS. Preventing heart disease in the 21st century: implications of the Pathobiological Determinants Of Atherosclerosis in Youth (PDAY) study. Circulation 2008;117(9):1216–27.
2. Gibbons R, Abrams J, Chatterjee K, et al. ACC/AHA 2002 Guideline update for the management of patients with chronic stable angina: a report of the American College of Cardiology/American Heart Association Task Force on practice guidelines (Committee to update the 1999 guidelines for the management of patients with chronic stable angina). 2002. Available at: www.acc.org/clinical/guidelines/stable/stable.pdf. Accessed October 20, 2010.
3. Yusuf S, Hawken S, Ounpuu S, et al. INTERHEART study investigators. Effect of potentially modifiable risk factors associated with myocardial infarction in 52 countries (the INTERHEART study): case-control study. Lancet 2004;364(9438):937–52.
4. Ford E, Ajani U, Croft J, et al. Explaining the decrease in U.S. deaths from coronary disease, 1980–2000. N Engl J Med 2007;356:2388–98.
5. Pepine C, Cohn P, Deedwania P, et al. Effects of treatment on outcome in mildly symptomatic patients with ischemia during daily life. The Atenolol Silent Ischemia Study (ASIST). Circulation 1994;90:762–8.
6. Dargie H, Ford I, Fox K. Total Ischaemic Burden European Trial (TIBET). Effects of ischaemia and treatment with atenolol, nifedipine SR and their combination on outcome in patients with chronic stable angina. Eur Heart J 1996;17:104–12.
7. Rehnqvist N, Hjemdahl P, Billing E. Effects of metoprolol vs verapamil in patients with stable angina pectoris. The Angina Prognosis Study in Stockholm (APSIS). Eur Heart J 1996;17:76–81.
8. Poole-Wilson P, Lubsen J, Kirwan B, et al. A coronary disease trial investigating outcome with nifedipine gastrointestinal therapeutic system investigators. Effect of long-acting nifedipine on mortality and cardiovascular morbidity in patients with stable

angina requiring treatment (ACTION trial): randomised controlled trial. Lancet 2004;364:849–57.

9. MacMahon D, Peto R, Cutler J, et al. Blood pressure, stroke, and coronary heart disease. Part I, prolonged differences in blood pressure; prospective observational studies corrected for the regression dilution bias. Lancet 1990;335:765.

10. The health benefits of smoking cessation. A report of the Surgeon General. Washington, DC: US Department of Health and Human Services; 1990.

11. Rose G, Hamilton P, Colwell L, et al. A randomised controlled trial of antismoking advice: 10 year results. J Epidemiol Community Health 1982;36:102–8.

12. Multiple Risk Factor Intervention Trial Research Group. Multiple risk factor intervention trial. Risk factor changes and mortality results. JAMA 1982; 248:1465–77.

13. Hjermann I, Velve K, Holme I, et al. Effect of diet and smoking intervention on the incidence of coronary heart disease. Report from the Oslo Study Group of a randomised trial in healthy men. Lancet 1981; 2:1303–10.

14. Writing on behalf of the 2002 Chronic Stable Angina Writing Committee Fraker TD Jr, Fihn SD. 2007 chronic angina focused update of the ACC/AHA 2002 Guidelines for the management of patients with chronic stable angina: a report of the American College of Cardiology/American Heart Association Task Force on Practice Guidelines Writing Group to develop the focused update of the 2002 Guidelines for the management of patients with chronic stable angina. Circulation 2007;116:2762–72.

15. Yusuf S, Sleight P, Pogue J, et al. The Heart Outcomes Prevention Evaluation Study Investigators. Effects of an angiotensin-converting-enzyme inhibitor, ramipril on cardiovascular events in high-risk patients. N Engl J Med 2000;342:145–53.

16. The EURopean trial On reduction of cardiac events with Perindopril in stable coronary Artery disease Investigators. Efficacy of perindopril in reduction of cardiovascular events among patients with stable coronary artery disease: randomised, double-blind, placebo-controlled, multicentre trial (the EUROPA study). Lancet 2003;362:782–8.

17. Yusuf S, Teo KK, Pogue J, et al. Telmisartan, ramipril, or both in patients at high risk for vascular events. ONTARGET investigators. N Engl J Med 2008;358: 1547–59.

18. Deedwania PC, Carbajal EV, Bobba VR. Trials and tribulations associated with angina and traditional therapeutic approaches. Clin Cardiol 2007; 30(2 Suppl 1):16–24.

19. Hueb W, Soares P, Almeida DeOliveira S, et al. Five-year follow-op of the medicine, angioplasty, or surgery study (MASS): a prospective, randomized trial of medical therapy, balloon angioplasty, or bypass surgery for single proximal left anterior descending coronary artery stenosis. Circulation 1999;100(Suppl 19):II107–13.

20. Hueb W, Lopes N, Gersh B, et al. Five-year follow-up of the medicine, angioplasty, or surgery study (MASS II): a randomized controlled clinical trial of 3 therapeutic strategies for multivessel coronary artery disease. Circulation 2007;115:1082–9.

21. Boden W, O'Rourke R, Teo K, et al. Optimal medical therapy with or without PCI for stable coronary disease. COURAGE Trial Research Group. N Engl J Med 2007;356:1503–16.

22. Frye R, August P, Brooks M, et al. A randomized trial of therapies for type 2 diabetes and coronary artery disease. BARI 2D Study Group. N Engl J Med 2009; 360:2503–15.

23. McFalls E, Ward H, Moritz T, et al. Coronary-artery revascularization before elective major vascular surgery. N Engl J Med 2004;351:2795–804.

24. Hueb W, Bellotti G, deOliveira S, et al. The Medicine, Angioplasty or Surgery Study (MASS): a prospective, randomized trial of medical therapy, balloon angioplasty or bypass surgery for single proximal left anterior descending artery stenoses. J Am Coll Cardiol 1995;26:1600–5.

Index

Note: Page numbers of article titles are in **boldface** type.

A

Acute myocardial infarction (AMI), ARBs after, 144

Acyl-coenzyme A cholesterol acyl transferase inhibitors, in atherosclerosis management and prevention, 125

Alcohol, in CVD prevention, 27–28

Aldosterone antagonists, in CVD prevention, 149

AMI. See *Acute myocardial infarction (AMI).*

Angiotensin receptor blockers (ARBs)
  ACE inhibitors with, in CVD prevention, 146–149
  after AMI, 144
  in congestive heart failure, 144
  in CVD prevention, 144–146
  in hypertension, 144
  in stroke, 144, 146

Angiotensin-converting enzyme (ACE) inhibitors
  ARBs with, in CVD prevention, 146–149
  in congestive heart failure, 143
  in CVD prevention, 141–143
  in hypertension, 141, 143
  in postmyocardial infarction, 143
  in stroke, 143

Anticoagulation, antiplatelet therapy for coronary heart disease prevention and, 81

Antiplatelet nonprescription, as barrier to antiplatelet therapy for coronary heart disease prevention, 82

Antiplatelet therapy
  described, 71–72
  in coronary heart disease prevention, **71–85**
    anticoagulation and, 81
    aspirin, 72–73
    barriers to, 82
    cangrelor, 77–79
    clopidogrel, 73–77
    comorbidities and, 80–81
    elinogrel, 77–79
    GPIIB/IIIA inhibitors, 79
    heart failure and, 81
    in diabetics, 80–81
    in low-income countries, 81
    in special populations, 79–81
    in the elderly, 80
    in women, 80
    intravenous formulations, 77–79
    nonthienopyridine $P2Y_{12}$ inhibitors, 77
    phosphodiesterase inhibitors, 79
    prasugrel, 77
    protease activated receptor inhibitors, 79
    thienopyridine $P2Y_{12}$ inhibitors, 73–77
    ticagrelor, 77
    toward personalized therapy, 81–82
  nonadherence to, as barrier to antiplatelet therapy for coronary heart disease prevention, 82

Antisense to Apo-B-100, in atherosclerosis management and prevention, 125–126

Apnea, sleep, CVD in women related to, 39

ApoA-1
  HDL and, 127
  wild-type, in atherosclerosis management and prevention, 129

ApoA-1 gene transcription, small-molecule stimulator of, in atherosclerosis management and prevention, 128

ApoA-1 mimetic peptides, in atherosclerosis management and prevention, 128–129

ARBs. See *Angiotensin receptor blockers (ARBs).*

Aspirin, in coronary heart disease prevention, 72–73

Atherosclerosis
  lipids and, 87–88
  management and prevention of
    emerging therapies for, **123–135**
      described, 123–124
      HDL–based therapies, 126–129
      LDL-C–lowering agents, 124–126
    inflammation- or immune-modulation therapies in, 130–131
  RAAS in, 140–141

B

ß-blockers, in prevention of coronary events in patients with stable CAD, 158–159

BI204, in atherosclerosis management and prevention, 130–131

Biomarker(s), CVD events related to, 7–9

C

CAD. See *Coronary artery disease (CAD).*

Calcium channel blockers (CCBs), in prevention of coronary events in patients with stable CAD, 159

Calibration, as criterion for vascular disease risk algorithm, 4

Cangrelor, in coronary heart disease prevention, 77–79

Cardiovascular disease (CVD)

Cardiol Clin 29 (2011) 167–171
doi:10.1016/S0733-8651(10)00131-1
0733-8651/11/$ – see front matter © 2011 Elsevier Inc. All rights reserved.

Moving?

Make sure your subscription moves with you!

To notify us of your new address, find your **Clinics Account Number** (located on your mailing label above your name), and contact customer service at:

Email: journalscustomerservice-usa@elsevier.com

800-654-2452 (subscribers in the U.S. & Canada)
314-447-8871 (subscribers outside of the U.S. & Canada)

Fax number: 314-447-8029

Elsevier Health Sciences Division
Subscription Customer Service
3251 Riverport Lane
Maryland Heights, MO 63043

*To ensure uninterrupted delivery of your subscription, please notify us at least 4 weeks in advance of move.

LIBRARY OF
TEXAS HEART INSTITUTE